Stem Cell Biology and Regenerative Medicine

Series Editor
Kursad Turksen, Ph.D.
kursadturksen@gmail.com

More information about this series at http://www.springer.com/series/7896

Essam M. Abdelalim
Editor

Recent Advances in Stem Cells

From Basic Research to Clinical Applications

Humana Press

Editor
Essam M. Abdelalim
Qatar Biomedical Research Institute
Hamad Bin Khalifa University
Doha, Qatar

ISSN 2196-8985 ISSN 2196-8993 (electronic)
Stem Cell Biology and Regenerative Medicine
ISBN 978-3-319-33268-0 ISBN 978-3-319-33270-3 (eBook)
DOI 10.1007/978-3-319-33270-3

Library of Congress Control Number: 2016943088

Printed on acid-free paper

This Humana Press imprint is published by Springer Nature
The registered company is Springer International Publishing AG Switzerland

Preface

Stem cells, including pluripotent stem cells (PSCs) and adult stem cells (ASCs), have the ability to differentiate into several cell types, raising the hope for potential understanding and treating incurable human diseases. Despite the short history of human embryonic stem cells (hESCs) and human induced pluripotent stem cells (hiPSCs), they are already in clinical trials for some diseases, suggesting a considerable progress in the field of PSCs. The discovery of iPSC technology as well as the recent success in establishment of ESCs using somatic cell nuclear transfer (SCNT) has allowed for the generation of PSCs from somatic cells and has led to the production of in vitro patient-specific PSCs, which have several applications, such as in vitro modeling of different diseases, drug screening, and eventually providing a personalized medicine. On the other hand, ASCs have been in research use for more than 50 years and have been discovered in many organs and tissues. ASCs such as hematopoietic stem cells (HSCs) and mesenchymal stem cells (MSCs) have been used for transplantation-based therapies for several years. Recently, our knowledge about ASCs has greatly expanded, and there is an increased interest in their use as a therapy for certain diseases, such as blood disorders and repair of cartilage and bone defects.

This volume in the important Springer series of cutting-edge contributions in stem cell research represents a collection of chapters, focusing on some of the important topics currently being addressed in stem cell field. hESCs have a great therapeutic potential. However, there are controversies surrounding their use in research because their generation includes the human embryo destruction. This issue and others related to ethics and patents in stem research are covered in Chapter One. Stem cells can differentiate into different cell types, allowing screening and testing new drugs. This topic is covered in details in Chapter Two. Chapter Three discusses a genome editing technology, which has recently attracted more attention in the stem cell field, particularly modifying genomes in patient-specific iPSCs for disease modeling and transplantation therapy. Chapters Four and Five describe the potential use of PSCs for modeling of kidney and motor neuron diseases. The recent progress in the differentiation of PSCs into functional pancreatic β cells in vitro as well as their use to model and treat different forms of diabetes is also covered in Chapter Six. Furthermore, how iPSCs are clinically applied in cancer is discussed in Chapter Seven. There are several chapters about ASCs. Chapter Eight summarizes the current knowledge on banking of umbilical cord blood stem cells. Chapters Nine and Ten discuss the use of MSCs for bone repair and their cellular interactions during fracture repair stages. Furthermore, the applications of neural crest stem cells are highlighted and summarized in Chapter Eleven. Finally, the recent progress in lung stem cell research is discussed in Chapter Twelve. The chapters were written by world-renowned scientists in the field of PSCs and ASCs, presenting cutting-edge studies of interest to academics, physicians, and readers with general interests in the stem cell and regenerative medicine fields. Thus, this book is valuable for a broad audience.

I would like to extend my gratitude to the authors, who contributed chapters in this volume. I would also like to thank Kursad Turksen (Series Editor) for inviting me to edit this volume. I would like to express my appreciation to Aleta Kalkstein and Michael Koy (at Springer) for assisting me to complete this project.

Doha, Qatar Essam M. Abdelalim

Contents

Contributors

Basem M. Abdallah Molecular Endocrinology Laboratory (KMEB), Department of Endocrinology, Institute of Clinical Research, Odense University Hospital and University of Southern Denmark, Odense, Denmark

Department of Biological Sciences, College of Science, King Faisal University, Hofuf, Saudi Arabia

Essam M. Abdelalim Qatar Biomedical Research Institute, Hamad Bin Khalifa University (HBKU), Qatar Foundation, Doha, Qatar

Abdullah AlDahmash Molecular Endocrinology Laboratory (KMEB), Department of Endocrinology, Institute of Clinical Research, Odense University Hospital and University of Southern Denmark, Odense, Denmark

Stem Cell Unit, Department of Anatomy, Faculty of Medicine, King Saud University, Riyadh, Saudi Arabia

Asma Al-Shammary Molecular Endocrinology Laboratory (KMEB), Department of Endocrinology, Institute of Clinical Research, Odense University Hospital and University of Southern Denmark, Odense, Denmark

Deanship of Scientific Research, University of Hail, Hail, Saudi Arabia

Tomoko Betsuyaku Division of Pulmonary Medicine, Department of Medicine, Keio University School of Medicine, Tokyo, Japan

Delphine Bohl French Institute of Health and Medical Research, Sorbonne University Paris, Brain and Spine Institute, France

Liuhong Cai Center for Reproductive Medicine, The Third Affiliated Hospital, Sun Yat-sen University, Guangzhou, China

Elina Davé Union College, Schenectady, NY, USA

Neil Davey Harvard University, Cambridge, MA, USA

Sonya Davey Perelman School of Medicine at the University of Pennsylvania, Philadelphia, PA, USA

Ahmed El-Hashash Stem Cells, Regenerative Medicine and Developmental Biology Program, Children's Hospital Los Angeles, Keck School of Medicine and Ostrow School of Dentistry, University of Southern California, Los Angeles, CA, USA

Jehan J. El-Jawhari Leeds Institute of Rheumatic and Musculoskeletal Medicine, St. James University Hospital, University of Leeds, Leeds, UK

NIHR, Leeds Biomedical Research Unit, Chapel Allerton Hospital, University of Leeds, Leeds, UK

Mohamed M. Emara Qatar Biomedical Research Institute, Hamad Bin Khalifa University (HBKU), Qatar Foundation, Doha, Qatar

Cecília de Souza Fernandez Institute of Mathematics and Statistics, Federal Fluminense University (UFF), Niterói, RJ, Brazil

Teresa de Souza Fernandez Laboratory Division, National Cancer Institute (INCA), Bone Marrow Transplantation Center (CEMO), Rio de Janeiro, RJ, Brazil

Peter V. Giannoudis Leeds Institute of Rheumatic and Musculoskeletal Medicine, St. James University Hospital, University of Leeds, Leeds, UK

NIHR, Leeds Biomedical Research Unit, Chapel Allerton Hospital, University of Leeds, Leeds, UK

Navin R. Gupta Division of Renal Medicine, Department of Medicine, Brigham and Women's Hospital, Harvard Medical School, Boston, MA, USA

Ahmed E. Hegab Division of Pulmonary Medicine, Department of Medicine, Keio University School of Medicine, Tokyo, Japan

Yoon-Young Jang Department of Oncology and Institute for Cell Engineering, Johns Hopkins University School of Medicine, Baltimore, MD, USA

Dunia Jawdat Cord Blood Bank, King Abdullah International Medical Research Center (KAIMRC), King Saud bin Abdulaziz University for Health Sciences, Ministry of National Guard Health Affairs, Riyadh, Saudi Arabia

Eui-Bae Jeung Laboratory of Veterinary Biochemistry and Molecular Biology, College of Veterinary Medicine, Chungbuk National University, Cheongju, Chungbuk, Republic of Korea

Elena Jones Leeds Institute of Rheumatic and Musculoskeletal Medicine, St. James University Hospital, University of Leeds, Leeds, UK

NIHR, Leeds Biomedical Research Unit, Chapel Allerton Hospital, University of Leeds, Leeds, UK

Hee Young Kang Laboratory of Veterinary Biochemistry and Molecular Biology, College of Veterinary Medicine, Chungbuk National University, Cheongju, Chungbuk, Republic of Korea

Moustapha Kassem Molecular Endocrinology Laboratory (KMEB), Department of Endocrinology, Institute of Clinical Research, Odense University Hospital and University of Southern Denmark, Odense, Denmark

Stem Cell Unit, Department of Anatomy, Faculty of Medicine, King Saud University, Riyadh, Saudi Arabia

Hany M. Khattab Department of Oral Implantology and Regenerative Dental Medicine, Tokyo Medical and Dental University, Tokyo, Japan

Albert Q. Lam Division of Renal Medicine, Department of Medicine, Brigham and Women's Hospital, Harvard Medical School, Boston, MA, USA

Harvard Stem Cell Institute, Cambridge, MA, USA

Dennis McGonagle Leeds Institute of Rheumatic and Musculoskeletal Medicine, St. James University Hospital, University of Leeds, Leeds, UK

NIHR, Leeds Biomedical Research Unit, Chapel Allerton Hospital, University of Leeds, Leeds, UK

André Luiz Mencalha Laboratory of Cancer Biology (LABICAN), State University of Rio de Janeiro (UERJ), Roberto Alcantara Gomes Biology Institute (IBRAG), Rio de Janeiro, RJ, Brazil

Na Xu George Washington University School of Law, Washington, DC, USA

Zhaohui Ye Department of Medicine, Johns Hopkins University School of Medicine, Baltimore, MD, USA

About the Editor

Essam M. Abdelalim is a Scientist at Qatar Biomedical Research Institute (QBRI) in Doha, Qatar, and an Assistant Professor at Hamad Bin Khalifa University (HBKU) in that city. He is also Associate Professor at the Suez Canal University in Ismailia, Egypt, where he received his B.Sc. degree and his M.Sc. degree. He received his Ph.D. in Medical Science from Shiga University of Medical Science in Otsu, Japan, and was later appointed Assistant Professor at that university. Dr. Abdelalim was awarded a Postdoctoral Fellowship from the Japan Society for Promotion of Science, where he studied the roles of natriuretic peptides and p53 in the regulation of self-renewal, pluripotency, and differentiation of embryonic stem cells (ESCs).

Dr. Abdelalim's research interests focus on understanding the molecular mechanisms controlling unique characteristics of pluripotent stem cells (PSCs) and establishing their differentiation into specific cell types. His current research focuses on the potential use of PSCs to study diabetes, insulin resistance, and pancreatic beta cell development.

Chapter 1
Ethics and Patents in Stem Cell Research

Elina Davé, Na Xu, Neil Davey, and Sonya Davey

1.1 Introduction

Henrietta Lacks was a poor African-American woman born in Roanoke, Virginia in 1920 [1]. When she was 31, she had abnormal pain and bleeding and felt a mass in her cervix. She became a patient at Johns Hopkins' Hospital where physicians diagnosed her with cervical cancer [1]. During one of Henrietta's radiation treatments, a doctor removed samples of her cancer cells, without her knowledge. Despite receiving radiation and transfusions, she died of uremic poisoning while at the hospital at the age of 31 [1].

Henrietta's cancer cell samples were taken to Dr. George Gey's lab. Gey noticed that these cells, when preserved under appropriate conditions, did not die, giving them an "immortal" characteristic [1]. The cells were named HeLa. Gey continued to distribute HeLa cells to other scientists to help them make advances in their research [1]. These cells were cloned and shared with many scientists across the

E. Davé
Union College, Schenectady, NY, USA
e-mail: dave.elina@gmail.com

N. Xu
George Washington University School of Law, Washington, DC, USA
e-mail: naxu.mail@gmail.com

N. Davey
Harvard University, Cambridge, MA, USA
e-mail: ndavey@college.harvard.edu

S. Davey (✉)
Perelman School of Medicine at the University of Pennsylvania,
3400 Civic Boulevard, Philadelphia, PA 19104, USA
e-mail: Sonya.davey@uphs.upenn.edu; davey.sonya@gmail.com

E.M. Abdelalim (ed.), *Recent Advances in Stem Cells*, Stem Cell Biology and Regenerative Medicine, DOI 10.1007/978-3-319-33270-3_1

world [2, 3]. HeLa cells are commercially available and are the basis for 60,000 research papers as well as medical achievements including the polio vaccine created by Salk.

The telomeres in HeLa cells are not incrementally shortened during cell division, thereby circumventing the Hayflick Limit and not undergoing senescence. Although there is much debate about how to classify HeLa cells, various studies have been conducted to identify cancer stem cell-like populations within HeLa cells [4]. The story of Henrietta Lacks introduced the complicated and delicate topic of ethics in immortal cancer cell lines and stem cells.

Lacks' family was unaware of all the research that involved the usage of HeLa cells [2, 3]. Later in 2013, without the Lacks family's knowledge, researchers sequenced and published the complete genome of the HeLa cell line [2, 3]. Because of concerns from the Lacks family, the data was initially withheld until the Director of the National Institutes of Health [5] reached an agreement with the family—the HeLa Genome Data Use Agreement—where the genome sequence could be accessed by approved researchers (National Institutes of Health).

In addition, there are 11,000 patents involving HeLa cells. The issue of commercializing a person's cells was brought to the Supreme Court of California in the case Moore versus Regents of the University of California, where the court ruled that a person's discarded cells are no longer the property of that person and can be commercialized [6].

Overall, HeLa cells have raised many ethical questions. While scientists dispute their categorization as a cancer stem cell, they provide an excellent test case of the first usage of "immortal" cell lines in research.

1.2 Stem Cell Research

1.2.1 Types of Stem Cells

Stem cells are defined as a class of undifferentiated cells that can differentiate into various specialized cell types. Noncancerous human stem cells can be categorized into human embryonic stem cells (hESCs), induced pluripotent stem cells (iPSCs), and human parthenogenetic stem cells (hpSCs) [7]. hESCs come from 4 to 5-day-old human embryos that are in the blastocyst phase of development. iPSCs are generated from adult somatic cells through the induction of four transcription factors (Oct4, Sox2, cMyc, Klf4) [7]. hpSCs are formed by parthenogenesis (chemical stimulation of an ovum without fertilization of oocytes that form blastocysts) [7]. iPSCs and hpSCs do not involve the destruction of human embryos, and for this reason the usage of hESCs has specifically been ethically questioned.

1.2.2 History of Stem Cell Research

In 1981, Martin Evans from the University of Cambridge located the first ESCs in mice [8]. Evans was able to demonstrate that embryonic cells were able to regenerate fertile breeding mice from tissue culture cells and could carry out mutations that were introduced to the cells [8]. This concept is the basis of targeted genetic manipulation and newer developments that have created unique ways to experiment with mammalian genetics.

In 1998, James Thomson and John Gearhart individually isolated hESCs and grew hESCs in a lab [9]. Thomson was able to derive and maintain hESCs from human blastocysts that were produced through in vitro fertilization [9]. Gearhart was able to derive embryonic germ cell lines [10]. Thomson and Gearhart furthered their research by conducting animal studies on mice and monkeys, respectively, using hESCs. hESCs are particularly useful as they can be differentiated into all cell types in the body.

Embryonic stem cells have various therapeutic potentials including the creation of tissue that is immunocompatible with the recipient. In January 2009, the Food and Drug Administration (FDA) approved the first Phase I clinical trial of hESC-derived tissues for the transplantation of oligodendrocytes derived from hESCs into spinal cord injured individuals [11].

Later in 2006, Shinya Yamanaka discovered a way to bypass the destruction of human embryos, and invented iPSCs [12]. Yamanaka converted somatic cells into iPSCs by insertion of specific transcription factors into skin fibroblast cells [12]. In 2014, Masayo Takahashi successfully began conducting the world's first ever trial of a therapy based on iPSCs, in hopes to treat age-related blindness [13]. Overall, all of these discoveries have opened many doors for new therapies, but have also raised interesting ethical questions.

1.2.3 Ethics of Stem Cell Research

Stem cells offer great promise for new medical treatments as they generate viable cells to replace diseased cells and thus this principle can be applied to regenerate damaged tissue in humans. However, there is controversy on both the research and patentability of hESCs. A hESC is extracted from an embryo when it consists of approximately 250 cells in the trophoblast. The hESCs are taken from the 40 cells located in the inner layer of the blastocyst. To access the cells, the trophoblast must be removed, thus preventing further development of the embryo. The notion of destroying an embryo invited opposition to the research of hESCs because opponents believed that an embryo is a human life. Questions about stem cell research have subsequently been raised. For example, is a human embryo at 5 days old equivalent to a human life? When does a life begin—is it at fertilization, in the womb, or at birth? Will the potential use of hESCs to cure many human diseases justify the destruction of single embryos? Will such hESCs be patent-eligible even though US patent law has no morality ban on patenting biological materials? The three key parts behind the ethics of stem cell research are divided into destroying the human embryo, using the human embryo in research, and creating human embryos [14].

1.2.3.1 Ethics of Destroying Human Embryos for Research

An argument in favor of hESCs is that there are many therapeutic benefits, in which case the value of research exceeds the destruction of the embryo. The most basic argument for why it is unethical to destroy human embryos is that it is equivalent to the destruction of a human being because of the embryo's capacity to become a human being. This has led to various debates about what constitutes a human being, ranging from fertilization of a one-cell zygote to 15 days after (when monozygotic twinning occurs) to birth [14]. Right to life groups in the United States believe that embryonic stem cell research violates the embryo's sanctity of life. An opposing argument for why early human embryos are not human beings is that the cells that constitute the early embryo are homogeneous and within the same membrane, therefore not a human being. Overall, there is no clear conclusion about when an embryo becomes a human being [14].

1.2.3.2 Ethics of Using Human Embryonic Stem Cells in Research

There are many situations in which researchers are not directly involved in the destruction of embryos—in fact, the embryos used in the USA for research today are from in vitro fertility clinics where the embryos were created but not used [14]. However, there is a concern that research on hESCs will lead to future mass destruction of embryos as the results from therapeutic research could lead to possible breakthrough medical treatments and thereby increase the demand for hESCs.

1.2.3.3 Ethics of Creating Stem Cell Banks

Most hESCs are derived from leftover embryos which were not utilized during infertility treatments. However, these leftover embryos are not genetically diverse enough to address the issue of immune rejection by recipients of stem cell transplants [14]. There could be ways to create embryos by cloning technologies and through the creation of stem cell banks. However, both these approaches have ethical concerns. In the case of stem cell banks, for example, there is a concern that there will be a need to obtain thousands of eggs to prepare cloned embryos, which in turn could result in abuse of women who provide the eggs [14].

1.3 US Governmental Guidelines on Stem Cell Research

The ethical debate over research involving embryonic stem cells began in 1973 when the Supreme Court ruled in *Roe vs. Wade*, 410 U.S. 113 (1973), that a fetus is not considered a person with rights, under the 14th Amendment, and legalized abortion [15]. This historic decision activated opponents as they considered abortion to be destruction of life and later opposed stem cell research. In 1974, Congress initiated a temporary suspension on federally funded clinical research that used human embryos until national guidelines could be established [15]. The U.S. Department of Health and Human Services also mandated regulations and denied funding for therapeutic research using human embryos. Federal government policymakers provided limited funding for any research with human embryos due to the conception and birth of the first "test tube" baby, Louise Brown, by in vitro fertilization (IVF) in 1978 [15].

Almost two decades later, under the National Institutes of Health Revitalization Act, President Clinton and Congress gave the NIH direct authority to fund human embryo research for the first time in 1993 [16]. NIH established a Human Embryo Research Panel consisting of scientists, ethicists, public policy experts, and patient advocates to establish the eligibility criteria for providing federal funding [16]. The panel proposed that federal funding should be provided for research to obtain stem cells from the destruction of spare embryos from fertility clinics. President Clinton, however, rejected parts of these recommendations; he directed NIH to allocate no funding for experiments that would create new embryos specifically for research. In 1996, due to the Dickey–Wicker Amendment, the U.S. Congress passed a rider attached to the appropriation bill banning the use of federal funds for either creating or destroying human embryos [16]. President Clinton signed this bill, thus limiting embryo research to the private sector.

In 1998, James Thomson of the University of Wisconsin and John Gearhart of Johns Hopkins University successfully cultured and created the first hESC lines using private funds [16]. This was an historic achievement and the NIH realized the value of this milestone to revolutionize the practice of medicine to treat conditions like Parkinson's, heart disease, diabetes, and spinal cord injury [16]. However, the research to treat these conditions required long-term federal funding, which was blocked by the Dickey–Wicker Amendment.

Harriet Rabb, the General Counsel at the Department of Health and Human Services, provided a legal opinion to the NIH in favor of the funding of human stem cell research [16]. She maintained that if the derivation of the hESC lines was funded privately, then federal funding of later research would not pose a problem regarding the creation of embryos. She concluded that a hESC was not legally an organism, as it cannot develop into a viable embryo outside the uterus, and therefore not covered by the Dickey–Wicker Amendment [16]. In 1999, President Clinton strongly endorsed the new guidelines and the NIH began to accept research proposals from scientists. Therefore, the Clinton Administration first opened the door for federal funding at this time [16].

President George W. Bush adopted a conservative interpretation of Harriet Rabb's opinion. He announced that federally funded embryonic stem cell research would be allowed only on stem cell lines that were derived prior to August 9, 2001, the date of his address [16]. The Bush Administration ordered an official withdrawal of federal funding guidelines that the Clinton Administration had authorized and reduced the funding for stem cell research [16]. The policy was restrictive as only 21 cell lines were viable over the period of President Bush's two terms, reducing access to basic material required to conduct stem cell research. During the period from 2005 to 2007, Congress tried twice to overturn the ban on federal funding but President Bush vetoed the bill both times [16].

In the meantime, stem cell research continued in private sectors and shifted from federal funding to state or overseas funding for research initiatives. In 2004, California and New Jersey were the first two states that approved stem cell research funding. They were followed by Connecticut, Illinois, Maryland, New York, and Wisconsin over a period of 2 years [17]. The federal funding restrictions also provided a motivation for scientists to use adult cells that did not require destruction of the embryo.

In 2009, President Obama lifted the ban on federal funding of newly created cell lines as long as the embryos used were not created solely for the purpose of conducting research and ethical guidelines set by NIH were followed [17].

A few weeks after the new NIH guidelines were in effect, a few plaintiffs, including two adult stem cell researchers, James Sherley and Theresa Deisher, filed a lawsuit against the Department of Health and Human Services and the NIH claiming that the federal funding is in violation of the Dickey–Wicker Amendment [16]. They were both against embryonic stem cell research and believed adult stem cell research funding would decrease due to an increase in embryonic stem cell funding. The Chief Judge Royce Lamberth dismissed the case, but after an appeal, the case was reversed and was sent back to him for reconsideration. After reviewing the case in 2010, Chief Judge Lamberth granted an injunction stopping government funding of hESC research; he decided that Rabb's logic against Dickey–Wicker Amendment was not correct. In the meantime, the NIH put a hold on new research grants and renewals until the appeal was resolved by the Justice Department. The Washington D.C. Court of Appeals blocked the temporary injunction by Judge Lamberth and allowed federal funding to continue in the interim [16].

On July 27, 2011, Judge Lamberth issued a ruling that the US Government can continue funding embryonic stem cell research and threw out the 2009 lawsuit. The Lamberth ruling was a relief for many scientists. During the 2011 fiscal year, by the NIH's estimates, federal funding for human non-embryonic stem cell research and hESC research was $358 million and $126 million, respectively [16].

Since the ruling in 2011, there have been several attempts to overturn the decision and stop federal funding for stem cell research. On August 24, 2012, the U.S. Court of Appeals for the D.C. Circuit upheld a lower court ruling that dismissed a lawsuit challenging the Obama administration's expansion of federal funding for stem cell research. In addition, the Supreme Court declined to hear the case on January 7, 2013, by Sherley and Deisher, and upheld the previous ruling of the D.C. Circuit Court's ruling in 2011 [17]. This was a major victory for the scientific community pursuing innovative research on stem cells.

Currently, the NIH has invested more than $500 million in hESC research. Scientists conducting the research maintain that continued federal funding will be necessary to make progress in this field. In particular, they would have greater flexibility to conduct collaborative work within labs, across labs, and around the world on the latest treatments and breakthroughs.

1.4 Debates on Patenting of Stem Cells in the United States

A hot debate on the ethics of patenting human embryonic stem cells ("human ESCs" or "hESCs") started in 1998 after the University of Wisconsin obtained its US patent on the isolation and culture of hESCs. Although moral dilemmas, federal funding of stem cell research, and media attention all have fueled the intense debate, since the inception of the debate, the focus has always been the source of hESCs, impediment to research, and control of the hESCs market.

1.4.1 Impediment to Research

One aspect of the debate is the impediment that stem cell patents impose on stem cell research. The United States Patent and Trademark Office (USPTO) has granted hundreds of stem cell-related patents over the years. The owners of these patents have a legal right to prevent others from making, using, selling, offering to sell, or importing the inventions claimed in these patents.

Patent owners, such as universities or private companies, may use their patents themselves, license or control the use of their patents by others, sell their patents, or enforce their legal rights against potential infringers in a court. Patent owners may often contract to provide a license to another party to use the patented material or technology, and may require in return a payment of an up-front fee plus royalties from sales of any products derived from the licensed technology. Patent owners may also impose a material transfer agreement governing the transfer of research material, and may limit the scope of relevant research, publication, and ownership of resulting technology developed.

Tensions between patent owners and the scientific community have accumulated. With the increase of stem cell-related patents, it is obviously becoming more and more difficult and expensive for researchers to use stem cell lines and technologies that are protected by patents. Patent owners therefore have been accused of restricting the research of stem cells. Particularly, academic researchers who have less resources to negotiate a patent license are limited to the use of government funding and stem cell lines from the NIH. In a highly competitive area such as stem cell research, the availability of public funding is extremely limited and highly sought after. Hence, there is an increasing tension between researchers interested in using patented stem cells and patent owners of stem cell-related patents.

On the other hand, patent owners often argue that their patent right is a legal right, which the US Constitution recognizes as a way to promote innovations of new technology. Patents reward inventors with incentives and legal protection. One can imagine that without patent protection, innovators and investors are less likely to devote substantial amounts of time and resources into developing new technologies. In fact, stem cell technologies progressed relatively slowly at first, as it took 17 years from the first successful derivation of the mouse ESC in 1981 to the breakthrough derivation of human ESCs in 1998 [9, 18]. However, afterwards, with the increase of stem cell-related patents, it only took 11 years for stem cell technologies to progress to the first hESC human trial.

Society should, however, put onus on patent owners on how they should exercise their rights. Patent owners may exert their patent right, but they also need to loosen their stronghold and share social responsibilities. In an example, patent owner Wisconsin Alumni Research Foundation (WARF) began in 2007 to permit academic institutions to carry out industry-sponsored research involving its stem cells without a license, and it reduced restrictions on stem cell material transfers between researchers. If more patent owners join the effort to exert less control, require reduced cost on their patent licenses, and facilitate rapid exchange of research material, then the positive and negative effects of patent rights would become more balanced.

1.4.2 Control of Stem Cells Market Through Broad Patents

Another aspect in the debate is how the control of ESC market by some patent owners affects the long-term development of the stem cell therapies. Once a patent owner acquires enough resources and becomes a dominant player in the market, the patent owner may choose to crush small competitors in the courtroom, rather than having to compete with their products and services. The potential of developing successful stem cell therapies may therefore be limited due to the restrictions on competition by the various stem cell-related patents.

It is also foreseeable that businesses and investors may be less inclined to invest in the long-term development of the stem cell therapies in the USA, as compared to other foreign countries, due to the existing patent laws in the USA. Over the years, patents on stem cells have accumulated rapidly in the USA. They cover broad and diverse aspects of stem cell technologies, such as culturing methods including methods of differentiating stem cells and methods of treatment of stem cells, alternatives to ESCs including tissue stem cells (e.g., Published US Patent Application 20050176707), converting differentiated cells to undifferentiated states (e.g., WO2001085917), and adult stem cells and ectopic stem cell factors. Because of the number of method patents on stem cells, businesses and investors who intend to develop a stem cell therapy but have no patents of their own will have to obtain multiple licenses to multiple blocking patents and complementary patents so as to avoid the risk of infringing these patents. The foreseeable complexity of the multiple licensing scheme and royalty payments are bottlenecks to the future development of new technologies in the stem cell market.

1.5 Laws on Patent Eligibility of Stems Cells Worldwide

In a study on the global stem cell patent landscape, it was shown that top three sources of stem cell patent and applications are through the PCT (19 %), USA (21 %), and European Patent Office (EPO) (14 %). Other most active countries for stem cell patent filings were Australia (12 %), Canada (7 %), Japan (7 %), Germany (3 %), China (2 %), the United Kingdom (UK, 2 %), and Israel (1 %). The remaining 12 % of global stem cell filings were thinly dispersed across 53 additional countries [19]. The laws in a few countries on patent eligibility of stem cells are examined below.

1.5.1 The US Law on Patent Eligibility of Stem Cells

USPTO has issued a wide range of hESC-related patents in the past. US law presents no morality-based prohibition to patenting mammalian stem cells (Public Law 104-99 §128 (1996). In the USA, "any new and useful process, machine, manufacture, or composition of matter, or any new and useful improvement thereof" is patent eligible subject matter. 35 U.S.C. § 101. In 1981, the Supreme Court noted in *Diamond v. Diehr* that there are three exceptions to patent eligible subject matter: laws of nature, natural phenomena, and abstract ideas [20].

For a mammalian stem cell to be eligible for patents, it must not fall under any of the three exceptions, the most relevant of which is the natural phenomena exception. In *Diamond v. Chakrabarty*, the U.S. Supreme Court established the precedent that living biological material is not necessarily excluded from patent eligible subject matter under § 101 [21]. This decision provides support to patent eligibility of a wide scope of biological materials in all fields of biotechnology, including human stem cells.

The AIA, passed in September 2011, presents no direct barrier to patenting stem cells, but generally provides that "[n]o patent may issue on a claim directed to or encompassing a human organism [22]." The AIA is the most significant change in the US patent law since 1952. In terms of stem cells, the legislative history of AIA provides that under this Act, stem cells are patent eligible, but patent claims directed to or encompassing a human organism including "human embryo" are prohibited [23]. However, the AIA does not define the term "human organism."

In the future, if the U.S. Supreme Court construes "human organism" to include "human stem cells," human stem cells would be patent ineligible.

In *Ass'n for Molecular Pathology versus Myriad Genetics, Inc.* (569 U.S. ___ June 13, 2013) (hereafter referred to as the "*Myriad* decision"), the Supreme Court ruled that cDNAs are patent eligible, but genes are not [24]. The Myriad decision states, "We merely hold that genes and the information they encode are not patent eligible under §101 simply because they have been isolated from the surrounding genetic material." Following this case, one argument is that a stem cell is merely "isolated" from the body, and thus not patent eligible. For example, although the USPTO held the patents as valid, the Consumer Watchdog and the Public Patent Foundation challenged the WARF patents in court on grounds of patent eligibility. In this case, comparisons were made between the original stem cells and naturally occurring DNA, and the cultured stem cells and artificial cDNA. Thus far, the US Court of Appeals of the Federal Circuit, which rather than ruling on the validity of the patents, ruled that as a third party not directly harmed by the decision, Consumer Watchdog did not have the legal standing [25].

1.5.2 The European Law on Patent Eligibility of Stem Cells

The restriction on patenting human stem cells in the European Union (EU) is based on the morality ground. Directive 98/44/EC on the Legal Protection of Biotechnological Inventions (the "Biotech Directive") regulates the legal protection of biotechnological inventions across the EU. The Biotech Directive prohibits patenting any products that used human embryos for industrial or commercial purposes on a morality ground [26].

In denying WARF a patent on its hESCs, the EPO cited Article 53(a) of the European Patent Convention (EPC) and Rule 28(c) of the Implementing Regulations. Article 53(a) of the EPC excludes from patentability "inventions that commercial exploitation of which would be contrary to 'ordre public' or morality." Specific to stem cells, Rule 28(c) declares "uses of human embryos for industrial or commercial purposes" not patentable. In the decision, the EPO emphasized that it was not ruling out all patents on stem cells, but only patent filings necessarily involved destruction of human embryos. The EPO determined the WARF patent application violated Article 53(a) and Rule 28(c).

In *Brüstle v. Greenpeace* [27], the Court of Justice of the European Union (CJEU) interpreted the term "human embryo." The CJEU included into the scope of "human embryo" not only fertilized human ovum, but also "non-fertilized human ovum" that is "capable of commencing the process of development of a human being just as an embryo created by fertilization of an ovum can do so." In view of the difficulty in patenting human stem cells in the EU, it is no surprise that there is a trend for EU inventors to assign their invention for filing for patent protection abroad [19].

1.5.3 The UK Law on Patent Eligibility of Stem Cells

The UK patent law also contains a morality exception clause that closely follows the EPC rule. Recently, this changing scope of "human embryo" due to new scientific development recently affected a case involving International Stem Cell Corporation (ISCC). ISCC applied in the UK for two patents relating to methods where parthenogenesis is used to activate a human oocyte. The UK IPO concluded using the *Brüstle* decision that because the parthenogenetically derived structure (parthenote) was analogous to the blastocyst stage of normal embryonic development, this fell within the definition of "human embryo," and so are not patent eligible. ISCC appealed to the English High Court and argued that a parthenogenetically stimulated human oocyte was not capable of producing an embryo due to its inherent biological limitation, explaining that a parthenote contains only the maternal nuclear chromosome but no paternal DNA and is known not to undergo full development to give rise to an embryo. Thus, the CJEU concluded "that unfertilized human ovum whose division and further development had been stimulated by parthenogenesis does not constitute a 'human embryo'" [28]. By narrowing the definition of "human embryo," the CJEU indirectly reduced the reach of the WARF decision and the *Brüstle* decision and opened the door of patenting human parthenote stem cells.

1.5.4 Australia, Canada, Germany, China, and Japan on Patent Eligibility of Stem Cells

In Australia, Section 18 of Patents Act 1990 [29] provides that a "patentable invention" under Australian law is one that is a "manner of manufacture," is novel, involves an inventive step, is useful, and is not expressly excluded from patentability under the Act. In general, inventions involving biological materials may be patented if they have been isolated from their natural state. IP Australia has indicated that human cell lines are patentable on this basis. However, section 18 (2) of the Patents Act excludes "human beings and the biological processes for their generation" from patentability under Australian law. It has been suggested that this provision may prevent patent protection being available for inventions involving hESCs, but the Act does not define "human beings" or "biological processes for their generation." To date, there has been no judicial consideration of this provision. IP Australia narrowly interprets Section 18(2). As a matter of practice, IP Australia has developed a policy according to which examiners must refer patent applications that might fall within a "grey area" to supervising examiners, who then discuss the matter with a Deputy Commissioner. Currently, this policy covers inventions involving hESCs.

Canada, like the USA, has no morality exception in its patent law. The Canadian Intellectual Property Office (CIPO) has issued WARF a patent (Patent

No. 2190528) for primate embryonic stem cells mirroring the broad claims in the US patents.

China's patent law has allowed patents of all stem cells. Recently, China has made an amendment on the morality clause in its patent law to include an additional statement that "no patent will be granted for an invention based on genetic resources if the access or utilization of the said genetic resources is in violation of any law or administrative regulation." So far, the impact of this language on stem cell line patents remains unclear.

German patent law contains a morality exception clause that is virtually identical to that of the EPC and UK. In contrast to the UK, Germany has interpreted the morality language more strictly concerning stem cell line patentability.

Japanese patent law has a morality exception provision as well, but notwithstanding the provision, Japan has liberally granted many stem cell patents, including hESCs.

1.6 Summary

In sum, the stem cell field is a rapidly developing and exciting field that presents numerous opportunities. Countries around the globe have different positions regarding the patentability of stem cell lines. Besides differences in specifics of patent law, legal and ethical considerations all continue to shape the landscape of the stem cell patent policies.

References

1. Skloot R. The immortal life of Henrietta lacks. New York: Crown; 2010.
2. Callaway E. HeLa publication brews bioethical storm. Nature. 2013. doi:10.1038/nature.2013.12689.
3. Callaway E. Most popular human cell in science gets sequenced. Nature. 2013. doi:10.1038/nature.2013.12609.
4. Wang K, Zeng J, Luo L, Yang J, Chen J, Li B, Shen K. Identification of a cancer stem cell-like side population in the HeLa human cervical carcinoma cell line. Oncol Lett. 2013;6(6):1673–80.
5. National Institutes of Health. NIH, Lacks family reach understanding to share genomic data of HeLa cells. ScienceDaily. ScienceDaily, 7 August 2013. <www.sciencedaily.com/releases/2013/08/130807134010.htm>
6. Dorney M. Moore v. the Regents of the University of California: balancing the need for biotechnology innovation against the right of informed consent. Berekley Technol Law J. 1990. doi:10.15779/Z385957.
7. Davey S, Davey N, Gu Q, Xu N, Vatsa R, Devalraja S, Harris P, Gannavaram S, Dave R, Chakrabarty A. Interfacing of science, medicine and law: the stem cell patent controversy in the United States and the European Union. Front Cell Dev Biol. 2015;3:71.
8. Martin GR. Isolation of a pluripotent cell line from early mouse embryos cultured in medium conditioned by teratocarcinoma stem cells. Proc Natl Acad Sci U S A. 1981;78(12):7634–8.

9. Thomson J, Itskovitz-Eldor J, Shapiro S, Waknitz M, Swiergiel J, Marshall V, Jones J. Embryonic stem cell lines derived from human blastocysts. Science. 1998;282(5391):1145.
10. Gearhart J. New human embryonic stem-cell lines—more is better. N Engl J Med. 2004;350(13):1275–6.
11. Kimbrel EA, Lanza R. Current status of pluripotent stem cells: moving the first therapies to the clinic. Nat Rev Drug Discov. 2015;14(10):681–92. doi:10.1038/nrd4738. http://www.nature.com/nrd/journal/v14/n10/fig_tab/nrd4738_T1.html.
12. Takahashi K, Yamanaka S. Induction of pluripotent stem cells from mouse embryonic and adult fibroblast cultures by defined factors. Cell. 2006;126(4):663–76. doi:10.1016/j.cell.2006.07.024.
13. Cyranoksi D. Japanese women is first recipient of next-generation stem cells. Nature News. 2014.
14. Siegel A. Ethics of stem cell research. In: Zalta EN, editor. The stanford encyclopedia of philosophy. Spring 2013 Edition.
15. Wertz DC. Embryo and stem cell research in the United States: history and politics. Gene Ther. 2002;9(11):674–8.
16. Dunn K. The politics of stem cells. NOVA ScienceNOW. 2005. http://www.pbs.org/wgbh/nova/body/stem-cells-politics.html.
17. Wert G, Mummery C. Human embryonic stem cells: research, ethics and policy. Hum Reprod. 2003;18(4):672–82.
18. Evans M, Kaufman M. Establishment in culture of pluripotent cells from mouse embryos. Nature. 1981;292(5819):154–6.
19. Bergman K, Graff GD. The global stem cell patent landscape: implications for efficient technology transfer and commercial development. Nat Biotechnol. 2007;25:419–24. doi:10.1038/nbt0407-419.
20. Diamond v. Diehr, 450 U.S. 175, 185. 1981.
21. Diamond v. Chakrabarty, 447 U.S. 303. 1980.
22. Leahy-Smith America Invents Act (AIA), Pub. L. 112-29, sec. 33(a), 125 Stat. 284.
23. 157 Cong. Rec. E1177-04 Testimony of Representative Dave Weldon previously presented in connection with the Consolidated Appropriations Act, 2004, Pub. L. 108-199, '634, 118 Stat. 3, 101, and later resubmitted with regard to the AIA; see 149 Cong. Rec. E2417-01.
24. Association for Molecular Pathology v. Myriad Genetics, Inc., 133 S.Ct. 2107, 2116-17. 2013.
25. Consumer Watchdog v. Wisconsin Alumni Research Foundation, No. 2013-1377 (Fed. Cir. 2014).
26. Directive 98/44/EC, Article 6(2)(c).
27. Brüstle v. Greenpeace eV (C-34/10) [2012] 1 C.M.L.R. 41 (the "Brüstle decision").
28. International Stem Cell Corporation versus Comptroller General of Patents, CJEU, 18 December 2014, Case C-364/13.
29. Australia: PATENTS ACT 1990 No. 83, 1990 - Section 18 (Principal Act).

Chapter 2
Stem Cells for Drug Screening

Hee Young Kang and Eui-Bae Jeung

2.1 Introduction

2.1.1 General Concepts About Stem Cells

Stem cells are distinguished from other cells by two essential abilities. Specifically, they can generate identical copies of themselves, or self-renew, and are able to differentiate into any of the three germ layers (endoderm, mesoderm, and ectoderm). Differentiation is the process through which cells acquire new morphological and functional characteristics [1]. Terminally differentiated cells, which account for most cells in the body, do not have the ability to self-renew or differentiate (referred to as stemness).

Stem cells can be classified as totipotent, pluripotent, multipotent, and unipotent according to their lineage potentials. Totipotent cells proceed from early embryonic cells within the first couple of cell divisions after fertilization, and are capable of forming all cell types, including extraembryonic, or placental cells. Pluripotent cells can differentiate into every type of cell found in the body, except for placenta and amniotic sac cells. Multipotent cells can only give rise to more than one type within a related group of cell types, and are therefore more limited than pluripotent cells. Unipotent cells are only able to differentiate into one type of cell.

H.Y. Kang • E.-B. Jeung (✉)
Laboratory of Veterinary Biochemistry and Molecular Biology, College of Veterinary Medicine, Chungbuk National University, 1 Chungdae-ro, Seowon-gu, Cheongju, Chungbuk 28644, Republic of Korea
e-mail: nannaingir@hanmail.net; ebjeung@chungbuk.ac.kr

E.M. Abdelalim (ed.), *Recent Advances in Stem Cells*, Stem Cell Biology and Regenerative Medicine, DOI 10.1007/978-3-319-33270-3_2

2.1.2 Classification of Stem Cells

Stems cells are categorized as embryonic, adult, and induced pluripotent stem cells based on their developmental status. (1) Embryonic stem cells (ESCs) are pluripotent cells isolated from the inner cell mass of the blastocyst stage [2]. ESCs have long-term self-renewal, being able to divide and proliferate for a year or longer in the laboratory while remaining in their undifferentiated state. Appropriate conditions and environmental factors are required during culture to maintain an undifferentiated state of ESCs. (2) Adult stem cells (ASCs), which are also known as multipotent adult progenitor cells (MAPCs), are undifferentiated cells found within various tissues of the body that function in homeostasis and repair of tissue when needed. Microenvironments in which ASCs are found are known as stem cell niches. ASCs contain the major limitation of only being able to differentiate into cell types of the original tissue/organ-related group. Mesenchymal stem cells (MSCs) are a special type of ASC that have been found in approximately 30 other tissues, including bone marrow [3], brain [4], liver [5], skin [6], adipose [7], skeletal muscle [8], and blood [9]. MSCs can differentiate into other somatic cell types or mesenchymal tissues, including osteoblasts, adipocytes, chondrocytes, endothelial cells, skeletal myocytes, glia, neurons, and cardiac myocytes. For these reasons, the definition and potential of MSCs remain controversial. (3) Induced pluripotent stem cells (iPSCs) are adult cells that have been reprogrammed to an embryonic stem cell-like state by introducing and inducing expression of certain embryonic genes (e.g., OCT4, SOX2, KLF4, and c-MYC). These cells also have pluripotency. Nuclear reprogramming has been conducted using techniques such as somatic cell nuclear transfer (SCNT) [10], altered nuclear transfer (ANT) [11], cell fusion (i.e., fusion of skin cells with hESCs) [12], and virus-mediated transfection of four defined transcription factors [13].

2.1.3 General Application of Stem Cells

Stem cells have been applied to gain (1) a basic mechanistic understanding of how a stem cell regulates the genome and cellular functions (e.g., cell proliferation in a symmetrical or asymmetrical fashion, differentiation, apoptosis, immortality, and senescence), as well as for (2) regenerative medicine or stem cell therapy, (3) drug discovery, (4) toxicity testing of pharmaceuticals and stem cell therapy, (5) genetic therapy, and (6) to determine the role of stem cells in stem cell-derived diseases and the aging process [14]. In this study, we investigated the use of stem cells in the field of toxicology. In this field, multiple scientific disciplines as well as specific concepts and techniques have been employed to examine specific mechanisms of drugs or agents that induce acute or chronic effects. Toxicity tests contain multiple end points (e.g., molecular, biochemical, cellular, physiological, and pathological), or morbidity and mortality of the organism.

2.2 Necessity for Alternative Tests Using Stem Cells

Industries that are required to perform toxicity tests pay attention to alternative methods for replacing and screening methods used to investigate developmental and reproductive toxicity instead of animal-based toxicity tests. Research regarding alternative methods has been conducted in response to two European regulations. In 2003, the EU passed a law banning the testing of cosmetics and their ingredients on animals, which was reinforced by marketing bans with different deadlines. The Cosmetics Directive was conducted to protect and improve the welfare of animals used for experimental purposes, as well as to promote the development and use of alternative testing [15]. Six years after this directive became effective, animal experiments for cosmetic products and ingredients were completely banned, which was reinforced with a marketing ban in the EU in 2009, except for purposes such as toxicokinetics, repeated dose toxicity (RDT), skin sensitization, carcinogenicity, and reproductive toxicity [16].

In addition, the REACH (Registration, Evaluation, Authorization and Restriction of Chemical substances) legislation was implemented to reduce the increased use of animals for toxicity induced by environmental factors such as industrial chemicals, food additives, and cosmetics, especially for developmental toxicity testing [17]. Therefore, it is essential to develop and validate in vitro and in silico alternative methods for replacement of in vivo developmental toxicity studies [18]. Many in vitro methods such as the embryonic stem cell test (EST), rodent whole embryo culture assay, and chicken embryotoxicity test [19, 20] have been developed to evaluate the toxic potential of chemical substances during the development. Alternative tests of developmental toxicity should be able to assess potential effects over the various stages [21]. Toxicity tests using stem cells are suited to evaluation of toxic effects on early embryo development and do not require the use of primary animal tissues.

2.3 Production of Stem Cell-Derived Cell Types for Pharmacological and Toxicological Screening

The derivation of mESCs was first reported in 1981 [22, 23], but the derivation of hESC lines was not reported until 1998. hESC lines are derived from extra embryos produced by in vitro fertilization (IVF). The generation of hiPSCs from human skin cells in 2007 provided opportunities for scientists to overcome the ethical concerns associated with human embryos.

The unique ability of stem cells to regenerate themselves and different tissues of the body has fascinated scientists, and allowed pharmacological and toxicological screening. ESCs are expected to dramatically improve the ability to screen for side effects of new drugs much earlier in the developmental process, and ESCs and iPSCs differentiated along particular pathways are useful for screening cell type-specific toxicities such as cardiotoxicity, hepatotoxicity, nephrotoxicity (Chap. 4), and neurotoxicity (Chap. 5) as preclinical models. However, the concept of large-scale/high-throughput stem cell-based toxicity screens has several limitations that have hindered the establishment of these cells.

2.3.1 Reprogramming

Owing to development of methods introducing reprogramming factors (e.g., OCT4, SOX2, KLF4, C-MYC, NANOG, LIN28, and REX1) to the cells, somatic cells from a patient (e.g., skin fibroblasts, hair follicles, or whole blood) can easily be used to establish iPSC lines that are free from viral transgenes and genetically identical to the patient via non-integrating genomic approaches [24–27]. The following methods considering cell permeability, non-immunogenicity, easy synthesis, cost-effectiveness, and reversible effects of transfection reagents and genetic materials have been used in the reprogramming process: single/multiple transient transfections, excisable and non-integrating vectors, proteins and direct protein transduction, modified RNA, mRNA-based transcription factor delivery, microRNA transfections, plasmid and episomal vectors, chemical compounds, and small molecules.

2.3.2 Differentiation Reproducibility of Stem Cells

Reliable and reproducible differentiation protocols are important to obtaining specific cell types for drug development or safe pharmacology. Providing a continuous supply of well-defined and differentiated cells without variable contamination by precursor cells remains a significant hurdle that has only been achieved with a few cell types. Improvements in methods to increase the yield of differentiated cells are continuously being reported [28].

2.3.3 Achieving Mature Phenotypes

A major unresolved problem is caused by the fact that cells differentiated from pluripotent stem cells using currently available protocols are immature compared to their adult counterparts. In PSCs-derived cardiomyocytes, the cells are more similar to fetal than adult cardiomyocytes in that they lack a fully developed transverse tubule system [29], and they undergo spontaneous contractions not found in adult ventricular cardiomyocytes. Similarly, genomic expression profiling and functional screening of hiPSC-derived hepatocytes, cardiomyocytes, and neuronal cells have shown that an immature or fetal phenotype is typically obtained [30–32].

2.3.4 *Heterogeneity and Purification of PSCs-Derived Cells*

Differentiated cardiomyocytes are a mixture of cells consisting of atrial-, ventricular-, and nodal-like phenotypes, as well as heterogeneous populations undergoing differentiation into hepatocytes including sinusoidal endothelial cells, hepatic stellate cells, Kupffer cells, and cholangiocytes [33]. While this heterogeneity is an advantage owing to the possibility to assess physiological properties in multiple cell types, it acts as a disadvantage in that changes occurring in only one subpopulation of cells may be diluted. Accordingly, it is essential to collect differentiated cell subtypes of high purity for high-throughput application. Fluorescence-activated cell sorting (FACS) or magnetic bead sorting enables isolation of highly enriched populations from heterogeneous cell populations.

2.4 Developmental Toxicity Screening Using ESCs

2.4.1 *Mouse Embryonic Stem Cell Test Validated by the European Center for Validation of Alternative Methods (ECVAM)*

Developmental toxicology is an important area that investigates undesirable effects on the development of an organism. Developmental toxicity must consider influences by exposure before conception, during the period of prenatal development, or postnatally during the time of sexual maturation, as well as manifestation of malformations, growth retardation, embryo lethality, and malfunction [34] (Fig. 2.1). In vitro systems for testing developmental toxicity fall into three classes: cell cultures (e.g., EST, organ cultures (e.g., micromass assay), and embryo cultures (e.g., whole embryo culture). The most important advantages of cell cultures are ease of performance and reduced or no experimental animal use.

During stem cell-based drug screening, formation of embryonic bodies (EBs) [35] and morphological differences in differentiated cells offer indirect information on malformation. Growth retardation and embryo lethality can also be assessed by cytotoxicity tests using MTT, XTT or CCK, and DNA damage tests using comet assay. Moreover, influences of drugs on function can be evaluated by tissue-specific features, such as contraction of differentiated myocardial cells (EST), expression of mature lineage markers (FACS-EST) [36], and promoter activity of specific genes (Hand1-EST) [37].

The EST [38] is an in vitro validated system designed to screen potential embryo toxic chemicals during differentiation. This test is based on ESCs, which permit the classification of chemicals as strongly, weakly, or non-embryo toxic. The EST has been improved to include supplementary endpoints able to identify effects on the nervous system [39], skeletal system [40], and cardiovascular system [41] as suggested by the ECVAM committee. The ability of ES cells to differentiate into

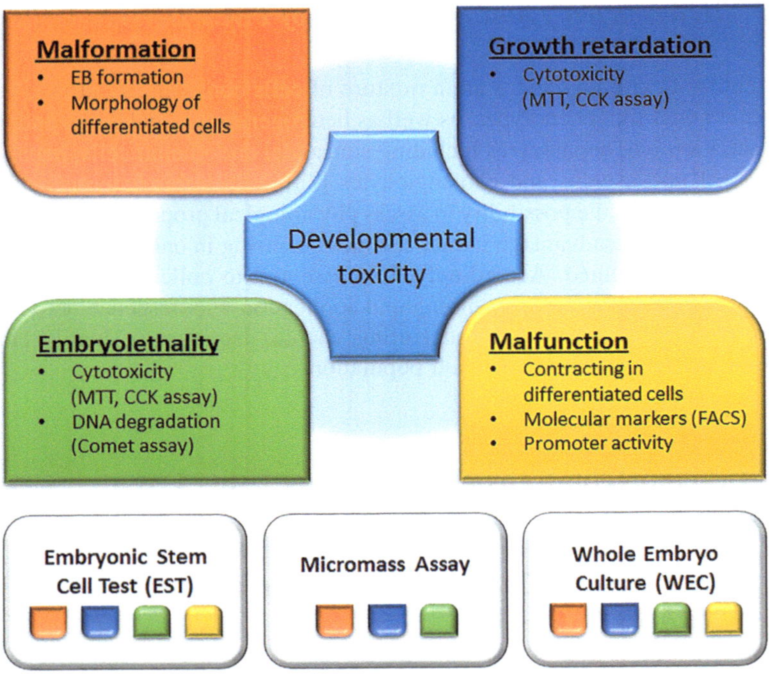

Fig. 2.1 Principal parameters in developmental toxicity. In developmental toxicity screening, malformation, growth retardation, embryo lethality, and malfunction are important manifestations that should be considered during in vitro screening. EST to screen the developmental toxicity of chemicals observes the formation of embryonic bodies and differences in morphology of differentiated cells to evaluate whether to induce malformation. Growth and lethality are assessed by cytotoxicity using MTT, XTT, or CCK. Impairment in function of differentiated cells is detected by contraction of differentiated myocardial cells, expression of tissue-specific lineage markers, and promoter activity assay. In particular, micromass assays were designed to screen embryo toxic and teratogenic agents, and the whole embryo culture method is useful for evaluating teratogenicity, delayed growth, embryo lethality, and impairment in partial function

various tissues is capable of screening chemical compounds with teratogenic effects [42, 43]. Furthermore, experts have advised that metabolic competences be added to the EST [34].

Mouse ESTs employ mESCs (D3) to represent embryonic tissue and fibroblasts (3T3 cells), as well as adult tissue. These tests assess three toxicological endpoints: (1) inhibition of growth (cytotoxicity) of undifferentiated ESCs (IC_{50} D3) and (2) 3T3 cells (IC_{50} 3T3), which represent differentiated cells after 10 days of treatment. This cytotoxicity is determined by the MTT assay, which is a colorimetric assay that reflects the number of viable cells present. This assay utilizes dehydrogenase enzymes present in the mitochondria of living cells to convert yellow soluble substrate, 3-(4,5-dimethylthiazol-2-yl)-2,5-diphenyl tetrazolium bromide (MTT), into purple insoluble formazan product, which becomes sequestered within the cells and is measured quantitatively at 500–600 nm using a microplate ELISA reader after solubilizing the cell membrane. (3) Inhibition of ESC differentiation into cardiac myoblasts (ID_{50}) after 10 days of treatment. To release from the undifferentiated stage, ESCs form EBs and differentiate into cardiomyocytes under appropriate conditions. Contracting cardiomyocytes mean to differentiate into the specialized cell types such as sinoatrial node, atrial, and ventricular cells, and to contain the intact functional interplay between these cell types. Spontaneous contraction of differentiated cells is measured by light microscopy and is an endpoint of EST. Concentration–response relationships are recorded and 50 % inhibition concentrations including IC_{50} D3, IC_{50} 3T3, and ID_{50} are determined for the three endpoints.

To validate in vitro embryotoxicity tests, the EST applies 20 potentially embryo toxic chemicals selected from a published list recommended by the US Teratology Society. These are then categorized into three classes of in vivo embryo toxicity, strong, weak, and non-embryo toxic [44]. These chemicals were selected according to high quality in vivo data obtained from both animal tests and human pregnancies. The embryotoxicity potential of chemicals is classified by statistical models using the half-maximal inhibition (ID50) value of inhibited differentiation of ESCs and IC50 values of decreased viability of 3T3 and ESCs after 10 days of exposure. These EST provided a correct classification of the embryo toxic potential of 78 % of the test chemicals, as well as a predictivity of 100 % when only strong embryo toxic chemicals were considered. In the prevalidation study, the standard operating procedure (SOP) of the EST was successfully transferred to other laboratories in Europe and the United States [45].

2.4.2 Hand1-Luc EST Based on a Luciferase Reporter Assay

The EST by ECVAM evaluates cardiac differentiation toxicity by counting the beating of embryonic bodies. However, this EST undergoes laborious manipulations, requires experimental expertise, and requires a minimum of 10 days to obtain results. Therefore, a new EST based on a luciferase reporter gene assay was established by successful stable transfection of mESCs (D3) containing the promoter region of the **h**eart **and** **n**eural crest **d**erivatives expressed transcript **1** (Hand1) or **c**ardio**my**opathy **a**ssociated **1** (Cmya1) gene at the upstream of the luciferase reporter gene. These tests were found to be capable of assessment 6 days after treatment with test chemicals [46] in 2011. These ESTs are more rapid and easier, called Hand1-Luc EST and Cmya1-Luc EST, respectively.

Hand1 is a basic helix-loop-helix transcription factor known to be essential for heart development and to show dynamic and spatially restricted expression patterns during development of the heart [47]. Cmya1, which is found in chicken striated muscle, is an intercalated disk protein related to cardiac morphogenesis [48]. Up- or downregulation of these genes was also observed during differentiation of mESCs into cardiomyocytes and neurons by DNA microarray analysis, and altered by embryo toxic chemicals [49]. Hand1/Cmya1-Luc EST using a 96-well plate with

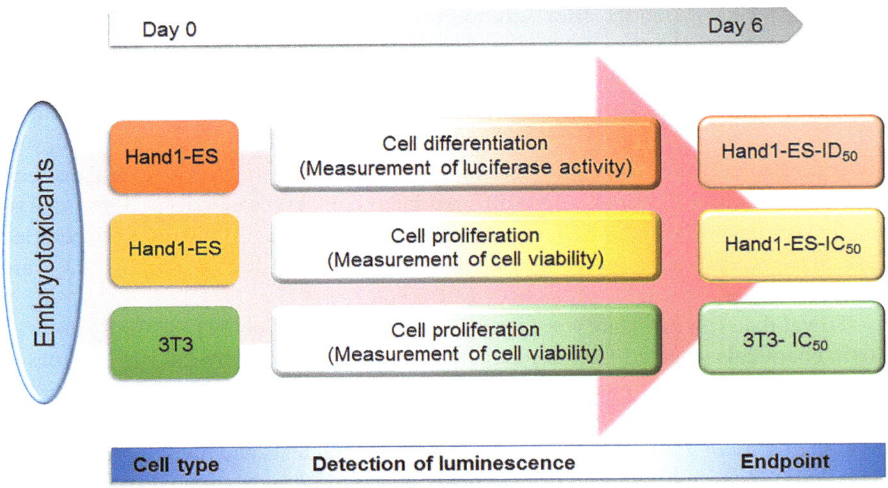

Fig. 2.2 Schema of the Hand1-Luc EST. To evaluate the developmental toxicity potential of embryotoxicants, Hand1-Luc EST has three endpoints with a 96-well microplate system and uses Hand1 promoter-transgenic mouse ESCs (Hand1-ES). Inhibitory effects (Hand1-ES-ID50) on cardiac differentiation are measured by chemiluminescence according to the luciferase activity of Han1-promoter. Cytotoxic effects on 3T3 fibroblasts (3T3-IC50) and transgenic mouse ESCs (Hand1-ES-IC50) were assessed by chemiluminescence

Hand- or Cmya1-ESCs consists of three endpoints (Fig. 2.2). Inhibitory effects on (1) differentiation of the transgenic ESCs and cytotoxic effects on (2) transgenic ESCs and (3) differentiated 3T3 cells were measured by detection of chemiluminescence. First, 24 chemicals that had been well characterized as embryotoxicants in vivo were evaluated by these EST at day 6 [46]. The reproducibility of Hand1- and Cmya1-ESTs was then investigated by comparing a set of six well-known chemicals at four different laboratories [50]. Consequently, the luciferase signal obtained with Hand1 was found to be much higher than that obtained with the Cmya1 gene. Adopted Hand1-Luc EST reduced the incubation time from 6 to 5 days (120 h). This method can be more easily performed without complex (e.g., formation of EB) and delicate (e.g., observation of beating) manipulation.

2.4.3 Limitations and Improvement of EST

The EST classified 20 test chemicals as non-, weakly, or strongly embryo toxic, and provided 78 % accuracy for estimation of embryo toxic potential based on a prediction model reflecting ESC (D3) viability, ESC (D3) differentiation, and 3T3 cell viability. However, it showed low predictability in a second study, with only 2 out of 13 test chemicals correctly classified. Therefore, the consortium of the ReProTect project questioned the applicability of this prediction model and recommended other test systems to assess the embryo toxic potential of compounds containing toxicity by metabolic activation [51]. EST also has several limitations; specifically, it consists of laborious and time-consuming steps such as hanging-drops to form EBs for differentiation initiation, exclusion of molecular endpoints to determine cardiac differentiation [52], and lack of information about the morphological changes induced by the teratogen.

Tissue-specific proteins are expressed in the process of ESC differentiation in patterns similar to those observed during mouse embryogenesis [43]. For example, cardiac-specific transcription factor Nkx2.5 is expressed in parallel to the α1-subunit of the L-type Ca2+ channel, followed by the expression of α- and β-myosin heavy chain isoforms during EB development [53]. As previously described, the improved EST has applied reporter gene assays using tissue-specific genes [46, 54]. The EST has also employed the quantifying cardiac markers α-myosin heavy chain and α-actin via FACS, which is known as FACS-EST. This method includes molecular endpoints, has the same sensitivity as the validated EST when applied for classification of ten compounds into three classes, and decreased test duration [36]. Accordingly, FACS-EST has been suggested as a new EST toxicological endpoint. Other potential biomarker genes include *Pnpla6*, *a-fetoprotein*, *nestin*, and *Vgfa*, which can be useful for evaluating embryotoxicity in early developmental stages [55].

Transcriptomics and proteomics are also used as endpoints of the EST. Embryotoxic chemicals elicit changes in the expression profiles of genes and proteins involved in development or differentiation [56–58]. This method requires 4 days, while EB requires 3 days with EB exposed for one additional day to evaluate chemicals, and shows 83 % accuracy for 12 tested chemicals (ten correct and two wrong predictions) [56]. In the same study, assessment using EST biomarker genes showed 67 % correct prediction (8 of the 12 tested chemicals). Protein markers are capable of being used to detect embryotoxicity of chemicals [56].

In a recent study, an EST reflecting inhibitory effects of embryotoxicants on EB growth or size was proposed [35]. The EB size-based EST assesses five toxic chemicals during formation of EBs, indomethacin, dexamethasone, hydroxyurea, 5-fluorouracil, and cytosine arabinoside, which act as an initiation point of differentiation. This EST microscopically demonstrated that EBs are dose-dependently reduced at 3 days after treatment with chemicals, and that the morphology of EB was distorted. However, this EST has not been validated, and therefore only suggests a cytotoxic point of view for differentiation potential during early embryonic development.

The ESC (D3) differentiation assays used in most studies are stand-alone, and have shown in vitro potency classification of chemicals. Any incorrect classification by an in vitro assay was likely due to the lack of in vivo kinetic processes. Some chemicals may be tested at higher concentrations in the EST than could be achieved in vivo. Therefore, it is important to combine the in vitro model with data describing in vivo kinetics to better predict developmental toxic potencies. One of the key in vivo kinetic processes during pregnancy or embryo development is placental transfer. The transport of compounds through the placental barrier may lead to different final concentrations of compounds reaching the fetus. The human ex vivo placental perfusion model has been used to investigate transport of compounds across the maternal–fetal barrier [59–62]. However, this method is laborious and dependent on fresh human placenta. In addition, it is difficult to assess large numbers of compounds using this method.

Conversely, placental transfer using the in vitro BeWo transport model is easy, rapid, and inexpensive [63]. When the human choriocarcinoma BeWo b30 cells were grown on a transwell insert, the cells became polarized and formed a cell layer, separating an apical compartment from a basolateral compartment, representing maternal and fetal compartments in vivo, respectively [64]. This model is designed so that compounds can be transported across the BeWo cell layer via active transport or paracellular diffusion excluding transmembrane diffusion. The EST combining the ESC (D3) differentiation assay with the in vitro BeWo transport model is used to predict the relative in vivo developmental toxicity of five antifungal reagents, ketoconazole, tebuconazole, propiconazole, prothioconazole, and fenarimol, which cause increased embryo lethality, cleft palate, reduced fetal weight, and skeletal malformations in animal studies [65]. This combination EST provides the possibility to better predict the in vivo developmental toxicity of chemicals than a stand-alone assay.

2.4.4 False-Negative Effects Due to Species Differences

Human embryos are dramatically or specifically different from mouse embryos in the formation, structure, and function of the fetal membranes and placenta [66]. For example, humans form embryonic discs instead of a mouse egg cylinder. The human yolk sac serves important functions such as the initiation of hematopoiesis during the early stages of gestation, then becomes vestigial during later stages. However, the mouse yolk sac is a well-vascularized, robust, and extraembryonic organ throughout gestation. Thus, mice have a limited capacity as a model system to understand events including the initiation and maintenance of human pregnancy.

Differences in species have been reported in developmental toxicology. For example, corticosteroids are embryo toxic in mice, but not humans [67]. Conversely, drugs such as thalidomide and 13-cis retinoic acid cause severe malformations during human development, but not in mice or rats [68]. These differences may be caused by species differences in DNA methylation, DNA repair, and the expression of genes related to drug metabolism [69]. The risk of false negatives as a result of interspecies variations in biochemical pathways has been a primary reason to humanize these developmental toxicity assays. However, cell-based in vitro assays with high human relevance are urgently needed for preclinical activities. Such studies should include target identification and validation, screening of compound efficacy, and safety assessment studies [70]. Since primary cells or cell lines rapidly lose important functional systems or already lack these properties, they have limitations when applied to drug screening. Moreover, many human primary cell types such as cardiomyocytes and neuronal cells are inaccessible for various reasons, including ethical problems [70]. Human pluripotent stem cells provide an important new in vitro model to understand processes such as infertility, pregnancy loss, and birth defects. [28].

Thus, humanization of EST requires establishment of a hESCs-based cytotoxicity test. The cytotoxic effects of well-characterized chemicals including 5-fluorouracil (5-FU) and retinoic acid (RA) on hESCs, differentiated hESCs, and MRC5 cells (human embryonic lung fibroblasts) were investigated under various media compositions [71]. In this study, hESCs (H1) expressed specific RA receptors to a greater extent than MRC-5 cells. These findings demonstrate that pluripotent cells show a higher sensitivity to well-known teratogens than fibroblast cultures, and that the hESCs-based system can reproduce the results previously obtained from mouse EST. While all-trans retinoic acid and 13-cis RA showed comparable cytotoxic effects on hESCs, only all-trans RA showed cytotoxic effects in mESCs in previous analyses [72]. These findings suggest that development of a hESC-based EST requires evaluation of human-specific developmental toxicity.

In 2014, the developmental toxic effects of embryotoxicants (5-FU and indomethacin) and non-embryotoxicants (penicillin G) on undifferentiated hESCs (H9) were studied using Affymetrix GeneChips. The results showed a remarkable conversion in expression profiles of genes related to development, cell cycle, and apoptosis [73]. These findings provide information regarding drug-dependent changes in undifferentiated hESCs.

In the field of toxicity testing or drug screening, the application of hESCs is promising since hESCs undergo unlimited proliferation during in vitro culture (self-renewal) and are pluripotent [74]. However, when employing hESCs in in vitro test methods, it is important to consider the culture conditions since they are still not completely standardized. It is also necessary to overcome several limitations. Specifically, hESCs are generally unable to form new colonies from single cells, have high variances and a relatively long population-doubling time, and undergo slower and less organized cardiac differentiation in hESCs than in mESCs [75].

2.5 Tissue-Specific Drug Screening Using iPSCs

Human ESCs, or reprogrammed iPSCs, have unlimited proliferation capacity and can differentiate into different mature cell types (cardiomyocytes, hepatocytes, neurons, etc.) through forced directed differentiation protocols. Thus, they offer a cost-effective and invaluable in vitro human cellular model for assessment of RDT and toxicity in human target organs (cardiotoxicity, hepatotoxicity, neurotoxicity, etc). This application prevents the need to sacrifice animals for experimentation purposes, allows the use of human cells, and avoids false negatives owing to interspecies differences. Since hESCs recapitulate the most essential steps of embryonic development, they are useful for embryo toxic studies of how these differentiation processes are changed by exposure to the tested chemicals.

However, as mentioned above, the differentiation procedure of hESCs requires difficult manipulation and standardized protocols. Therefore, iPSC application in toxicology and drug screening suggests new alternative tests and provides new chemical safety assessment strategies [76, 77].

2.5.1 Cardiotoxicity Test Using hSCs

Cardiovascular (CV) toxicity contributed to more than a third of safety-related drug withdrawals from 1990 to 2006 [78], which emphasizes the urgent need for transformation of preclinical CV toxicity screening cascades. The most general drug-induced cardiovascular toxicities based on frequency of post-approval adverse events include arrhythmia, coronary artery disorder, hyper/hypotension, cardiac disorder, and heart failure [79]. Since these toxicities are all characterized by disturbance of organ-specific functions, preclinical screening cascades targeting these risks have been forced to depend overwhelmingly on in vivo models [28].

However, existing preclinical models of in vivo and in vitro cardiotoxicity of drug candidates have some limitations. For example, telemetrized animals offer insight into the effects of drugs on heart function, but are expensive and show suboptimal sensitivity. Additionally, in vitro models that employ Purkinje fibers or cloned human ion channels show poor accuracy when applied to predict the effects of drug candidates. Therefore, hSC-derived cardiomyocytes are useful for screening of new chemical entities for potential cardiotoxicants and QT interval prolongation. The QT interval is the time from the start of the Q wave to the end of the T wave, and the portion of an electrocardiograph (ECG) that means the time from the beginning of ventricular depolarization to the end of ventricular repolarization. Thus, to detect potential effects of drug candidates, prolongation of the QT interval is a type of disease marker for acquired long QT syndrome and a cardiotoxic marker in drug discovery and development.

Human ESCs can be differentiated into functional cardiomyocytes by several protocols [80]. hESC-cardiomyocytes show expected morphological characteristics such as Z bands and intercalated disks, express various cardiac proteins including α-cardiac actin, atrial myosin light chain, ventricular myosin light chain, α-myosin heavy chain, atrial natriuretic peptide, and cardiac troponin T and I, and rhythmically contract with a longer action potential duration (APD), characteristic of cardiomyocytes. However, the use of hESCs has limited the potential source of cardiomyocyte progenitors or immature cells.

Differentiation of iPSC into cardiovascular cells is achieved via a multistep process that is tightly regulated by developmental signals, epigenetic programs, and extracellular microenvironments [81], and involves diverse pathways including BMP, TGF-β/activin/nodal, WNT/b-catenin, and FGF signaling. Global transcriptional profiles of human ESCs and iPSCs are very similar between the beating clusters derived from them. However, some fibroblasts-specific transcripts are retained in the iPSCs derived from them. In addition, a large number of these genes are expressed at the same level in iPSC-derived, but not ESC-derived, beating clusters [82]. These findings indicate that the differentiated and highly enriched iPSC derivatives retain epigenetic memory or specificity of the original cells.

Disease-specific human iPSC-cardiomyocytes act as more accurate predictors of drug-induced cardiotoxicity than standard human ether-a-go-go-related gene (hERG, Kv11.1 potassium channel) expressing HEK293 cells (Table 2.1) [83]. They are also able to analyze phenotypic and functional features manifested from changes in the individual genome. In particular, investigations of monogenic diseases in which a single genetic aberration causes severe deleterious effects on cellular function have been preferred iPSCs. For example, patient-specific iPSCs with long-QT syndrome caused by a mutation in the gene encoding the potassium channel (KCNQ1, KCNH2), sodium channel (SCN5A) or calcium channel (CACNA1C), or catecholaminergic polymorphic ventricular tachycardia (CPVT) by a mutation in the gene encoding the calcium channel (RYR2) or calcium-binding protein (CASQ2) have allowed investigation of the cell-autonomous pathophysiology (Table 2.1) and demonstrated that these in vitro disease models recapitulate key characteristics of the disorder and are suitable models to assess drug safety and efficacy [84].

2.5.2 Hepatotoxicity Test Using hSCs

Hepatotoxicity of new therapeutic agents is considered in preclinical and early clinical development [85, 86], FDA non-approval of new chemical entities, black box warnings, and withdrawals from the market [87]. The mechanisms responsible for drug-induced liver injury are only partly understood [86, 88]. Drug-induced liver injury is often detected after marketing approval when causality is difficult to identify, financial investment is high, and implications for individual patients are greatest. Development of methods to predict and prevent hepatotoxicity is needed, and such methods would reduce drug development conflict and the incidence of adverse drug reactions.

Various preclinical models are used during drug discovery, such as in silico tools to predict the chemical reactivity of the parent compound and metabolites, in vitro cytotoxicity screens using cell lines and primary hepatocytes, and in vivo preclinical models. Cell-based assays assess endpoints for cell health, including mitochondrial integrity and function, redox status, membrane integrity, and ATP generation. However, drug-induced liver injury is not predicted well by the current preclinical models because GLP toxicology studies, which investigate the relationship between dose and effects of chemicals on the exposed organism, are not completely concordant with the adverse effects of phase 1 clinical trials [89]. Unexpected adverse effects in liver are particularly dependent on metabolism and result from idiosyncratic toxicities or interspecies differences [85]. For these reasons, the development of in vitro screens of human liver function is highly desired.

Table 2.1 Patient-specific iPSCs derived from somatic cells with genetic disease

Name	Disease	Defect	Donor cell	
iPSC lines derived from patients with heart disease				
LQT1	Long-QT syndrome	KCNQ1 c.G569A (p.R190Q)	Fibroblast	Moretti et al., 2010 [102]
LQT1	Long-QT syndrome	KCNQ1 c.1893 del C (p.P631fs/33)	Fibroblast	Egashira et al., 2012 [103]
LQT2	Long-QT syndrome	KCNH2 c.C1841T (p.A614V)	Fibroblast	itzhaki et al., 2011 [104]
LQT2	Long-QT syndrome	KCNH2 c.G1681A (p.A561T)	Fibroblast	Matsa et al., 2011 [105]
LQT2	Long-QT syndrome	KCNH2 c.C526T (p.R176W)	Fibroblast	Lahti et al., 2012 [106]
LQT3	Long-QT syndrome, Brugada Syndrome	SCN5A c.5387_5389 in. TGA (p.1795 in. D)	Fibroblast	Davis et al., 2012 [107]
LQT8	Long-QT syndrome, Timothy Syndrome	CACNA1C c.G1216A (p.G406R)	Fibroblast	Yazawa et al., 2011 [108]
CPVT1	Catecholaminergic polymorphic ventricular tachycardia	RYR2 c.T7447A (p.F2483I)	Fibroblast	Fatima et al., 2011 [109]
CPVT1	Catecholaminergic polymorphic ventricular tachycardia	RYR2 c.C1217T (p.S406L)	Fibroblast	Jung et al., 2012 [110]
CPVT1	Catecholaminergic polymorphic ventricular tachycardia	RYR2 c.T12056G (p.M4109R)	Fibroblast	Itzhaki et al., 2012 [111]
CPVT2	Catecholaminergic polymorphic ventricular tachycardia	CASQ2 c.G1183C (p.D307H)	Fibroblast	Novak et al., 2012 [112]
DCM	Cardiomyopathies	TNTT2 p.R173W	Fibroblast	Sun et al., 2012 [113]
HCM	Cardiomyopathies	MYH7 c.G1988A (p.R663H)	Fibroblast	Lan et al., 2013 [114]
LS	LEOPARD syndrome	PTPN11 c.C140T (p.T468M)	Fibroblast	Carvajal-Vergara et al., 2010 [115]
ARVC	Arrhythmogenic right ventricular cardiomyopathy	PKP2 c.T1841C (p.L614P)	Fibroblast	Ma et al., 2013 [116]
ARVC	Arrhythmogenic right ventricular cardiomyopathy	PKP2 c.C2484T, Δ2483_2489, c.Δ2013 (p.R672fsX683)	Fibroblast	Kim et al., 2013 [117]
ARVC	Arrhythmogenic right ventricular cardiomyopathy	PKP2 c.972 insT/N (p.A324fsX335) PKP2 c.Δ148_151 (p.T50SfsX110)	Fibroblast	Caspi et al., 2013 [118]

(continued)

Table 2.1 (continued)

Name	Disease	Defect	Donor cell	
iPSC lines derived from patients with inherited metabolic disorders				
A1ATD	α1-antitrypsin deficiency	SERPINA1 p.E342K	Fibroblast	Rashid et al., 2010 [119]
GSD1a	Glycogen storage disease type 1 a	G6PC Deficiency	Fibroblast	
FH	Familial hypercholesterolemia	LDLR Deficiency	Fibroblast	
CNS	Crigler–Najjar syndrome	UGT1A1 Δ13bp in exon 2	Fibroblast	
Tyrosinemia	Hereditary tyrosinemia type 1	FAH p.V166G	Fibroblast	
Tyrosinemia	Hereditary tyrosinemia type 1	FAH p.Q64H	Fibroblast	
Tyrosinemia	Hereditary tyrosinemia type 1	FAH p.Q64H	Fibroblast	Ghodsizadeh et al., 2010 [120]
GSD1a	Glycogen storage disease type 1 a	SLC37A, c.A1124G	Fibroblast	
PFIC	Progressive familial hereditary cholestasis	Multifactorial	Fibroblast	
CNS	Crigler–Najjar syndrome	UGT1A1 p.L413P	Fibroblast	
WD	Wilson's disease (WD)	ATP7B p.R778L	Fibroblast	
iPSC lines derived from patients with genetic disease				
ADA	ADA-SCID	ADA p.G216R, fsΔGAAGA	Fibroblast	Park et al., 2008 [98]
GD	Gaucher disease type III	GBA c.A1226G (p.N370S), ins 84GG	Fibroblast	
DMD	Duchenne muscular dystrophy	DMD Δexon 45-52	Fibroblast	
BMD	Becker muscular dystrophy	DMD	Fibroblast	
DS1, DS2	Down syndrome	Trisomy 21	Fibroblast	
PD	Parkinson disease	Multifactorial	Fibroblast	
JDM	Juvenile diabetes mellitus	Multifactorial	Fibroblast	
SBDS	Shwachman–Bodian–Diamond syndrome	SBDS intron2, intron3	Bone marrow mesenchymal cells	
HD	Huntington disease	HTT 72 repeats of CAG	Fibroblast	
LNSc	Lesch–Nyhan syndrome (carrier)	Heterozygosity of HPRT1	Fibroblast	

c chromosome, *p* protein, *Δ* deletion, *ins* insertion, *fs* frame shift

To develop in vitro screens, multiple research groups have generated directed differentiation protocols toward human SC-derived hepatocytes (hESC-Hep and hiPSC-Hep), recapitulating key stages of natural liver development, including definitive endoderm, foregut, hepatic endoderm, bipotential hepatoblasts, and hepatocyte-like cells [90, 91]. hESCs and hiPSCs are differentiated into hepatocytes through a three-stage protocol consisting of a first phase of definitive endoderm induction, a second phase of hepatic lineage specification, and a third phase of hepatic maturation. These approaches based on hepatic embryogenesis involve a variety of pathways including fibroblast growth factor (FGF10), bone morphogenetic protein (BMP4), Wnt, activin, and hepatocyte growth factor (HGF) signaling.

Differentiated hESC-Hep and hiPSC-Hep have been analyzed by expression profiles of transcripts and protein and functional assays. The results of these analyses showed significant similarities to primary hepatocytes in transcriptional profile and functional properties, such as albumin and apolipoprotein B100 (ApoB100) secretion, functional bile transport, low density lipoprotein (LDL) uptake, urea synthesis, cytochrome P450 (CYP) activity (Cyp3A4), and glycogen storage [92]. However, when hESC-Hep and hiPSC-Hep were compared to fresh human fetal and adult hepatocytes, both cells were fetal-like, fell short of the adult phenotype, and upregulated expression of 81 % of phase 1 enzymes, such as alpha-fetoprotein (AFP, fetal markers) and Cyp3A7 (embryonic P450 activity). Half of these enzymes are statistically the same as human fetal hepatocytes. These differentiated cells also secrete albumin and metabolize testosterone (CYP3A) and dextrorphan (CYP2D6), similar to fetal hepatocytes [93].

In another study, hepatic disorder models using disease-specific human iPSCs closely resembled their native counterparts, recapitulated key aspects of the disease in question, and demonstrated measurable responses to therapeutic agents. The hiPSC-Hep can be generated from patients with inherited liver disease [94]. Moreover, pathogenic processes such as accumulation of misfolded proteins (α1-antitrypsin deficiency (A1ATD), familial transthyretin amyloidosis (TTR)), disruption of enzymatic activity (glycogen storage disease type 1a (GSD1a), Wilson's disease (WD)), receptor dysfunction (familial hypercholesterolemia (FH)), and infection by *hepatitis C virus* are reproduced in culture (Table 2.1). This hiPSC-Hep offers a new avenue to investigate the pathogenesis of these diseases. Each established individual stem cell population can be treated with environmentally induced variability in function and used to assess how much of the variability in drug toxicity is caused by genetic and environmental variations. Moreover, a library of hiPSC-Hep would be an invaluable model to enable detection of the potential risk of new therapeutics. Although the development of stem cell-based hepatocyte toxicity assays reflects the early stage, proof of concept and feasibility studies have been fulfilled using known toxicants [95]. Determination of the mechanistic basis of liver toxicity will permit more appropriate testing [28, 96].

2.5.3 *Other Disease-Specific iPSCs*

Generation of disease-specific iPSCs obtained from patients should consider processes such as reprogramming, differentiation and maturity, heterogeneity, and purification of iPSCs. Tissue cultures of immortal cell strains from patients are essential to medical research, but primarily restricted to tumor cell lines or transformed derivatives of native tissues. Strategies to accomplish nuclear reprogramming include SCNT, ANT, fusion of somatic cells with ESCs, and transfection of four defined transcription factors. Among these, methods for producing autologous, patient-derived pluripotent stem cells include SCNT and transfection of four transcription factors. hiPSCs and disease-specific hiPSCs are necessary complements to research using animal models of disease. Although murine models of human congenital and acquired diseases are valuable, they offer a limited representation of human pathophysiology and are not sufficient to mimic human diseases.

For these reasons, researchers have established disease-specific hiPSCs from patients with various genetic diseases and epigenetic-related disease. Genetic diseases are classified as monogenic by a single genetic aberration and polygenic disorders by multifactors or unknown causes [97]. Like iPSC-based models of cardiovascular disease, including LQT interval and arrhythmias, the following iPSC-based disease models have been generated and tested in drug development and discovery: adenosine deaminase deficiency-related severe combined immunodeficiency (ADA-SCID), Shwachman–Bodian–Diamond syndrome (SBDS), Gaucher disease (GD) type III, Duchenne (DMD) and Becker muscular dystrophy (BMD), Parkinson's disease (PD), Huntington's disease (HD), juvenile-onset, type 1 diabetes mellitus (JDM), Down syndrome (DS)/trisomy 21, the carrier state of Lesch–Nyhan syndrome (Table 2.1) [98]. Unlike genetic diseases based on the DNA sequence, the most important epigenetic phenomenon is genomic imprinting. Abnormal imprinting mechanisms during development provoke epigenetic diseases such as Beckwith–Wiedemann syndrome, Silver–Russell syndrome, Angelman syndrome, and Prader–Willi syndrome. The methylation status in imprinting genes is maintained during iPSC production via reprogramming and subsequent cultivation for differentiation [97]. Thus, by comparison of normal and pathologic tissues and evaluation of the reparative effects of suitable drug treatment for patients in vitro, hiPSCs obtained from patients can offer an opportunity to recapitulate pathologic human tissue in vitro and a new platform for drug screening.

2.6 Future Directions

The field of stem cell research represents one of the most exciting areas in life science and is showing rapid and dynamic expansion. (1) In basic scientific research, stem cells are an attractive system utilized in studies of gene functions and physiological processes during development. (2) Stem cells are useful in

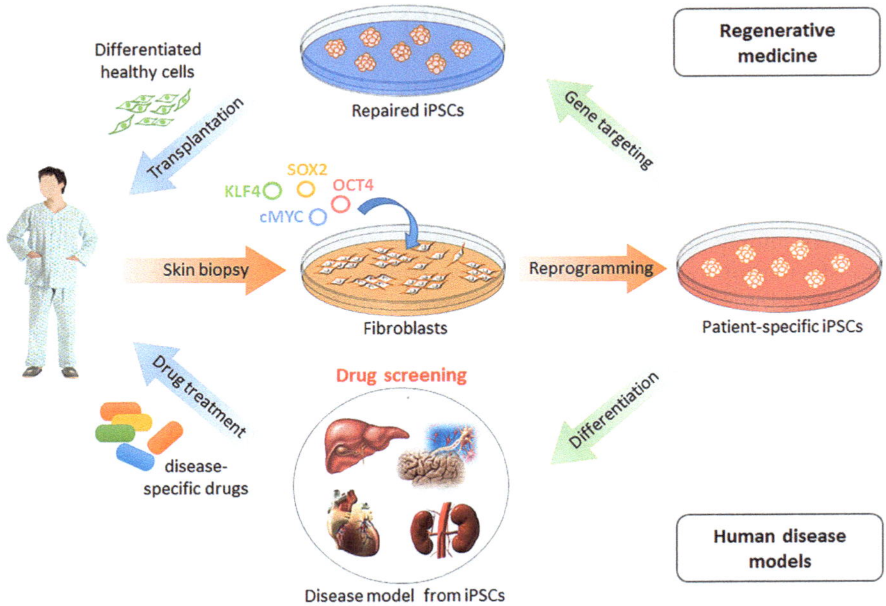

Fig. 2.3 Future direction of SCs: personalized therapy. Patient-specific iPSCs have the potential for use in modeling and treatment of human disease. iPSCs are derived by co-expression of transcription factors such as OCT4, SOX2, KLF4, and c-MYC in fibroblasts isolated from skin. The iPSCs can be applied to cell therapy through gene-targeting and drug screening. Gene-repaired patient-specific iPSCs can be differentiated into normal cell types and transplanted into defective organs. Moreover, differentiated cardiomyocytes, hepatocytes, renal cells, and neuronal subtypes from patient-specific iPSCs would be useful for in vitro disease models, and screening of potential drugs or discovery of novel therapeutic compounds [121]

biomedical research because of their inherent plasticity. Their ability to differentiate into specialized cell types may be useful for regenerative medicine to replace tissues damaged by injury, disease, or congenital defects. Various stem cell types such as mesenchymal cells, cord blood cells, adipose tissue cells, and adult stem cells have been successfully applied in wound healing and tissue regeneration. The US Food and Drug Administration (FDA) recently approved clinical trials using stem cells to treat heart disease [99]. iPSCs provide some distinct advantages in a clinical setting. Since iPSCs are autologous cells from the patient, they do not pose the same immune rejection risks in medical therapy. (3) In pharmaceutical and toxicological research, stem cells are powerful tools to evaluate the efficacy, safety, and hazards of drugs or compounds including developmental toxicity, tissue specificity, and disease-specific responses.

Similarly, SCs have tremendous potential for use in regenerative medicine and creation of human disease models for research, therapeutic testing, and drug screening (Fig. 2.3) [100]. Regenerative medicine is an exciting and rapidly expanding field that enables replacement of damaged tissues in the human body through gene editing or cellular transplantation. Patient-derived hiPSCs are able to offer customized models of several genetic diseases, disease progression, and epigenetic-related disease, and to recapitulate different aspects associated with pathologies after differentiation. Human ESCs and iPSCs are extremely valuable tools that can be used to discover novel drugs with potential therapeutic applications and to develop and screen drugs in pharmaceutical and toxicological studies. Especially, hiPSCs enable personalized therapy through modeling of patient-specific disease and screening of patient customized drugs.

2.7 Conclusions

Toxicological screening is necessary to assess the safety or hazards presented by candidate chemicals during drug development. Many toxicological screening methods have used laboratory animals; however, this poses ethics problems, is time-consuming and expensive, and has a low success-rate. Various alternatives such as ex vivo, in vitro, and in silico methods have been proposed to overcome the disadvantages of animal testing and are being applied to address the 3Rs (*R*eduction, *R*efinement, and *R*eplacement). In vitro methods using cell lines can provide more rapid, precise, and relevant information than animal studies, and enable low-cost assessment of pharmaco-toxicological profiling of target drugs because of their low compound and time requirements [101]. These methods also overcome interspecies differences and enable assays of high human relevance. Many in vitro tests deal with primary human cells, immortalized cells, or cancer cell lines; however, primary human cells are difficult to obtain and cannot predict effects in early development.

Stem cells have the capacity to self-renew and the ability to differentiate into all cell types. As previously stated, in vitro assays based on embryonic stem cells have been introduced and validated, such as the mouse EST suggested by ECVAM, Hand-Luc EST based on a luciferase reporter assay, EST using hESCs and hiPSCs, and disease-specific EST using hiPSCS that originated from patients. Drug screening methods using ESCs are useful for evaluating the toxicity of new candidate drugs during embryonic development, and methods using differentiated ESCs and iPSCs are suitable for assessing tissue-specific toxicity, although expression profile is still more similar to fetal than adult cells. Moreover, disease-specific iPSCs obtained from patients provide an extraordinary opportunity to recapitulate traits and differences between normal and pathologic human tissue. Additionally, hiPSC can overcome false-negative effects due to interspecies differences. Overall, these tests are capable of investigating diseases, developing drugs, and evaluating or identifying the effectiveness and availability of medication. Although protocols for differentiation of stem cells into adult like-cell should be developed, drug screening using stem cells is clearly the most powerful tool for pharmaceutical development.

Acknowledgments This research was supported by a grant (15182MFDS460) from Ministry of Food and Drug Safety in 2016.

References

1. Theise ND, Krause DS. Toward a new paradigm of cell plasticity. Leukemia. 2002;16 (4):542–8. doi:10.1038/sj.leu.2402445.
2. Nagy A, Gocza E, Diaz EM, Prideaux VR, Ivanyi E, Markkula M, Rossant J. Embryonic stem cells alone are able to support fetal development in the mouse. Development. 1990;110 (3):815–21.
3. Pittenger MF, Mackay AM, Beck SC, Jaiswal RK, Douglas R, Mosca JD, Moorman MA, Simonetti DW, Craig S, Marshak DR. Multilineage potential of adult human mesenchymal stem cells. Science. 1999;284(5411):143–7.
4. Clarke DL, Johansson CB, Wilbertz J, Veress B, Nilsson E, Karlstrom H, Lendahl U, Frisen J. Generalized potential of adult neural stem cells. Science. 2000;288(5471):1660–3.
5. Yang L, Li S, Hatch H, Ahrens K, Cornelius JG, Petersen BE, Peck AB. In vitro trans-differentiation of adult hepatic stem cells into pancreatic endocrine hormone-producing cells. Proc Natl Acad Sci U S A. 2002;99(12):8078–83. doi:10.1073/pnas.122210699.
6. Toma JG, Akhavan M, Fernandes KJ, Barnabe-Heider F, Sadikot A, Kaplan DR, Miller FD. Isolation of multipotent adult stem cells from the dermis of mammalian skin. Nat Cell Biol. 2001;3(9):778–84. doi:10.1038/ncb0901-778.
7. Zuk PA, Zhu M, Mizuno H, Huang J, Futrell JW, Katz AJ, Benhaim P, Lorenz HP, Hedrick MH. Multilineage cells from human adipose tissue: implications for cell-based therapies. Tissue Eng. 2001;7(2):211–28. doi:10.1089/107632701300062859.
8. Jackson KA, Mi T, Goodell MA. Hematopoietic potential of stem cells isolated from murine skeletal muscle. Proc Natl Acad Sci U S A. 1999;96(25):14482–6.
9. Zhao Y, Glesne D, Huberman E. A human peripheral blood monocyte-derived subset acts as pluripotent stem cells. Proc Natl Acad Sci U S A. 2003;100(5):2426–31. doi:10.1073/pnas. 0536882100.
10. French AJ, Adams CA, Anderson LS, Kitchen JR, Hughes MR, Wood SH. Development of human cloned blastocysts following somatic cell nuclear transfer with adult fibroblasts. Stem Cells. 2008;26(2):485–93. doi:10.1634/stemcells.2007-0252.
11. Hurlbut WB. Altered nuclear transfer: a way forward for embryonic stem cell research. Stem Cell Rev. 2005;1(4):293–300. doi:10.1385/SCR:1:4:293.
12. Cowan CA, Atienza J, Melton DA, Eggan K. Nuclear reprogramming of somatic cells after fusion with human embryonic stem cells. Science. 2005;309(5739):1369–73. doi:10.1126/ science.1116447.
13. Takahashi K, Yamanaka S. Induction of pluripotent stem cells from mouse embryonic and adult fibroblast cultures by defined factors. Cell. 2006;126(4):663–76. doi:10.1016/j.cell. 2006.07.024.
14. Kang KS, Trosko JE. Stem cells in toxicology: fundamental biology and practical considerations. Toxicol Sci. 2011;120 Suppl 1:S269–89. doi:10.1093/toxsci/kfq370.
15. Hartung T. Food for thought . . . on alternative methods for cosmetics safety testing. ALTEX. 2008;25(3):147–62.
16. Basketter DA, Clewell H, Kimber I, Rossi A, Blaauboer B, Burrier R, Daneshian M, Eskes C, Goldberg A, Hasiwa N, Hoffmann S, Jaworska J, Knudsen TB, Landsiedel R, Leist M, Locke P, Maxwell G, McKim J, McVey EA, Ouedraogo G, Patlewicz G, Pelkonen O, Roggen E, Rovida C, Ruhdel I, Schwarz M, Schepky A, Schoeters G, Skinner N, Trentz K, Turner M, Vanparys P, Yager J, Zurlo J, Hartung T. A roadmap for the development of alternative (non-animal) methods for systemic toxicity testing—t4 report*. ALTEX. 2012;29 (1):3–91.
17. Hartung T, Hoffmann S. Food for thought . . . on in silico methods in toxicology. ALTEX. 2009;26(3):155–66.
18. Hofer T, Gerner I, Gundert-Remy U, Liebsch M, Schulte A, Spielmann H, Vogel R, Wettig K. Animal testing and alternative approaches for the human health risk assessment under the

proposed new European chemicals regulation. Arch Toxicol. 2004;78(10):549–64. doi:10.1007/s00204-004-0577-9.
19. Adler S, Basketter D, Creton S, Pelkonen O, van Benthem J, Zuang V, Andersen KE, Angers-Loustau A, Aptula A, Bal-Price A, Benfenati E, Bernauer U, Bessems J, Bois FY, Boobis A, Brandon E, Bremer S, Broschard T, Casati S, Coecke S, Corvi R, Cronin M, Daston G, Dekant W, Felter S, Grignard E, Gundert-Remy U, Heinonen T, Kimber I, Kleinjans J, Komulainen H, Kreiling R, Kreysa J, Leite SB, Loizou G, Maxwell G, Mazzatorta P, Munn S, Pfuhler S, Phrakonkham P, Piersma A, Poth A, Prieto P, Repetto G, Rogiers V, Schoeters G, Schwarz M, Serafimova R, Tahti H, Testai E, van Delft J, van Loveren H, Vinken M, Worth A, Zaldivar JM. Alternative (non-animal) methods for cosmetics testing: current status and future prospects-2010. Arch Toxicol. 2011;85(5):367–485. doi:10.1007/s00204-011-0693-2.
20. Louisse J, Verwei M, Woutersen RA, Blaauboer BJ, Rietjens IM. Toward in vitro biomarkers for developmental toxicity and their extrapolation to the in vivo situation. Expert Opin Drug Metab Toxicol. 2012;8(1):11–27. doi:10.1517/17425255.2012.639762.
21. Spielmann H. Predicting the risk of developmental toxicity from in vitro assays. Toxicol Appl Pharmacol. 2005;207(2 Suppl):375–80. doi:10.1016/j.taap.2005.01.049.
22. Evans MJ, Kaufman MH. Establishment in culture of pluripotential cells from mouse embryos. Nature. 1981;292(5819):154–6.
23. Martin GR. Isolation of a pluripotent cell line from early mouse embryos cultured in medium conditioned by teratocarcinoma stem cells. Proc Natl Acad Sci U S A. 1981;78(12):7634–8.
24. Jia F, Wilson KD, Sun N, Gupta DM, Huang M, Li Z, Panetta NJ, Chen ZY, Robbins RC, Kay MA, Longaker MT, Wu JC. A nonviral minicircle vector for deriving human iPS cells. Nat Methods. 2010;7(3):197–9. doi:10.1038/nmeth.1426.
25. Seki T, Yuasa S, Oda M, Egashira T, Yae K, Kusumoto D, Nakata H, Tohyama S, Hashimoto H, Kodaira M, Okada Y, Seimiya H, Fusaki N, Hasegawa M, Fukuda K. Generation of induced pluripotent stem cells from human terminally differentiated circulating T cells. Cell Stem Cell. 2010;7(1):11–4. doi:10.1016/j.stem.2010.06.003.
26. Yakubov E, Rechavi G, Rozenblatt S, Givol D. Reprogramming of human fibroblasts to pluripotent stem cells using mRNA of four transcription factors. Biochem Biophys Res Commun. 2010;394(1):189–93. doi:10.1016/j.bbrc.2010.02.150.
27. Narsinh KH, Jia F, Robbins RC, Kay MA, Longaker MT, Wu JC. Generation of adult human induced pluripotent stem cells using nonviral minicircle DNA vectors. Nat Protoc. 2011;6(1):78–88. doi:10.1038/nprot.2010.173.
28. Scott CW, Peters MF, Dragan YP. Human induced pluripotent stem cells and their use in drug discovery for toxicity testing. Toxicol Lett. 2013;219(1):49–58. doi:10.1016/j.toxlet.2013.02.020.
29. Lieu DK, Liu J, Siu CW, McNerney GP, Tse HF, Abu-Khalil A, Huser T, Li RA. Absence of transverse tubules contributes to non-uniform Ca(2+) wavefronts in mouse and human embryonic stem cell-derived cardiomyocytes. Stem Cells Dev. 2009;18(10):1493–500. doi:10.1089/scd.2009.0052.
30. Israel MA, Yuan SH, Bardy C, Reyna SM, Mu Y, Herrera C, Hefferan MP, Van Gorp S, Nazor KL, Boscolo FS, Carson CT, Laurent LC, Marsala M, Gage FH, Remes AM, Koo EH, Goldstein LS. Probing sporadic and familial Alzheimer's disease using induced pluripotent stem cells. Nature. 2012;482(7384):216–20. doi:10.1038/nature10821.
31. Jozefczuk J, Prigione A, Chavez L, Adjaye J. Comparative analysis of human embryonic stem cell and induced pluripotent stem cell-derived hepatocyte-like cells reveals current drawbacks and possible strategies for improved differentiation. Stem Cells Dev. 2011;20(7):1259–75. doi:10.1089/scd.2010.0361.
32. Mummery C, Ward-van Oostwaard D, Doevendans P, Spijker R, van den Brink S, Hassink R, van der Heyden M, Opthof T, Pera M, de la Riviere AB, Passier R, Tertoolen L. Differentiation of human embryonic stem cells to cardiomyocytes: role of coculture with

visceral endoderm-like cells. Circulation. 2003;107(21):2733–40. doi:10.1161/01.CIR.0000068356.38592.68.
33. Kmiec Z. Cooperation of liver cells in health and disease. Adv Anat Embryol Cell Biol. 2001;161:III–XIII, 1–151.
34. Pellizzer C, Bremer S, Hartung T. Developmental toxicity testing from animal towards embryonic stem cells. ALTEX. 2005;22(2):47–57.
35. Hong EJ, Choi Y, Yang H, Kang HY, Ahn C, Jeung EB. Establishment of a rapid drug screening system based on embryonic stem cells. Environ Toxicol Pharmacol. 2015;39(1):327–38. doi:10.1016/j.etap.2014.12.003.
36. Buesen R, Genschow E, Slawik B, Visan A, Spielmann H, Luch A, Seiler A. Embryonic stem cell test remastered: comparison between the validated EST and the new molecular FACS-EST for assessing developmental toxicity in vitro. Toxicol Sci. 2009;108(2):389–400. doi:10.1093/toxsci/kfp012.
37. Le Coz F, Suzuki N, Nagahori H, Omori T, Saito K. Hand1-Luc embryonic stem cell test (Hand1-Luc EST): a novel rapid and highly reproducible in vitro test for embryotoxicity by measuring cytotoxicity and differentiation toxicity using engineered mouse ES cells. J Toxicol Sci. 2015;40(2):251–61. doi:10.2131/jts.40.251.
38. Scholz G, Genschow E, Pohl I, Bremer S, Paparella M, Raabe H, Southee J, Spielmann H. Prevalidation of the embryonic stem cell test (EST)-a new in vitro embryotoxicity test. Toxicol In Vitro. 1999;13(4–5):675–81.
39. Strubing C, Ahnert-Hilger G, Shan J, Wiedenmann B, Hescheler J, Wobus AM. Differentiation of pluripotent embryonic stem cells into the neuronal lineage in vitro gives rise to mature inhibitory and excitatory neurons. Mech Dev. 1995;53(2):275–87.
40. zur Nieden NI, Kempka G, Ahr HJ. In vitro differentiation of embryonic stem cells into mineralized osteoblasts. Differentiation. 2003;71(1):18–27. doi:10.1046/j.1432-0436.2003.700602.x.
41. Boheler KR, Czyz J, Tweedie D, Yang HT, Anisimov SV, Wobus AM. Differentiation of pluripotent embryonic stem cells into cardiomyocytes. Circ Res. 2002;91(3):189–201.
42. Scholz G, Pohl I, Genschow E, Klemm M, Spielmann H. Embryotoxicity screening using embryonic stem cells in vitro: correlation to in vivo teratogenicity. Cells Tissues Organs. 1999;165(3–4):203–11. doi:10.1159/000016700.
43. Rohwedel J, Guan K, Hegert C, Wobus AM. Embryonic stem cells as an in vitro model for mutagenicity, cytotoxicity and embryotoxicity studies: present state and future prospects. Toxicol In Vitro. 2001;15(6):741–53.
44. Genschow E, Spielmann H, Scholz G, Pohl I, Seiler A, Clemann N, Bremer S, Becker K. Validation of the embryonic stem cell test in the international ECVAM validation study on three in vitro embryotoxicity tests. Altern Lab Anim. 2004;32(3):209–44.
45. Tandon S, Jyoti S. Embryonic stem cells: an alternative approach to developmental toxicity testing. J Pharm Bioallied Sci. 2012;4(2):96–100. doi:10.4103/0975-7406.94808.
46. Suzuki N, Ando S, Yamashita N, Horie N, Saito K. Evaluation of novel high-throughput embryonic stem cell tests with new molecular markers for screening embryotoxic chemicals in vitro. Toxicol Sci. 2011;124(2):460–71. doi:10.1093/toxsci/kfr250.
47. Cross JC, Flannery ML, Blanar MA, Steingrimsson E, Jenkins NA, Copeland NG, Rutter WJ, Werb Z. Hxt encodes a basic helix-loop-helix transcription factor that regulates trophoblast cell development. Development. 1995;121(8):2513–23.
48. Wang DZ, Reiter RS, Lin JL, Wang Q, Williams HS, Krob SL, Schultheiss TM, Evans S, Lin JJ. Requirement of a novel gene, Xin, in cardiac morphogenesis. Development. 1999;126(6):1281–94.
49. Suzuki N, Ando S, Sumida K, Horie N, Saito K. Analysis of altered gene expression specific to embryotoxic chemical treatment during embryonic stem cell differentiation into myocardiac and neural cells. J Toxicol Sci. 2011;36(5):569–85.
50. Suzuki N, Yamashita N, Koseki N, Yamada T, Kimura Y, Aiba S, Toyoizumi T, Watanabe M, Ohta R, Tanaka N, Saito K. Assessment of technical protocols for novel

embryonic stem cell tests with molecular markers (Hand1- and Cmya1-ESTs): a preliminary cross-laboratory performance analysis. J Toxicol Sci. 2012;37(4):845–51.
51. Marx-Stoelting P, Adriaens E, Ahr HJ, Bremer S, Garthoff B, Gelbke HP, Piersma A, Pellizzer C, Reuter U, Rogiers V, Schenk B, Schwengberg S, Seiler A, Spielmann H, Steemans M, Stedman DB, Vanparys P, Vericat JA, Verwei M, van der Water F, Weimer M, Schwarz M. A review of the implementation of the embryonic stem cell test (EST). The report and recommendations of an ECVAM/ReProTect Workshop. Altern Lab Anim. 2009;37(3):313–28.
52. Piersma AH. Validation of alternative methods for developmental toxicity testing. Toxicol Lett. 2004;149(1–3):147–53. doi:10.1016/j.toxlet.2003.12.029.
53. Fassler R, Rohwedel J, Maltsev V, Bloch W, Lentini S, Guan K, Gullberg D, Hescheler J, Addicks K, Wobus AM. Differentiation and integrity of cardiac muscle cells are impaired in the absence of beta 1 integrin. J Cell Sci. 1996;109(Pt 13):2989–99.
54. Bremer S, Worth AP, Paparella M, Bigot K, Kolossov E, Fleischmann BK, Hescheler J, Balls M. Establishment of an in vitro reporter gene assay for developmental cardiac toxicity. Toxicol In Vitro. 2001;15(3):215–23.
55. Pamies D, Vicente-Salar N, Sogorb MA, Roche E, Reig JA. Specific effect of 5-fluorouracil on alpha-fetoprotein gene expression during the in vitro mouse embryonic stem cell differentiation. Int J Toxicol. 2010;29(3):297–304. doi:10.1177/1091581810366312.
56. van Dartel DA, Pennings JL, de la Fonteyne LJ, Brauers KJ, Claessen S, van Delft JH, Kleinjans JC, Piersma AH. Evaluation of developmental toxicant identification using gene expression profiling in embryonic stem cell differentiation cultures. Toxicol Sci. 2011;119 (1):126–34. doi:10.1093/toxsci/kfq291.
57. van Dartel DA, Pennings JL, Robinson JF, Kleinjans JC, Piersma AH. Discriminating classes of developmental toxicants using gene expression profiling in the embryonic stem cell test. Toxicol Lett. 2011;201(2):143–51. doi:10.1016/j.toxlet.2010.12.019.
58. Osman AM, van Dartel DA, Zwart E, Blokland M, Pennings JL, Piersma AH. Proteome profiling of mouse embryonic stem cells to define markers for cell differentiation and embryotoxicity. Reprod Toxicol. 2010;30(2):322–32. doi:10.1016/j.reprotox.2010.05.084.
59. Mose T, Mathiesen L, Karttunen V, Nielsen JK, Sieppi E, Kummu M, Morck TA, Myohanen K, Partanen H, Vahakangas K, Knudsen LE, Myllynen P. Meta-analysis of data from human ex vivo placental perfusion studies on genotoxic and immunotoxic agents within the integrated European project NewGeneris. Placenta. 2012;33(5):433–9. doi:10.1016/j.placenta.2012.02.004.
60. Myllynen P, Mathiesen L, Weimer M, Annola K, Immonen E, Karttunen V, Kummu M, Morck TJ, Nielsen JK, Knudsen LE, Vahakangas K. Preliminary interlaboratory comparison of the ex vivo dual human placental perfusion system. Reprod Toxicol. 2010;30(1):94–102. doi:10.1016/j.reprotox.2010.04.006.
61. Myllynen P, Vahakangas K. An examination of whether human placental perfusion allows accurate prediction of placental drug transport: studies with diazepam. J Pharmacol Toxicol Methods. 2002;48(3):131–8. doi:10.1016/S1056-8719(03)00038-8.
62. Syme MR, Paxton JW, Keelan JA. Drug transfer and metabolism by the human placenta. Clin Pharmacokinet. 2004;43(8):487–514. doi:10.2165/00003088-200443080-00001.
63. Bode CJ, Jin H, Rytting E, Silverstein PS, Young AM, Audus KL. In vitro models for studying trophoblast transcellular transport. Methods Mol Med. 2006;122:225–39.
64. Cerneus DP, van der Ende A. Apical and basolateral transferrin receptors in polarized BeWo cells recycle through separate endosomes. J Cell Biol. 1991;114(6):1149–58.
65. Li H, Rietjens IM, Louisse J, Blok M, Wang X, Snijders L, van Ravenzwaay B. Use of the ES-D3 cell differentiation assay, combined with the BeWo transport model, to predict relative in vivo developmental toxicity of antifungal compounds. Toxicol In Vitro. 2015;29 (2):320–8. doi:10.1016/j.tiv.2014.11.012.
66. Castellucci M, Scheper M, Scheffen I, Celona A, Kaufmann P. The development of the human placental villous tree. Anat Embryol. 1990;181(2):117–28.

67. Larsen Jr JW, Greendale K. ACOG Technical Bulletin Number 84—February 1985: teratology. Teratology. 1985;32(3):493–6. doi:10.1002/tera.1420320319.
68. Nau H. Teratogenicity of isotretinoin revisited: species variation and the role of all-trans-retinoic acid. J Am Acad Dermatol. 2001;45(5):S183–7. doi:10.1067/mjd.2001.113720.
69. Krtolica A, Ilic D, Genbacev O, Miller RK. Human embryonic stem cells as a model for embryotoxicity screening. Regen Med. 2009;4(3):449–59. doi:10.2217/rme.09.13.
70. Jensen J, Hyllner J, Bjorquist P. Human embryonic stem cell technologies and drug discovery. J Cell Physiol. 2009;219(3):513–9. doi:10.1002/jcp.21732.
71. Adler S, Lindqvist J, Uddenberg K, Hyllner J, Strehl R. Testing potential developmental toxicants with a cytotoxicity assay based on human embryonic stem cells. Altern Lab Anim. 2008;36(2):129–40.
72. Adler S, Pellizzer C, Hareng L, Hartung T, Bremer S. First steps in establishing a developmental toxicity test method based on human embryonic stem cells. Toxicol In Vitro. 2008;22(1):200–11. doi:10.1016/j.tiv.2007.07.013.
73. Jung EM, Choi YU, Kang HS, Yang H, Hong EJ, An BS, Yang JY, Choi KH, Jeung EB. Evaluation of developmental toxicity using undifferentiated human embryonic stem cells. J Appl Toxicol. 2015;35(2):205–18. doi:10.1002/jat.3010.
74. Kaufman DS, Thomson JA. Human ES cells—haematopoiesis and transplantation strategies. J Anat. 2002;200(Pt 3):243–8.
75. Guan K, Furst DO, Wobus AM. Modulation of sarcomere organization during embryonic stem cell-derived cardiomyocyte differentiation. Eur J Cell Biol. 1999;78(11):813–23. doi:10.1016/S0171-9335(99)80032-6.
76. Laustriat D, Gide J, Peschanski M. Human pluripotent stem cells in drug discovery and predictive toxicology. Biochem Soc Trans. 2010;38(4):1051–7. doi:10.1042/BST0381051.
77. Trosko JE, Chang CC. Factors to consider in the use of stem cells for pharmaceutic drug development and for chemical safety assessment. Toxicology. 2010;270(1):18–34. doi:10.1016/j.tox.2009.11.019.
78. Shah RR. Can pharmacogenetics help rescue drugs withdrawn from the market? Pharmacogenomics. 2006;7(6):889–908. doi:10.2217/14622416.7.6.889.
79. Laverty H, Benson C, Cartwright E, Cross M, Garland C, Hammond T, Holloway C, McMahon N, Milligan J, Park B, Pirmohamed M, Pollard C, Radford J, Roome N, Sager P, Singh S, Suter T, Suter W, Trafford A, Volders P, Wallis R, Weaver R, York M, Valentin J. How can we improve our understanding of cardiovascular safety liabilities to develop safer medicines? Br J Clin Pharmacol. 2011;163(4):675–93. doi:10.1111/j.1476-5381.2011.01255.x.
80. Burridge PW, Keller G, Gold JD, Wu JC. Production of de novo cardiomyocytes: human pluripotent stem cell differentiation and direct reprogramming. Cell Stem Cell. 2012;10(1):16–28. doi:10.1016/j.stem.2011.12.013.
81. Moretti A, Laugwitz KL, Dorn T, Sinnecker D, Mummery C. Pluripotent stem cell models of human heart disease. Cold Spring Harb Perspect Med. 2013;3(11). doi:10.1101/cshperspect.a014027.
82. Gupta MK, Illich DJ, Gaarz A, Matzkies M, Nguemo F, Pfannkuche K, Liang H, Classen S, Reppel M, Schultze JL, Hescheler J, Saric T. Global transcriptional profiles of beating clusters derived from human induced pluripotent stem cells and embryonic stem cells are highly similar. BMC Dev Biol. 2010;10:98. doi:10.1186/1471-213X-10-98.
83. Liang P, Lan F, Lee AS, Gong T, Sanchez-Freire V, Wang Y, Diecke S, Sallam K, Knowles JW, Wang PJ, Nguyen PK, Bers DM, Robbins RC, Wu JC. Drug screening using a library of human induced pluripotent stem cell-derived cardiomyocytes reveals disease-specific patterns of cardiotoxicity. Circulation. 2013;127(16):1677–91. doi:10.1161/CIRCULATIONAHA.113.001883.
84. Sinnecker D, Laugwitz KL, Moretti A. Induced pluripotent stem cell-derived cardiomyocytes for drug development and toxicity testing. Pharmacol Ther. 2014;143(2):246–52. doi:10.1016/j.pharmthera.2014.03.004.

85. Guengerich FP. Mechanisms of drug toxicity and relevance to pharmaceutical development. Drug Metab Pharmacokinet. 2011;26(1):3–14.
86. Lee WM. Drug-induced hepatotoxicity. N Engl J Med. 2003;349(5):474–85. doi:10.1056/NEJMra021844.
87. Schuster D, Laggner C, Langer T. Why drugs fail—a study on side effects in new chemical entities. Curr Pharm Des. 2005;11(27):3545–59.
88. Kaplowitz N. Biochemical and cellular mechanisms of toxic liver injury. Semin Liver Dis. 2002;22(2):137–44. doi:10.1055/s-2002-30100.
89. Olson H, Betton G, Robinson D, Thomas K, Monro A, Kolaja G, Lilly P, Sanders J, Sipes G, Bracken W, Dorato M, Van Deun K, Smith P, Berger B, Heller A. Concordance of the toxicity of pharmaceuticals in humans and in animals. Regul Toxicol Pharmacol. 2000;32 (1):56–67. doi:10.1006/rtph.2000.1399.
90. Du Y, Wang J, Jia J, Song N, Xiang C, Xu J, Hou Z, Su X, Liu B, Jiang T, Zhao D, Sun Y, Shu J, Guo Q, Yin M, Sun D, Lu S, Shi Y, Deng H. Human hepatocytes with drug metabolic function induced from fibroblasts by lineage reprogramming. Cell Stem Cell. 2014;14 (3):394–403. doi:10.1016/j.stem.2014.01.008.
91. Si-Tayeb K, Lemaigre FP, Duncan SA. Organogenesis and development of the liver. Dev Cell. 2010;18(2):175–89. doi:10.1016/j.devcel.2010.01.011.
92. Ogawa S, Surapisitchat J, Virtanen C, Ogawa M, Niapour M, Sugamori KS, Wang S, Tamblyn L, Guillemette C, Hoffmann E, Zhao B, Strom S, Laposa RR, Tyndale RF, Grant DM, Keller G. Three-dimensional culture and cAMP signaling promote the maturation of human pluripotent stem cell-derived hepatocytes. Development. 2013;140(15):3285–96. doi:10.1242/dev.090266.
93. Baxter M, Withey S, Harrison S, Segeritz CP, Zhang F, Atkinson-Dell R, Rowe C, Gerrard DT, Sison-Young R, Jenkins R, Henry J, Berry AA, Mohamet L, Best M, Fenwick SW, Malik H, Kitteringham NR, Goldring CE, Piper Hanley K, Vallier L, Hanley NA. Phenotypic and functional analyses show stem cell-derived hepatocyte-like cells better mimic fetal rather than adult hepatocytes. J Hepatol. 2015;62(3):581–9. doi:10.1016/j.jhep.2014.10.016.
94. Fahad AS. Prevalence of Human Herpesvirus-8 (HHV-8) in untreated patients with early stage Mycosis Fungoides (A retrospective study). Int J Health Sci. 2010;4(2):128–38.
95. Kulkarni JS, Khanna A. Functional hepatocyte-like cells derived from mouse embryonic stem cells: a novel in vitro hepatotoxicity model for drug screening. Toxicol In Vitro. 2006;20 (6):1014–22. doi:10.1016/j.tiv.2005.12.011.
96. LeCluyse EL, Witek RP, Andersen ME, Powers MJ. Organotypic liver culture models: meeting current challenges in toxicity testing. Crit Rev Toxicol. 2012;42(6):501–48. doi:10.3109/10408444.2012.682115.
97. Santostefano KE, Hamazaki T, Biel NM, Jin S, Umezawa A, Terada N. A practical guide to induced pluripotent stem cell research using patient samples. Lab Invest. 2015;95(1):4–13. doi:10.1038/labinvest.2014.104.
98. Park IH, Arora N, Huo H, Maherali N, Ahfeldt T, Shimamura A, Lensch MW, Cowan C, Hochedlinger K, Daley GQ. Disease-specific induced pluripotent stem cells. Cell. 2008;134 (5):877–86. doi:10.1016/j.cell.2008.07.041.
99. Butler J, Fonarow GC, Zile MR, Lam CS, Roessig L, Schelbert EB, Shah SJ, Ahmed A, Bonow RO, Cleland JG, Cody RJ, Chioncel O, Collins SP, Dunnmon P, Filippatos G, Lefkowitz MP, Marti CN, McMurray JJ, Misselwitz F, Nodari S, O'Connor C, Pfeffer MA, Pieske B, Pitt B, Rosano G, Sabbah HN, Senni M, Solomon SD, Stockbridge N, Teerlink JR, Georgiopoulou VV, Gheorghiade M. Developing therapies for heart failure with preserved ejection fraction: current state and future directions. JACC Heart Fail. 2014;2(2):97–112. doi:10.1016/j.jchf.2013.10.006.
100. Ebben JD, Zorniak M, Clark PA, Kuo JS. Introduction to induced pluripotent stem cells: advancing the potential for personalized medicine. World Neurosurg. 2011;76(3–4):270–5. doi:10.1016/j.wneu.2010.12.055.

101. Kari G, Rodeck U, Dicker AP. Zebrafish: an emerging model system for human disease and drug discovery. Clin Pharmacol Ther. 2007;82(1):70–80. doi:10.1038/sj.clpt.6100223.
102. Moretti A, Bellin M, Welling A, Jung CB, Lam JT, Bott-Flugel L, Dorn T, Goedel A, Hohnke C, Hofmann F, Seyfarth M, Sinnecker D, Schomig A, Laugwitz KL. Patient-specific induced pluripotent stem-cell models for long-QT syndrome. N Engl J Med. 2010;363 (15):1397–409. doi:10.1056/NEJMoa0908679.
103. Egashira T, Yuasa S, Suzuki T, Aizawa Y, Yamakawa H, Matsuhashi T, Ohno Y, Tohyama S, Okata S, Seki T, Kuroda Y, Yae K, Hashimoto H, Tanaka T, Hattori F, Sato T, Miyoshi S, Takatsuki S, Murata M, Kurokawa J, Furukawa T, Makita N, Aiba T, Shimizu W, Horie M, Kamiya K, Kodama I, Ogawa S, Fukuda K. Disease characterization using LQTS-specific induced pluripotent stem cells. Cardiovasc Res. 2012;95(4):419–29. doi:10.1093/cvr/cvs206.
104. Itzhaki I, Maizels L, Huber I, Zwi-Dantsis L, Caspi O, Winterstern A, Feldman O, Gepstein A, Arbel G, Hammerman H, Boulos M, Gepstein L. Modelling the long QT syndrome with induced pluripotent stem cells. Nature. 2011;471(7337):225–9. doi:10.1038/nature09747.
105. Matsa E, Rajamohan D, Dick E, Young L, Mellor I, Staniforth A, Denning C. Drug evaluation in cardiomyocytes derived from human induced pluripotent stem cells carrying a long QT syndrome type 2 mutation. Eur Heart J. 2011;32(8):952–62. doi:10.1093/eurheartj/ehr073.
106. Lahti AL, Kujala VJ, Chapman H, Koivisto AP, Pekkanen-Mattila M, Kerkela E, Hyttinen J, Kontula K, Swan H, Conklin BR, Yamanaka S, Silvennoinen O, Aalto-Setala K. Model for long QT syndrome type 2 using human iPS cells demonstrates arrhythmogenic characteristics in cell culture. Dis Model Mech. 2012;5(2):220–30. doi:10.1242/dmm.008409.
107. Davis RP, Casini S, van den Berg CW, Hoekstra M, Remme CA, Dambrot C, Salvatori D, Oostwaard DW, Wilde AA, Bezzina CR, Verkerk AO, Freund C, Mummery CL. Cardiomyocytes derived from pluripotent stem cells recapitulate electrophysiological characteristics of an overlap syndrome of cardiac sodium channel disease. Circulation. 2012;125(25):3079–91. doi:10.1161/CIRCULATIONAHA.111.066092.
108. Yazawa M, Hsueh B, Jia X, Pasca AM, Bernstein JA, Hallmayer J, Dolmetsch RE. Using induced pluripotent stem cells to investigate cardiac phenotypes in Timothy syndrome. Nature. 2011;471(7337):230–4. doi:10.1038/nature09855.
109. Fatima A, Xu G, Shao K, Papadopoulos S, Lehmann M, Arnaiz-Cot JJ, Rosa AO, Nguemo F, Matzkies M, Dittmann S, Stone SL, Linke M, Zechner U, Beyer V, Hennies HC, Rosenkranz S, Klauke B, Parwani AS, Haverkamp W, Pfitzer G, Farr M, Cleemann L, Morad M, Milting H, Hescheler J, Saric T. In vitro modeling of ryanodine receptor 2 dysfunction using human induced pluripotent stem cells. Cell Physiol Biochem. 2011;28 (4):579–92. doi:10.1159/000335753.
110. Jung CB, Moretti A, Mederos y Schnitzler M, Iop L, Storch U, Bellin M, Dorn T, Ruppenthal S, Pfeiffer S, Goedel A, Dirschinger RJ, Seyfarth M, Lam JT, Sinnecker D, Gudermann T, Lipp P, Laugwitz KL. Dantrolene rescues arrhythmogenic RYR2 defect in a patient-specific stem cell model of catecholaminergic polymorphic ventricular tachycardia. EMBO Mol Med. 2012;4(3):180–91. doi:10.1002/emmm.201100194.
111. Itzhaki I, Maizels L, Huber I, Gepstein A, Arbel G, Caspi O, Miller L, Belhassen B, Nof E, Glikson M, Gepstein L. Modeling of catecholaminergic polymorphic ventricular tachycardia with patient-specific human-induced pluripotent stem cells. J Am Coll Cardiol. 2012;60 (11):990–1000. doi:10.1016/j.jacc.2012.02.066.
112. Novak A, Barad L, Zeevi-Levin N, Shick R, Shtrichman R, Lorber A, Itskovitz-Eldor J, Binah O. Cardiomyocytes generated from CPVTD307H patients are arrhythmogenic in response to beta-adrenergic stimulation. J Cell Mol Med. 2012;16(3):468–82. doi:10.1111/j.1582-4934.2011.01476.x.
113. Sun N, Yazawa M, Liu J, Han L, Sanchez-Freire V, Abilez OJ, Navarrete EG, Hu S, Wang L, Lee A, Pavlovic A, Lin S, Chen R, Hajjar RJ, Snyder MP, Dolmetsch RE, Butte MJ, Ashley EA, Longaker MT, Robbins RC, Wu JC. Patient-specific induced pluripotent stem cells as a

model for familial dilated cardiomyopathy. Sci Transl Med. 2012;4(130):130ra147. doi:10.1126/scitranslmed.3003552.
114. Lan F, Lee AS, Liang P, Sanchez-Freire V, Nguyen PK, Wang L, Han L, Yen M, Wang Y, Sun N, Abilez OJ, Hu S, Ebert AD, Navarrete EG, Simmons CS, Wheeler M, Pruitt B, Lewis R, Yamaguchi Y, Ashley EA, Bers DM, Robbins RC, Longaker MT, Wu JC. Abnormal calcium handling properties underlie familial hypertrophic cardiomyopathy pathology in patient-specific induced pluripotent stem cells. Cell Stem Cell. 2013;12(1):101–13. doi:10.1016/j.stem.2012.10.010.
115. Carvajal-Vergara X, Sevilla A, D'Souza SL, Ang YS, Schaniel C, Lee DF, Yang L, Kaplan AD, Adler ED, Rozov R, Ge Y, Cohen N, Edelmann LJ, Chang B, Waghray A, Su J, Pardo S, Lichtenbelt KD, Tartaglia M, Gelb BD, Lemischka IR. Patient-specific induced pluripotent stem-cell-derived models of LEOPARD syndrome. Nature. 2010;465(7299):808–12. doi:10.1038/nature09005.
116. Ma D, Wei H, Lu J, Ho S, Zhang G, Sun X, Oh Y, Tan SH, Ng ML, Shim W, Wong P, Liew R. Generation of patient-specific induced pluripotent stem cell-derived cardiomyocytes as a cellular model of arrhythmogenic right ventricular cardiomyopathy. Eur Heart J. 2013;34(15):1122–33. doi:10.1093/eurheartj/ehs226.
117. Kim C, Wong J, Wen J, Wang S, Wang C, Spiering S, Kan NG, Forcales S, Puri PL, Leone TC, Marine JE, Calkins H, Kelly DP, Judge DP, Chen HS. Studying arrhythmogenic right ventricular dysplasia with patient-specific iPSCs. Nature. 2013;494(7435):105–10. doi:10.1038/nature11799.
118. Caspi O, Huber I, Gepstein A, Arbel G, Maizels L, Boulos M, Gepstein L. Modeling of arrhythmogenic right ventricular cardiomyopathy with human induced pluripotent stem cells. Circ Cardiovasc Genet. 2013;6(6):557–68. doi:10.1161/CIRCGENETICS.113.000188.
119. Rashid ST, Corbineau S, Hannan N, Marciniak SJ, Miranda E, Alexander G, Huang-Doran I, Griffin J, Ahrlund-Richter L, Skepper J, Semple R, Weber A, Lomas DA, Vallier L. Modeling inherited metabolic disorders of the liver using human induced pluripotent stem cells. J Clin Invest. 2010;120(9):3127–36. doi:10.1172/JCI43122.
120. Ghodsizadeh A, Taei A, Totonchi M, Seifinejad A, Gourabi H, Pournasr B, Aghdami N, Malekzadeh R, Almadani N, Salekdeh GH, Baharvand H. Generation of liver disease-specific induced pluripotent stem cells along with efficient differentiation to functional hepatocyte-like cells. Stem Cell Rev. 2010;6(4):622–32. doi:10.1007/s12015-010-9189-3.
121. Robinton DA, Daley GQ. The promise of induced pluripotent stem cells in research and therapy. Nature. 2012;481(7381):295–305. doi:10.1038/nature10761.

Chapter 3
Genome Editing in Human Pluripotent Stem Cells

Liuhong Cai, Yoon-Young Jang, and Zhaohui Ye

3.1 Applications of Genome Editing in Human Pluripotent Stem Cells

Human embryonic stem cells (ESCs) and induced pluripotent stem cells (iPSCs) are playing increasingly important roles in biomedical research. The potentials of these cell types to give rise to all adult cell types greatly facilitate studies of human development. The fact that iPSCs carry the exact genetic information of the donor cells from which they are derived offers unprecedented opportunities to study disease mechanisms. Because their ability to expand while maintaining pluripotency, human ESCs and iPSCs also provide great alternatives to adult stem cells for regenerative medicine. To fully realize these potentials in research and medicine, the ability to efficiently and precisely modify genomes in pluripotent stem cells is required. Here are some major applications of human pluripotent stem cells that can be greatly aided by effective genome editing.

L. Cai
Center for Reproductive Medicine, The Third Affiliated Hospital, Sun Yat-sen University, Guangzhou, China
e-mail: cailh@mail.sysu.edu.cn

Y.-Y. Jang
Department of Oncology and Institute for Cell Engineering, Johns Hopkins University School of Medicine, Baltimore, MD, USA
e-mail: yjang3@jhmi.edu

Z. Ye, Ph.D. (✉)
Department of Medicine, Johns Hopkins University School of Medicine, Baltimore, MD, USA
e-mail: zye@jhmi.edu

E.M. Abdelalim (ed.), *Recent Advances in Stem Cells*, Stem Cell Biology and Regenerative Medicine, DOI 10.1007/978-3-319-33270-3_3

3.1.1 Better Developmental Biology Models

The developments of mouse ESCs and homologous recombination technologies have revolutionized studies of mammalian genetics and developmental biology [1–4]. Altering the sequence of a gene-of-interest with gene knockout, conditional knockout or precise mutation generation in mouse genome followed by analyzing the phenotypes has become a standard procedure to assess a new gene function. One of the most effective ways to monitor or to isolate cells of particular tissue types is to knock-in a reporter gene into the locus of a well-defined tissue-specific gene under the control of its endogenous promoter/enhancer elements. Expression of the reporter gene (e.g., green fluorescent protein) in tissue-specific manner facilitates advanced imaging and flow cytometry analyses. This gene tagging strategy is also great for tracking and evaluating the expression patterns of a target gene. Since the first report of human ESCs in 1998 [5], it has been anticipated that the human counterpart of mouse ESCs will provide a long-awaited system to uncover human-specific knowledge or to translate what we learned in mouse to human conditions. Indeed, the human ESCs and the later developed iPSCs have proven to be powerful systems for understanding normal developmental processes [6]. Varieties of tissue or cell types have been generated from them using two-dimensional or three-dimensional culture conditions. Therefore there will be tremendous demands for the creation of genetically modified pluripotent stem cells, similar to the more established mouse models, to study gene functions, dissect signal transduction pathways, and conduct cell lineage tracing (Fig. 3.1).

3.1.2 Disease Modeling and Functional Genomics

Pluripotent stem cells, particularly patient-specific iPSCs, offer enormous potential for modeling diseases [7]. Although animal studies have been instrumental in dissecting mechanisms of many diseases, there are fundamental differences between mouse and man. Human-relevant models are essential for understanding the basics of diseases and for developing safe and effective drug treatments. Immortalized cancer cell lines have so far been the main players in human-based biomedical research. Their limitations, which include significantly abnormal karyotype/ploidy and growth factor-independent proliferation, have already been realized. In addition, majority of the human diseases do not have disease-relevant cell lines established. In comparison, two main features of human iPSCs make them superior choices for disease modeling purposes. First is their unique ability to give rise to all functional cell types that may play important roles in diseases. Secondly iPSCs can be derived from various cell types from patients; therefore they retain the exact patient genetic information. Even for diseases caused by somatic mutations (i.e., mutations not existing in the patient's germline or other unaffected tissues/organs) that are acquired later in life, iPSC can be derived directly from the diseased tissues for research purposes [8]. Disease modeling using patient-specific iPSCs has

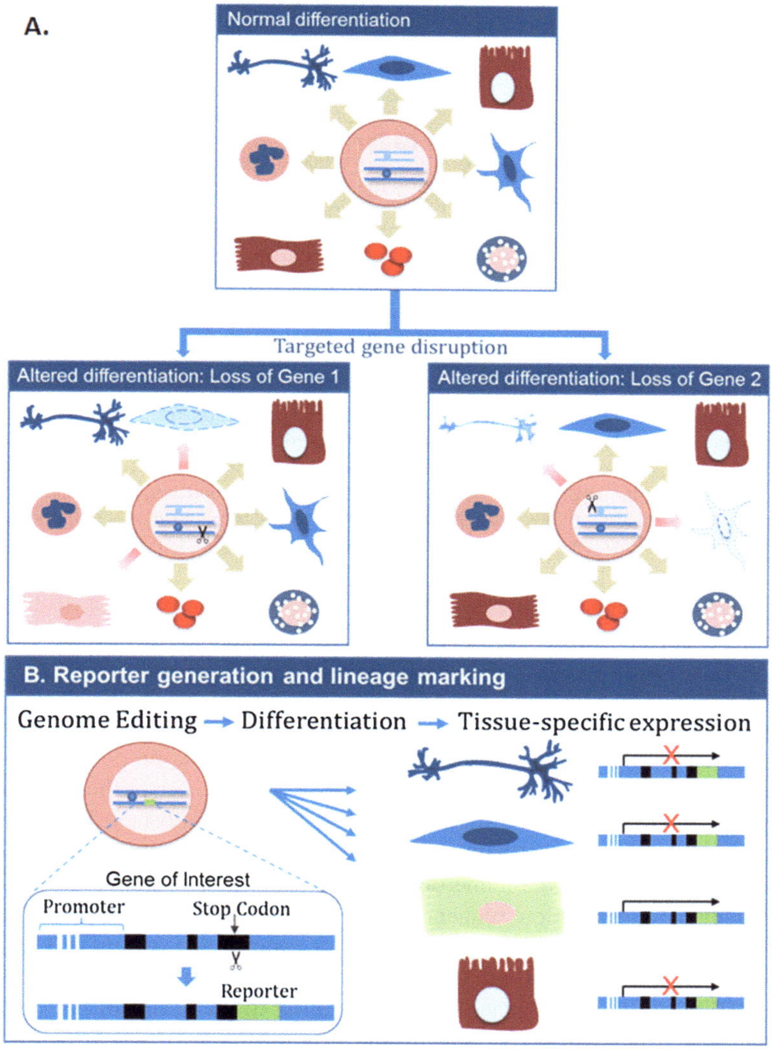

Fig. 3.1 Genome editing in human developmental biology and human genetics research. (**a**) The precision of genome editing and the pluripotency of ESCs and iPSCs can be combined for genetic studies of human developmental biology. Targeted modifications of gene-of-interest followed by differentiation can be used to evaluate gene function in development. (**b**) Gene editing can also be used to generate improved reporter systems to study tissue-specificity of genetic elements or to conduct lineage tracing experiment. Reporter/marker genes can be integrated into precise loci in the genome under the control of endogenous promoter/enhancer elements; expression patterns of the reporter gene therefore reflect the tissue-specificity of the gene-of-interest

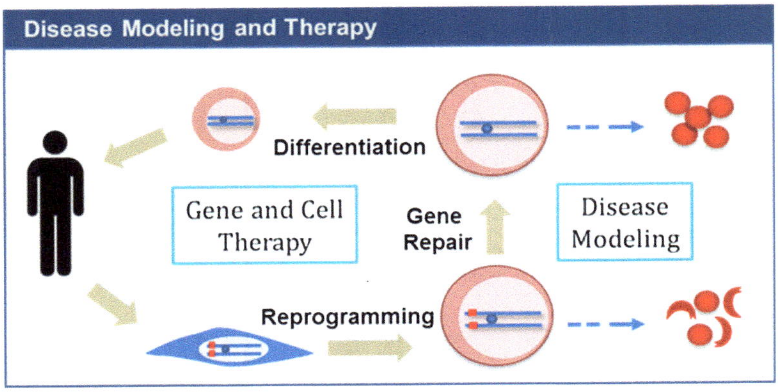

Fig. 3.2 Human iPSC-based disease modeling and therapy development. Patient-specific iPSCs carry genetic information of the patients and can be used for disease modeling to understand molecular and genetic basis of pathogenesis. By genome editing, the disease-related mutations can be repaired to generate isogenic cell lines to study their precise contributions to disease phenotypes. The gene-repaired iPSCs may also serve as sources for autologous cell therapies, if functional cell types (such as transplantable hematopoietic stem cells) can be derived

been reported in many diseases, with the differentiated cell types from iPSCs recapitulating disease features. These models provide unprecedented opportunities for dissecting the roles of each genetic mutation and/or polymorphism in disease predisposition or progression (Fig. 3.2).

An important research application of the patient-specific iPSCs is functional genomics. The iPSC system, with its tremendous differentiation potentials, serves as a powerful tool to study functionality of genetic variants such as those discovered from genome-wide association studies (GWAS). One major obstacle in iPSC-based functional genomics study is that the direct comparison between patient and control iPSCs is complicated by the numerous existing genomic polymorphisms as being revealed by next-generation sequencing [9]. It gets particularly complicated in studies of acquired or chronic diseases such as cancers and age-related diseases; the accumulated mutations (both driver and passenger mutations) may impede the interpretation of the target gene. The best solution to this problem is to generate isogenic iPSC lines that differ only in the gene-of-interest, similar to the well-established mouse genetic models (Fig. 3.2). This conceptually straightforward approach had been technically challenging until the recent breakthroughs in genome editing technologies.

3.1.3 Cell and Gene Therapy

Because of their unique differentiation capacity, human pluripotent stem cells have been anticipated to play important roles in regenerative medicine ever since the first report of human ESCs. The discovery of human iPSCs also paved the way for autologous cell therapies, which can avoid the complications associated with potential immune rejections. Although healthy tissues regenerated from the patients' own iPSCs would potentially serve the purposes of repairing the injured ones, this approach of simple replacement will not be effective if genetic conditions are the initial causes of the tissue injury. Examples of these diseases include sickle cell disease, thalassemias, duchenne muscular dystrophy, and amyotrophic lateral sclerosis (ALS), all of which have underlying genetic defects that prevent the direct use of patients' own cells, without genetic modification, for regenerative therapy. In these cases, the ability to genetically correct the mutations in these patient-specific iPSCs will be essential for developing therapeutic applications based on pluripotent stem cells (Fig. 3.2).

Strategies to genetically modify iPSCs include stable gene integration mediated by plasmid transfection, viral vector-based transduction, and DNA transposon-based gene transfer. These strategies have their limitations in medicine. For diseases that are caused by loss-of-function mutation of a single gene, supplying a functional and extra copy of the gene could effectively restore cellular functions and cure the disease. However, this strategy will not be suitable for diseases that are caused by the gain-of-function genetic mutations. In addition, the relatively random insertion of genetic elements in the genome presents risks for insertional mutagenesis, which has been responsible for cases of unexpected cancer development after gene therapy [10–12]. Additional concern regarding the effectiveness of this strategy is that the transgenes delivered through these methods are usually under the control of other promoters than their own endogenous locus control elements; therefore a more physiologically controlled transcriptional regulation is lacking, which may prevent the full therapeutic effect from being reached. For these reasons, on-site and more precise genome editing is a more preferred way for gene and cell therapy development.

3.2 Development of Genome Editing in Human Pluripotent Stem Cells

3.2.1 Conventional Strategies for Targeted Genome Editing in Human Pluripotent Stem Cells

Despite the tremendous success of homologous recombination in mouse ESCs and animal models, it was not straightforward to translate the technique into human pluripotent stem cells. Ever since the first establishment of human ESC lines in 1998 [5], investigators have been attempting to replicate the gene targeting success in human system. It turned out to be more challenging than original expected and few laboratories have succeeded before the advancement in designer endonucleases [13–17]. The main obstacle lies in the fundamental differences between mouse and human stem cells. These two types of ESCs vary significantly in their sizes and culture conditions; but more importantly the human ESCs have a much lower capacity of forming colonies from single cells than their murine counterpart [18]. The difference in intrinsic machineries that maintain genomic integrity is likely an even more significant contributor to the difficulty in human stem cell gene targeting. The first success of homologous recombination in human ESCs was achieved in 2003 in the laboratory that first derived them [13]. By modifying the mouse ESC electroporation conditions that were suboptimal for human cells [19], the investigators successfully deleted the last exons of hypoxanthine phosphoribosyltransferase 1 (*HPRT1*) gene on X-chromosome in human ESCs using homologous recombination. Using the same strategy, they also successfully generated knock-in cell lines in which an EGFP reporter gene is co-expressed with the OCT4-encoding gene *POU5F1*. Differentiation experiments showed that the EGFP reporter, linked to the last exon of OCT4 gene through an internal ribosome entry site (IRES) element, was expressed in the undifferentiated state and was subsequently turned off upon differentiation, demonstrating the potential of such engineered hESC lines in studying gene expression during development [13]. Although it was a significant technological achievement, the gene targeting efficiencies in these proof-of-principle experiments are substantially lower than that observed in mouse ESCs and other human cancer cell lines; 6–28 human ESC clones with homologous recombination events were obtained in the *HPRT1* and *OCT4* targeting experiments, respectively, after transfecting 1.5×10^7 cells [13]. Along with the technical challenges that were associated with human ESC culture in the early stage of stem cell research, such a low efficiency was almost prohibitive for most laboratories to perform homologous recombination in their favorite genes in human ESCs. Improving genome-editing conditions remained a priority in pluripotent stem cell research.

The genome editing efficiencies in human pluripotent stem cells had been steadily increasing in the past decade in part thanks to a better understanding of mechanisms underlying their survival and proliferation, which in turn resulted in the development of more advanced and simplified culturing conditions. Compared to the initial culture condition that required mouse embryonic fibroblasts (MEFs) as feeder cells, several more defined culture systems offer improved cell proliferation and elimination of feeder cells that can complicate the gene transfer and genomic DNA analysis procedures [20]. Among the technical developments, the discovery of the pro-survival effects of a specific rho-associated kinase (ROCK) inhibitor was one of the most significant in advancing human pluripotent stem cell research [21]. Addition of the ROCK inhibitor in culture medium overcomes the obstacle of poor single cell survival and recovery, which was one of the most serious impediments to advances in many human pluripotent stem cell-related applications including gene targeting. Higher level of single cell survival permits higher gene delivery efficiency through transfection. It also allows easier selection of single clones that have undergone successful genome editing. Improved gene targeting efficiencies have been observed by integrating ROCK inhibitors in the culture medium during the process [22]. Although the overall improvements in culturing conditions, together with enhanced transfection technologies, contribute to the higher efficiencies in genome editing in human ESCs and iPSCs, the most significant contributor is the development of engineered endonucleases.

3.2.2 *Engineered Endonuclease Technology for Improved Genome Editing*

Genome editing has become one of the most exciting frontiers in science thanks to the innovative tools that have elevated our ability to make precise changes in predetermined locations in genomes. The new tool set, which is still expanding, consists of several forms of engineered endonucleases that currently include zinc finger nucleases (ZFNs), transcription activator-like effector nucleases (TALENs), and clustered regularly interspaced short palindromic repeats (CRISPRs). Interestingly, none of these tools was designed to modify the cellular DNA repair machinery. Instead, they were all designed with a common purpose of making DNA strand breaks at precise genomic locations (Fig. 3.3). The desired modifications to the

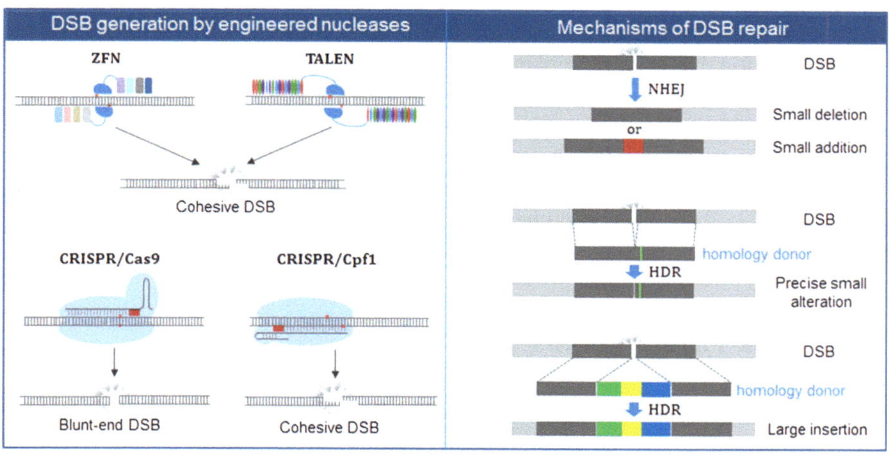

Fig. 3.3 Current designer endonuclease systems for enhancing genome editing. The common mechanism underlying the ability of designer endonucleases to enhance genome editing is the generation of DNA double strand breaks (DSBs) at precise genomic locations. ZFNs and TALENs are both fusion proteins that rely on the catalytic domain of FokI endonuclease to make DNA cleavage. Therefore they both generate the same type of cohesive-end DSBs with 5′-overhangs. CRISPR/Cas9 is a ribonuclease, in which the RNA component (single guide RNA) determines the DNA-binding specificity based on a 20-nucleotide sequence followed by the NGG PAM sequence (*red rectangle*). DSBs generated by Cas9 are blunt-ended. CRISPR/Cpf1 differs from Cas9 in their PAM sequence requirement (TTTN, *red rectangle*) and the cohesive DSBs after DNA cleavage. DSB repair by nonhomologous end joining (NHEJ) is error-prone and results in gene disruption by small insertion and/or deletion. When a homology donor is present, DSB can be repaired by the high fidelity homology-directed repair (HDR) pathways, which can introduce precise changes to the genomic location where the DSB was generated

genome will be generated during the subsequent repair by the cell's own DNA repair machinery. That is the basic principle underlying the development of the current designer endonucleases. In normal or physiological conditions, DNA damages caused by various factors such as radiation, UV lights, or reactive oxygen species occur constantly in cells particularly in those that are undergoing active DNA replication and division. The DNA damages, such as double strand DNA breaks, need to be repaired by the DNA repair machinery in order to maintain genomic integrity. DNA double strand breaks in mammalian cells are primarily repaired by either the error-prone nonhomologous end joining (NHEJ) or the high fidelity homology-directed repair (HDR) pathways. Although there are distinct repair mechanisms in either one of these pathways, for the purpose of this chapter, we will follow the tradition in stem cell research and use the term homologous recombination to describe the processes of homology-based gene targeting in human ESCs and iPSCs. The traditional homologous recombination-based gene targeting developed by Capecchi and colleagues was designed to introduce precise changes to the genome by introducing into the cell a "donor" DNA template that includes the desired changes flanked by DNA with identical or high-homology sequences to the intended site in genome [3]. In the rare events that DNA damages occur in the genomic region of interest and a DNA repair process is triggered, the externally introduced "donor" DNA may be used as a template for homologous recombination-based repair because of the high homology of its sequence to the genomic region that is being repaired (Fig. 3.3). The limitation of this approach lies in the rarity, and particularly so in human ESCs and iPSCs, of the DNA damage and repair events in any given genomic region. Based on experimental observations, it was hypothesized that if DNA breaks can be induced at desired location in the genome, the chances of introducing changes to that location will be significantly increased [23, 24]. This hypothesis is what motivated the efforts to engineer endonucleases for target-specific DNA strand break generation.

3.2.2.1 Zinc Finger Nucleases

The engineering of ZFNs is the first success in designer endonucleases aimed at enhancing genome editing [25–27]. The goal was to create an enzyme that can specifically bind and cut genomic DNA at a pre-designed location. Most of the natural endonucleases recognize specific DNA sequences; however, their specificity is generally defined by 4–6 nucleotides, too short to be unique within any mammalian genomes. One such example is the enzyme FokI, a bacterial type IIS restriction endonuclease consisting of an N-terminal DNA-binding domain and a nonspecific DNA cleavage domain at the C-terminus. The binding of the DNA by its DNA-binding domain, which has a specificity for 5′-GGATG-3′ sequence, will activate the DNA cleavage domain, which has no sequence specificity [28–30]. To take advantage of the DNA cleavage capacity of the natural enzymes, artificial proteins were created by combining the nonspecific cleavage domain of FokI endonuclease with DNA-binding domains of zinc finger proteins (ZFPs) that usually function as transcription factors. The zinc finger domain contains a tandem array of Cys2-His2 fingers with each finger recognizing a specific short stretch (3–4 nucleotide) of DNA [31]. A three- or four-finger protein will then be able to recognize 9 or 12 bp of DNA with specificity. An important feature of FokI that benefits targeting specificity is the requirement of protein dimerization for the formation of a catalytically active nuclease complex [29]. This means that in order to cleave the DNA, a pair of ZFNs must recognize and bind to neighboring regions with appropriate spacing for the FokI dimer to be formed. It further increases the sequence specificity of ZFNs to 18-bp or 24-bp for a pair of three-finger or four-finger ZFNs, offering a much higher probability of finding unique sequences in human genome. Further engineering has resulted in the development of variant ZFNs that cleave DNA only when paired as a heterodimer. These ZFNs modify a native endogenous locus as efficiently as the parental architecture, but with a reduced level of nonspecific genome-wide cleavage [32, 33].

It took several years for the technology to be successful in human pluripotent stem cells after the initial demonstrations of ZFN functionality in animal and human cells [25, 34]. One major reason is the poor hESC single cell survival and lack of efficient transfection in the earlier years of stem cell research. The first report of ZFN-mediated gene targeting in human ESCs utilized non-intergrading lentiviral vector as the delivery tool for ZFNs [35]. The improvement of single cell survival by ROCK inhibitor accelerated the research using nonviral delivery of plasmids encoding ZFNs and donor vectors [21]. In 2009, two reports using human ESCs and iPSCs demonstrated the utility of ZFNs in precise gene knockout and reporter cell line generation by simple DNA transfection [36, 37]. Using a human ES cell line that carries a chromosomally integrated mutant green fluorescent protein (GFP) reporter gene and a homologous donor vector that can repair the mutation upon homologous recombination, it was demonstrated that the ZFNs designed to target sequence inside the GFP gene enhanced gene correction by more than 1400-fold [36]. This study also demonstrated for the first time the generation of human ESC lines without detectable alterations in stem cell karyotypes or pluripotency after ZFN-mediated gene targeting. The enhanced efficiency facilitated the first gene knockout in human iPSCs at the endogenous phosphatidylinositol N-acetylglucosaminyltransferase subunit A (*PIG-A*) gene, a gene commonly mutated in a hematologic disease paroxysmal nocturnal hemoglobinuria (PNH) [36]. The ZFN technology also enhanced the capability of creating more faithful reporter cell lines by inserting reporter genes at desired endogenous loci. With ZFNs designed to target OCT4, a EGFP gene was inserted into human ESCs at the *POU5F1* locus with much enhanced efficiency [37]. Because the reporter cell lines are often used to monitor the differentiation status along human development, many of the potential targets will be the genes that are not expressed at pluripotent stem cell stage but rather upregulated upon differentiation. Therefore a key test for ZFNs is to target in human ESCs and iPSCs the transcriptionally inactive genes. Initial study showed that EGFP gene can be efficiently inserted into the paired-like homeodomain transcription factor 3 (*PITX3*) gene in human ESCs and iPSCs with the addition of ZFNs. Since PITX3 is a transcription factor only expressed in dopaminergic neurons and some other differentiated cell types, this study demonstrated that ZFN-mediated gene targeting is a robust tool for modifying genes, regardless of their expression status, to generate cell type-specific reporter systems [37].

The ZFN is a tremendous success as a proof-of-principle of designer endonuclease technology. It will remain a useful tool for genome editing in many systems including human ESCs and iPSCs. The available reagents that have shown great effectiveness will be valuable for future research and clinical applications [38–41]. The drawback of the technology is the difficulty in designing high-quality ZFNs. Although several strategies have been developed to engineer the Cys2His2 zinc fingers to bind various sequences [27, 42–45], vast majority of the research laboratories do not have the requisite expertise and resources to design and make them. Despite the reported success and the commercial sources that are devoted to ZFN generation, many researchers could not find the optimal ZFNs that target the desired genomic region(s) that best suit their research purposes. Therefore the search for additional tools continued.

3.2.2.2 Transcription Activator-Like Effector Nucleases (TALENs)

The TALEN technology was built upon a similar principle to ZFNs: a sequence-specific DNA binding domain fused to a nuclease domain that has no sequence specificity [46]. In fact, most of the available TALEN reagents use the same FokI nuclease as the catalytic domain. The fundamental difference between these two types of engineered nucleases is at the DNA binding domains. As the name implies, the DNA binding domain in TALENs originated from the transcription activator-like effector (TALE), a protein naturally made by *Xanthomonas* bacteria during their infection in plants. Once inside the plant cells, the bacterial TALE proteins bind promoter sequences in the plant genome to activate certain genes that are beneficial to bacterial infection. The DNA binding domain of TALE has been studied in detail; it recognizes plant DNA sequences through a variable number of repeats of around 34 amino acids [47, 48]. Three important features made the TALE a great template for protein engineering, particularly for the purposes of making a designer endonuclease. First, there is a one-to-one correspondence between each repeat and one single DNA base (i.e., a TALE domain of 16 repeats binds to a stretch of 16-bp DNA with specificity). Second, each repeat of the DNA binding domain has almost identical 34-amino acid sequences except the two residues at positions 12 and 13 (also termed repeat variable di-residues or RVDs), and these two residues appear to determine the binding specificity of each repeat to the DNA base. Third, the repeat motifs that have sufficient binding affinity and specificity for each of the four DNA bases (i.e., A, T, C, G) have already been naturally selected during bacterial evolution. This single-base recognition of TALE-DNA binding repeats offers far greater design flexibility than zinc finger's triplet recognition. Like ZFNs, optimal FokI domain dimerization and efficient DNA cleavage require sufficient spacer between the DNA binding sequences of the

TALEN pair. In general, TALENs prefer a longer spacer (13–30 bp) than ZFNs (<9 bp) [49, 50], in part due to the larger size of the TALE domain than that of the zinc fingers. An additional requirement in TALEN design is that each target sequence must be preceded by a T nucleotide. Due to these constraints, engineering a pair of high-quality TALENs is more than simple mix-and-match of the available individual repeat motifs. However, this is not a significant issue for potential TALEN users because web-based informatics programs have been developed to facilitate designing TALENs based on the sequence of the desired genomic regions [49, 51]. Additionally, most of the required reagents for TALEN assembly have been made readily available by the developing laboratories through the nonprofit global plasmid repository Addgene (website: http://www.addgene.org). It is therefore no longer a significant challenge to make functional TALENs by a regular research laboratory equipped with general molecular biology expertise.

TALENs have been shown to efficiently facilitate genome editing in many model systems including human ESCs and iPSCs [49, 52–58]. As with the earlier technologies, the first TALEN-mediated targeting in human ESCs and iPSCs was conducted at the *POU5F1* (OCT4) locus [53]. Similar to the ZFN experiment, TALENs significantly enhanced genome-editing efficiency. As observed in the ZFNs experiments [37], TALENs stimulated genome editing at both transcriptionally active and inactive loci [53]. Independent studies using ZFNs and TALENs to target the Z-mutation of alpha-1 antitrypsin (*AAT*) gene in AAT deficiency patient-specific iPSCs also demonstrated comparable efficiencies of these two systems in mediating homologous recombination-based gene repair [39, 59]. Since the single DNA base recognition of TALE binding repeats offers greater flexibility than zinc finger's triplet recognition, statistically there is a higher probability in finding suitable TALEN binding sequences than ZFN binding sequences in any given genomic region. This is a significant advantage of TALEN over the current ZFN technology; it provides a greater power to target disease-associated genetic elements across the entire human genome. TALEN-facilitated gene corrections have since been reported in various disease-specific human iPSCs [59–63], demonstrating the potential of this technology in developing iPSC-based cell and gene therapies. For research purposes, it is equally important to create disease-associated genetic variants in control iPSCs with normal genetic background. Such isogenic iPSC lines are essential for studying the functional consequences of the genetic variants [9]. Development of TALENs also contributed to the success of this type of research that has led to new disease models using human iPSCs [64–66].

3.2.2.3 Clustered Regularly Interspaced Short Palindromic Repeats (CRISPR)

Although TALEN provides a powerful alternative to ZFN technology, it is the discovery of CRISPR that placed genome editing at forefront of media and public attention [67]. The naturally occurring CRISPR, a type of repetitive DNA elements as its name suggests, was originally discovered in bacteria in 1987 [68].

Its biological functions remain mysterious until 2005 when studies suggested, and 2 years later proved, that it serves as a microbial adaptive immune system to destroy viral genetic elements [69–71]. Numerous studies have then been performed to detail the components of CRISPR complexes and the mechanisms of the adaptive immunity mediated by them [72, 73]. At the heart of the type II CRISPR system, where majority of the current genome editing tools are derived, there is a ribonuclease complex formed by the CRISPR-associated (Cas) enzyme, a CRISPR RNA (crRNA), and a trans-activating crRNA (tracrRNA) [74]. The crRNA directs the Cas9 enzyme to a specific region of DNA that has a complementary sequence of its own. A three-nucleotide (NGG for type II CRISPR, where "N" can be any one of the four nucleotides) protospacer adjacent motif (PAM) immediately following the complementary DNA sequence at the 3′ is required for the binding and cleavage activities of the CRISPR complex [75, 76]. Later it was shown that the crRNA and tracrRNA can be conjugated into a single guide RNA (sgRNA) that retains the Cas9 guiding function in vitro [77]. After this series of elegant biochemical experiments, a pair of studies demonstrated the feasibility of CRISPR, engineered from *Streptococcus pyogenes* type II CRISPR, in stimulating both NHEJ- and HDR-mediated genome editing in mammalian cells including human iPSCs [78, 79]. Both studies also demonstrated a unique advantage of CRISPR over ZFN and TALEN in mediating multiplexed genome editing; multiple guide RNAs can be delivered to the cells to target multiple loci simultaneously.

The major difference of CRISPR from the other two systems is that the protein/enzyme component (e.g., Cas9) does not need to be reengineered each time for a new target. The targeting specificity-determining component, the sgRNA, can be easily changed and synthesized. Although TALENs also have great flexibility in designing, each TALEN requires re-engineering and the assembly process is more complicated and time consuming. In comparison, the process of making CRISPRs is much simplified with significantly reduced costs. The simplicity and multiplicity had made the system an instant favorite among many research laboratories. Cas9 guide RNA libraries for genome scale loss-of-function screening were generated shortly after the first reports of CRISPR application in human cells [80, 81]. Data have been quickly generated to demonstrate the high efficiency of CRISPR/Cas9 in cell lines and animal models. In comparative studies conducted using human iPSCs, it has been shown that CRISPRs facilitate a higher genome editing efficiency than TALENs [79, 82, 83], providing more incentives for investigators to utilize this technology. However, studies have also suggested that the efficiency advantage of CRISPR/Cas9 over TALEN is more significant in inducing NHEJ-mediated gene disruption, and less significant in facilitating homologous recombination-based gene modification [83, 84]. The mechanism underlying this phenomenon is not yet fully understood, but the difference in the type of double strand breaks generated by these two nucleases (TALEN cleavage generates cohesive-ended DNA double strand breaks while Cas9 generates blunt-ended double strand breaks) may be a contributing factor.

Another advantage of CRISPR over ZFN and TALEN is the capability of specific targeting at a selected allele of a heterozygous gene. Humans are diploid organisms because there are two alleles at each genetic locus, with one allele inherited from each parent. In many genes there are minor DNA sequence differences, some of which are single nucleotide polymorphisms (SNPs), between the two alleles. Genetic mutations also often occur in only one allele of a given gene, which are termed heterozygous mutations. Because the specificity of CRISPR is determined by a 20-nucleotide sequence in the guide RNA and that single nucleotide changes in the 3′ region (closer to the PAM) of the guide RNA may significantly affect the CRISPR binding, it provides previously unavailable opportunities to design genome editing strategies that can target one allele with a specific genotype (e.g., a disease-causing point mutation) without interfering with the other allele (e.g., a wild-type allele without mutation). The feasibility of this strategy has been demonstrated in patient-specific iPSCs that carry either heterozygous or homozygous point mutations [83]. One current limitation of this strategy is that it can only apply to the genomic regions where the polymorphic nucleotide is within a short (in general $<=5$ bp) distance to the PAM, because nucleotide differences further away from PAM can be better tolerated by CRISPR/Cas9. However, different CRISPR systems with diverse PAM motifs are being developed [85, 86], which will make allele-specific targeting feasible in a larger portion of human genome.

The development of CRISPR technology has already provided more opportunities for research using human pluripotent stem cells, particularly for generating genetic models of diseases. So far researchers have successfully applied the CRISPR technology in human iPSCs to correct genetic mutations, generate mutations, delete a large genome fragment, and create targeted genome rearrangement [82, 83, 87–92]. In addition to these genome-editing purposes, CRISPR/Cas9 has been reengineered and repurposed for targeted transcriptional activation, transcriptional repression, and epigenetic regulations [93–102], making it a valuable and versatile tool.

3.2.3 Major Challenges in Improving Current Genome Editing Technologies

3.2.3.1 Maintaining Genome Integrity of Human Pluripotent Stem Cells After Genome Editing

Because human ESCs and iPSCs hold great therapeutic potentials, it is critical to minimize the negative effects of genome editing on genome integrity of these cells. The relatively hush conditions associated with gene delivery, whether chemical transfection or electroporation, together with a long culture period required for clonal expansion, selection cassette removal, and a secondary clonal expansion call for the concerns for potential compromise in genome integrity in the resultant cell lines. This concern has been addressed by cytogenetic analysis, array comparative genomic hybridization (aCGH), and genome-scale sequencing of gene targeted patient-specific iPSCs [22]. It has been shown that no additional mutations or copy number variations were identified after two subsequent clonal selection events. It is conceivable to estimate that there is no major increase in risk of accumulating genetic mutations during the cell culture time required for completing genome editing than any other routine cell culture [22].

A more relevant concern over the safety of the procedure lies in the potential off-target effects of the designer endonucleases. Since these nucleases enhance genome editing by creating DNA strand breaks at predetermined loci, it would be concerning if off-target binding and cutting occurs frequently at other unintended loci. In fact, the potential of nonspecific targeting by the earliest designer nuclease ZFNs has been speculated and observed soon after the first report ZFN-mediated genome modification in mammalian cells [50, 103]. Compared to ZFNs and TALENs, the CRISPR technology is far more user friendly for general laboratories to implement, therefore it is no surprise that the reports of substantial off-target effects by CRISPR/Cas9 attracted significant attention from both the research community and the general public [104–107]. These studies were mainly conducted in transformed or cancer cell lines that are commonly used in research laboratories for variety of biochemical studies. Because the traditional gene targeting efficiency in human ESCs and iPSCs is substantially low and therefore more dependent, than cancer cell lines, on the designer nucleases for precise genome editing, the question of the fidelity of these tools in pluripotent stem cells became an urgent one. The stem cell research field quickly moved to address this issue. By whole genome sequencing of gene targeted human pluripotent stem cell lines, several groups demonstrated that the off-target effects of both TALEN and CRISPR/Cas9 appear to be absent or minimal in selected human iPSC clones [108–110]. While there are technological limitations of these studies that may have prevented them from revealing the low level of off-targeting, it is reassuring to know that the fidelity of the current genome editing technologies in human stem cells is significantly higher than one would predict based on the results from other transformed cell lines.

In the meantime, various strategies have been developed to further enhance the specificity of CRISPR technology. One such strategy is to decrease the length of the gRNA-DNA interface, which is based on the observation that the mismatch at the 5′-end nucleotides of the complementary region is more tolerated and the hypothesis that truncating this region could result in lower affinity than what is required for an off-target binding and cutting. Experimental data supported this hypothesis and have shown that 5′-end truncated gRNAs are more sensitive to mismatches and thus more specific while maintaining the on-target activities [111]. Another popular approach is based on the further engineered CRISPR/Cas9, which has been mutated to possess only one catalytic domain instead of the original two functional domains [112, 113]. When two such Cas9-gRNA complexes, also termed "double nickase," bind to adjacent sequences at complementary strands, a DNA double strand break with 5′-overhang will be created. This double strand break will trigger cellular intrinsic DNA repair system similar to other double strand breaks created by ZFNs and TALENs do. However, in order to generate a double strand break, binding of two Cas9-gRNAs is required because each single complex can only generate a single strand nick that will be repaired using the complementary strand DNA as template. The requirement for two gRNA recognition sequence significantly lowers the frequency of potential off-target binding. A variant of this strategy is to create a fusion protein that contains a Cas9 with both catalytic domains mutated and a FokI catalytic domain, similar to the ZFN and TALEN technologies. In this case, only the co-binding of DNA by two adjacent Cas9-FokI complexes will result in dimerization of FokI which can generate double strand DNA breaks [114].

In addition, advance in bioinformatics will help users to design their TALENs or CRISPR guide RNAs with the lowest possibilities of off-target binding [107]. Multiple online programs have been developed by the leading laboratories in this research area to facilitate convenient and improved designer endonuclease design (at the time of writing, examples of some comprehensive web-based programs include: http://tools.genome-engineering.org, http://zifit.partners.org, http:/www.e-crisp.org). Potential on-target recognition sequences of the TALENs or guide-RNAs as well as their predicted off-target sites are generally provided by the programs. These readily available resources have contributed to the popularity of TALEN and CRISPR in research. One limitation of all these programs is that the predictions are made based on the sequence of a reference human genome (or reference genomes of other species of the user's choice), which has to be taken into consideration in each experimental design. SNPs occur normally throughout a person's DNA. Sequencing studies have demonstrated that on average there are at least a few million SNPs in the human genome [115], although most of these variations are found in the DNA between protein-coding genes. Changes in only a few nucleotides or, in the case of CRISPR, even a single nucleotide can have substantial effect on the binding affinity and specificity of the nucleases [116]. When designing experiments and interpreting data, one should take into consideration that the target cell line may have sequence differences from the reference genome. If possible, the genomic region of interest should be sequenced before the planning of experiments.

Although it is unlikely that the technologies will ever be improved to a perfect specificity, one advantage in human ESC or iPSC genome editing is that the clones can be fully analyzed by whole genome sequencing along with other functional assays. This feature will become even more useful when the sequencing technology is getting more advanced and affordable. Because off-target modifications by these designer endonucleases will occur as a low frequency event, it will be ideal to sequence and identify clones with minimal mutation load for downstream applications.

3.2.3.2 Improving Homologous Recombination Efficiency

For both research and clinical applications, it is often desired to perform homologous recombination-based genome editing. Precise correction or generation of genetic mutations and insertion of reporter genes to endogenous loci all require homologous recombination. Even though the development of ZFN, TALEN, and

CRISPR has significantly enhanced genome-editing efficiency and enabled many new applications, the percentages of cells that can undergo desired genome editing in each experiment remain low. The efficiency of homology donor plasmid-based gene targeting, currently a main gene targeting strategy in most biomedical laboratories, is another order of magnitude lower than NHEJ-mediated gene disruption efficiency. Data on the absolute efficiency (number of targeted clones/number of input cells) of homologous recombination are not yet extensive because majority of the studies in literature showed only the percentages of ESC/iPSC clones with targeted integration among selected drug-resistant clones. However, the level of improvement can still be estimated using data from limited studies. The absolute efficiency of homologous recombination events in human ESCs using the traditional gene targeting approach was originally shown to be 4–18 per 10 million input cells when *HPRT* and *POU5F1* loci were targeted [13]. When aided by the latest genome editing tools, it has been shown that the efficiencies of targeting adeno-associated virus integration site 1 (AAVS1), Janus kinase 2 (*JAK2*), or alpha-1 antitrypsin (*AAT*) loci in human iPSCs were at the ranges of 134–648 (TALEN-mediated) and 200–595 (CRISPR/Cas9-mediated) per 10 million input cells. The genomic loci targeted in these studies are different, but it is still reasonable to estimate that TALEN and CRISPR/Cas9 boost targeting efficiency by 10–100-fold. Even though the majority cells (>99.9 %) after transfection procedure remain un-targeted, it may not seem to be a big problem because the drug selection cassette that is generally included in the targeting donors will help to select the rare targeting events. With the improved human ESC and iPSC clonal culture conditions, this magnitude of improvement in efficiency is sufficient for experienced laboratories to achieve successful gene targeting on regular basis. However, this whole process including drug selection, clonal expansion, and a second round of clonal selection after drug selection cassette removal (e.g., Cre-lox recombination) can easily take several weeks or longer to complete. While this time frame is currently considered acceptable as routine laboratory practice, it will require significant improvement for patient-specific iPSC-based cell and gene therapy to become reality. A long wait-time for patients would not be the only problem; a lengthy and repeated clonal selection process also increases the possibility of the cells to accumulate and select for potentially tumorigenic somatic mutations. A significant improvement in homologous recombination will allow precise genome editing without drug selection, a process currently of low efficiency [38].

The contributing factors to an overall low homologous recombination frequency include ineffective gene transfer into the cells, inefficient DNA strand break generation, and an unfavorable preference for NHEJ repair over homologous recombination by the cellular DNA repair machinery following the DNA strand break. Therefore continued improvement in homologous recombination will require efforts in all these areas. Beside the transfection reagents (e.g., chemical transfection and electroporation) and transduction systems (e.g., lentivirus and adenovirus), the form of the endonucleases will also have an impact on the delivery efficiency. The current standard delivery form of the designer endonucleases is plasmid DNA that carry the expression cassettes of the protein (and small RNAs in the case of CRISPR). Using in vitro transcribed RNAs is an alternative approach that, with technology improvement in chemical modification of RNA molecules, may provide better cell survival and protein expression. It also reduces the risk of unwanted random integration of plasmid DNAs in the genome. More recently, it has also been demonstrated that preformed Cas9 ribonucleoproteins (i.e., functional complexes formed by Cas9 protein and guide RNA molecules) can be used for efficient genome editing [117, 118]. Continued improvement in the latter technology will have a positive impact on genome editing because it initiates genome editing quicker than other forms of delivery by eliminating the delay required for the Cas9 and guide RNA to be expressed and integrated inside the cells. And because there are no continuous transcription and translation processes to produce more CRISPR complexes after the desired DNA cleavage has been produced, using these preformed complexes could also lead to lower levels of nonspecific targeting.

In the near future, research on the balance between NHEJ and homologous recombination (or other forms of HDR) will likely draw significant interest from investigators in genome editing, as it may hold a key to an improved efficiency. A more complete understanding of the DNA repair pathways can lead to innovative strategies to tip the balance and promote homologous recombination. Small molecular compounds have already been identified that can affect the ratio of different types of DNA repair; these compounds, when added into the culture medium during genome targeting experiments, have been shown to increase either the homology-based gene repair or the NHEJ-mediated frameshift gene disruption [119–121]. As discussed in previous section, the type of DNA breaks also has an effect on the initiation of different type of DNA repair, with cohesive-end double strand breaks more effectively promoting homologous recombination than blunt-end strand breaks. The double nickase CRISPR system, which generates DNA double strand breaks with 5′-overhangs, is likely more efficient in stimulate homology-based repair than the single standard CRISPR/Cas9 [112, 113]. A new CRISPR family member CRISPR-Cpf1 has recently been reported [86]. It has been shown to generate DNA double strand breaks efficiently and has several distinct features from Cas9 including the generation of 5′ overhangs at DNA breaks. Whether Cpf1 is more effective than Cas9 in applications involving homologous recombination still remains to be determined. It is anticipated that other types of endonucleases with distinct DNA binding and cleavage mechanisms will be discovered or engineered in the future, providing diverse and more advanced tools for developing novel applications of human pluripotent stem cells.

3.3 Conclusions and Future Perspectives

The past few years have seen a rapid development in genome editing technologies. The engineered endonucleases such as ZFN, TALEN, and CRISPR provide unprecedented opportunities to introduce desired changes into genomes. While these technological developments are anticipated to have broad and revolutionary impacts on biomedicine as a whole, they are particularly significant in advancing human pluripotent stem cell research; the low efficiency of homologous recombination-based genetic engineering in human ESCs and iPSCs had been a major roadblock to translating stem cell technologies into effective research tools and therapies. With the improved genome editing efficiencies aided by these endonucleases, researchers now have more options to establish precise disease models, to evaluate links between genetic elements and functional outcomes, and to develop innovative gene and cell therapies.

There are significant ongoing efforts to further improve technologies critical for effective and safe genome editing. The designer nucleases, which rely on making DNA strand breaks to stimulate DNA repair, pose a unique risk of inducing unwanted mutations and genome instability. Strategies such as using CRISPR nickase systems and improved bioinformatics tools have been developed to reduce the rates of off-target mutagenesis. It is anticipated that continued re-engineering of the current designer endonucleases and discovery of novel types of nucleases will further improve genome editing specificity. In the meantime, it is still a labor-intensive process to introduce precise genetic modifications into the desired genome locations in human stem cells due to the lower efficiency of homologous recombination than that of the error-prone NHEJ DNA repair. Compared to the availability of DNA strand break-inducing tools, our current ability to control the balance between NHEJ and homologous recombination is limited. A better understanding of the cellular DNA repair mechanisms will no doubt contribute to the development of more efficient and precise genome editing.

References

1. Evans M, Kaufman M. Establishment in culture of pluripotential cells from mouse embryos. Nature. 1981;292:154–6.
2. Martin G. Isolation of a pluripotent cell line from early mouse embryos cultured in medium conditioned by teratocarcinoma stem cells. Proc Natl Acad Sci U S A. 1981;78:7634–8.
3. Thomas KR, Capecchi MR. Introduction of homologous DNA sequences into mammalian cells induces mutations in the cognate gene. Nature. 1986;324:34–8.
4. Thomas KR, Capecchi MR. Site-directed mutagenesis by gene targeting in mouse embryo-derived stem cells. Cell. 1987;51:503–12.
5. Thomson J, Itskovitz-Eldor J, Shapiro S, Waknitz M, Swiergiel J, Marshall V, Jones J. Embryonic stem cell lines derived from human blastocysts. Science. 1998;282:1145–7.
6. Yamanaka S. Induced pluripotent stem cells: past, present, and future. Cell Stem Cell. 2012;10:678–84.
7. Yoshida Y, Yamanaka S. Recent stem cell advances: induced pluripotent stem cells for disease modeling and stem cell-based regeneration. Circulation. 2010;122:80–7.
8. Ye Z, Zhan H, Mali P, Dowey S, Williams DM, Jang YY, Dang CV, Spivak JL, Moliterno AR, Cheng L. Human-induced pluripotent stem cells from blood cells of healthy donors and patients with acquired blood disorders. Blood. 2009;114:5473–80.
9. Soldner F, Jaenisch R. Medicine. iPSC disease modeling. Science. 2012;338:1155–6.
10. Hacein-Bey-Abina S, Von Kalle C, Schmidt M, McCormack M, Wulffraat N, Leboulch P, Lim A, Osborne C, Pawliuk R, Morillon E, Sorensen R, Forster A, Fraser P, Cohen J, de Saint

Basile G, Alexander I, Wintergerst U, Frebourg T, Aurias A, Stoppa-Lyonnet D, Romana S, Radford-Weiss I, Gross F, Valensi F, Delabesse E, Macintyre E, Sigaux F, Soulier J, Leiva L, Wissler M, Prinz C, Rabbitts T, Le Deist F, Fischer A, Cavazzana-Calvo M. LMO2-associated clonal T cell proliferation in two patients after gene therapy for SCID-X1. Science. 2003;302:415–9.
11. Hacein-Bey-Abina S, Garrigue A, Wang GP, Soulier J, Lim A, Morillon E, Clappier E, Caccavelli L, Delabesse E, Beldjord K, Asnafi V, MacIntyre E, Dal Cortivo L, Radford I, Brousse N, Sigaux F, Moshous D, Hauer J, Borkhardt A, Belohradsky BH, Wintergerst U, Velez MC, Leiva L, Sorensen R, Wulffraat N, Blanche S, Bushman FD, Fischer A, Cavazzana-Calvo M. Insertional oncogenesis in 4 patients after retrovirus-mediated gene therapy of SCID-X1. J Clin Invest. 2008;118:3132–42.
12. Howe SJ, Mansour MR, Schwarzwaelder K, Bartholomae C, Hubank M, Kempski H, Brugman MH, Pike-Overzet K, Chatters SJ, de Ridder D, Gilmour KC, Adams S, Thornhill SI, Parsley KL, Staal FJ, Gale RE, Linch DC, Bayford J, Brown L, Quaye M, Kinnon C, Ancliff P, Webb DK, Schmidt M, von Kalle C, Gaspar HB, Thrasher AJ. Insertional mutagenesis combined with acquired somatic mutations causes leukemogenesis following gene therapy of SCID-X1 patients. J Clin Invest. 2008;118:3143–50.
13. Zwaka T, Thomson J. Homologous recombination in human embryonic stem cells. Nat Biotechnol. 2003;21:319–21.
14. Irion S, Luche H, Gadue P, Fehling HJ, Kennedy M, Keller G. Identification and targeting of the ROSA26 locus in human embryonic stem cells. Nat Biotechnol. 2007;25:1477–82.
15. Davis RP, Ng ES, Costa M, Mossman AK, Sourris K, Elefanty AG, Stanley EG. Targeting a GFP reporter gene to the MIXL1 locus of human embryonic stem cells identifies human primitive streak-like cells and enables isolation of primitive hematopoietic precursors. Blood. 2008;111:1876–84.
16. Di Domenico AI, Christodoulou I, Pells SC, McWhir J, Thomson AJ. Sequential genetic modification of the hprt locus in human ESCs combining gene targeting and recombinase-mediated cassette exchange. Cloning Stem Cells. 2008;10:217–30.
17. Ruby KM, Zheng B. Gene targeting in a HUES line of human embryonic stem cells via electroporation. Stem Cells. 2009;27:1496–506.
18. Amit M, Carpenter MK, Inokuma MS, Chiu CP, Harris CP, Waknitz MA, Itskovitz-Eldor J, Thomson JA. Clonally derived human embryonic stem cell lines maintain pluripotency and proliferative potential for prolonged periods of culture. Dev Biol. 2000;227:271–8.
19. Eiges R, Schuldiner M, Drukker M, Yanuka O, Itskovitz-Eldor J, Benvenisty N. Establishment of human embryonic stem cell-transfected clones carrying a marker for undifferentiated cells. Curr Biol. 2001;11:514–8.
20. Amit M, Itskovitz-Eldor J. Maintenance of human embryonic stem cells in animal serum- and feeder layer-free culture conditions. Methods Mol Biol. 2006;331:105–13.
21. Watanabe K, Ueno M, Kamiya D, Nishiyama A, Matsumura M, Wataya T, Takahashi JB, Nishikawa S, Muguruma K, Sasai Y. A ROCK inhibitor permits survival of dissociated human embryonic stem cells. Nat Biotechnol. 2007;25:681–6.
22. Howden SE, Gore A, Li Z, Fung HL, Nisler BS, Nie J, Chen G, McIntosh BE, Gulbranson DR, Diol NR, Taapken SM, Vereide DT, Montgomery KD, Zhang K, Gamm DM, Thomson JA. Genetic correction and analysis of induced pluripotent stem cells from a patient with gyrate atrophy. Proc Natl Acad Sci U S A. 2011;108:6537–42.
23. Jasin M. Genetic manipulation of genomes with rare-cutting endonucleases. Trends Genet. 1996;12:224–8.
24. Vasquez KM, Marburger K, Intody Z, Wilson JH. Manipulating the mammalian genome by homologous recombination. Proc Natl Acad Sci U S A. 2001;98:8403–10.
25. Bibikova M, Carroll D, Segal DJ, Trautman JK, Smith J, Kim YG, Chandrasegaran S. Stimulation of homologous recombination through targeted cleavage by chimeric nucleases. Mol Cell Biol. 2001;21:289–97.

26. Durai S, Mani M, Kandavelou K, Wu J, Porteus MH, Chandrasegaran S. Zinc finger nucleases: custom-designed molecular scissors for genome engineering of plant and mammalian cells. Nucleic Acids Res. 2005;33:5978–90.
27. Urnov FD, Rebar EJ, Holmes MC, Zhang HS, Gregory PD. Genome editing with engineered zinc finger nucleases. Nat Rev Genet. 2010;11:636–46.
28. Wah DA, Hirsch JA, Dorner LF, Schildkraut I, Aggarwal AK. Structure of the multimodular endonuclease FokI bound to DNA. Nature. 1997;388:97–100.
29. Bitinaite J, Wah DA, Aggarwal AK, Schildkraut I. FokI dimerization is required for DNA cleavage. Proc Natl Acad Sci U S A. 1998;95:10570–5.
30. Wah DA, Bitinaite J, Schildkraut I, Aggarwal AK. Structure of FokI has implications for DNA cleavage. Proc Natl Acad Sci U S A. 1998;95:10564–9.
31. Wolfe SA, Nekludova L, Pabo CO. DNA recognition by Cys2His2 zinc finger proteins. Annu Rev Biophys Biomol Struct. 2000;29:183–212.
32. Miller JC, Holmes MC, Wang J, Guschin DY, Lee YL, Rupniewski I, Beausejour CM, Waite AJ, Wang NS, Kim KA, Gregory PD, Pabo CO, Rebar EJ. An improved zinc-finger nuclease architecture for highly specific genome editing. Nat Biotechnol. 2007;25:778–85.
33. Szczepek M, Brondani V, Büchel J, Serrano L, Segal DJ, Cathomen T. Structure-based redesign of the dimerization interface reduces the toxicity of zinc-finger nucleases. Nat Biotechnol. 2007;25:786–93.
34. Porteus MH, Baltimore D. Chimeric nucleases stimulate gene targeting in human cells. Science. 2003;300:763.
35. Lombardo A, Genovese P, Beausejour CM, Colleoni S, Lee YL, Kim KA, Ando D, Urnov FD, Galli C, Gregory PD, Holmes MC, Naldini L. Gene editing in human stem cells using zinc finger nucleases and integrase-defective lentiviral vector delivery. Nat Biotechnol. 2007;25:1298–306.
36. Zou J, Maeder M, Mali P, Pruett-Miller S, Thibodeau-Beganny S, Chou B, Chen G, Ye Z, Park I, Daley G, Porteus M, Joung J, Cheng L. Gene targeting of a disease-related gene in human induced pluripotent stem and embryonic stem cells. Cell Stem Cell. 2009;5:97–110.
37. Hockemeyer D, Soldner F, Beard C, Gao Q, Mitalipova M, DeKelver R, Katibah G, Amora R, Boydston E, Zeitler B, Meng X, Miller J, Zhang L, Rebar E, Gregory P, Urnov F, Jaenisch R. Efficient targeting of expressed and silent genes in human ESCs and iPSCs using zinc-finger nucleases. Nat Biotechnol. 2009;27:851–7.
38. Soldner F, Laganière J, Cheng AW, Hockemeyer D, Gao Q, Alagappan R, Khurana V, Golbe LI, Myers RH, Lindquist S, Zhang L, Guschin D, Fong LK, Vu BJ, Meng X, Urnov FD, Rebar EJ, Gregory PD, Zhang HS, Jaenisch R. Generation of isogenic pluripotent stem cells differing exclusively at two early onset Parkinson point mutations. Cell. 2011;146:318–31.
39. Yusa K, Rashid ST, Strick-Marchand H, Varela I, Liu PQ, Paschon DE, Miranda E, Ordóñez A, Hannan NR, Rouhani FJ, Darche S, Alexander G, Marciniak SJ, Fusaki N, Hasegawa M, Holmes MC, Di Santo JP, Lomas DA, Bradley A, Vallier L. Targeted gene correction of α1-antitrypsin deficiency in induced pluripotent stem cells. Nature. 2011;478:391–4.
40. Hoban MD, Cost GJ, Mendel MC, Romero Z, Kaufman ML, Joglekar AV, Ho M, Lumaquin D, Gray D, Lill GR, Cooper AR, Urbinati F, Senadheera S, Zhu A, Liu PQ, Paschon DE, Zhang L, Rebar EJ, Wilber A, Wang X, Gregory PD, Holmes MC, Reik A, Hollis RP, Kohn DB. Correction of the sickle-cell disease mutation in human hematopoietic stem/progenitor cells. Blood. 2015;125(17):2597–604.
41. Chang CJ, Bouhassira EE. Zinc-finger nuclease-mediated correction of α-thalassemia in iPS cells. Blood. 2012;120:3906–14.
42. Maeder ML, Thibodeau-Beganny S, Sander JD, Voytas DF, Joung JK. Oligomerized pool engineering (OPEN): an 'open-source' protocol for making customized zinc-finger arrays. Nat Protoc. 2009;4:1471–501.
43. Pruett-Miller SM, Connelly JP, Maeder ML, Joung JK, Porteus MH. Comparison of zinc finger nucleases for use in gene targeting in mammalian cells. Mol Ther. 2008;16:707–17.

44. Sander JD, Maeder ML, Reyon D, Voytas DF, Joung JK, Dobbs D. ZiFiT (Zinc Finger Targeter): an updated zinc finger engineering tool. Nucleic Acids Res. 2010;38:W462–8.
45. Doyon Y, Vo TD, Mendel MC, Greenberg SG, Wang J, Xia DF, Miller JC, Urnov FD, Gregory PD, Holmes MC. Enhancing zinc-finger-nuclease activity with improved obligate heterodimeric architectures. Nat Methods. 2011;8:74–9.
46. Joung JK, Sander JD. TALENs: a widely applicable technology for targeted genome editing. Nat Rev Mol Cell Biol. 2013;14:49–55.
47. Boch J, Scholze H, Schornack S, Landgraf A, Hahn S, Kay S, Lahaye T, Nickstadt A, Bonas U. Breaking the code of DNA binding specificity of TAL-type III effectors. Science. 2009;326:1509–12.
48. Moscou MJ, Bogdanove AJ. A simple cipher governs DNA recognition by TAL effectors. Science. 2009;326:1501.
49. Cermak T, Doyle EL, Christian M, Wang L, Zhang Y, Schmidt C, Baller JA, Somia NV, Bogdanove AJ, Voytas DF. Efficient design and assembly of custom TALEN and other TAL effector-based constructs for DNA targeting. Nucleic Acids Res. 2011;39:e82.
50. Gabriel R, Lombardo A, Arens A, Miller JC, Genovese P, Kaeppel C, Nowrouzi A, Bartholomae CC, Wang J, Friedman G, Holmes MC, Gregory PD, Glimm H, Schmidt M, Naldini L, von Kalle C. An unbiased genome-wide analysis of zinc-finger nuclease specificity. Nat Biotechnol. 2011;29:816–23.
51. Reyon D, Tsai SQ, Khayter C, Foden JA, Sander JD, Joung JK. FLASH assembly of TALENs for high-throughput genome editing. Nat Biotechnol. 2012;30:460–5.
52. Clark KJ, Voytas DF, Ekker SC. A TALE of two nucleases: gene targeting for the masses? Zebrafish. 2011;8:147–9.
53. Hockemeyer D, Wang H, Kiani S, Lai CS, Gao Q, Cassady JP, Cost GJ, Zhang L, Santiago Y, Miller JC, Zeitler B, Cherone JM, Meng X, Hinkley SJ, Rebar EJ, Gregory PD, Urnov FD, Jaenisch R. Genetic engineering of human pluripotent cells using TALE nucleases. Nat Biotechnol. 2011;29:731–4.
54. Mussolino C, Morbitzer R, Lütge F, Dannemann N, Lahaye T, Cathomen T. A novel TALE nuclease scaffold enables high genome editing activity in combination with low toxicity. Nucleic Acids Res. 2011;39:9283–93.
55. Bedell VM, Wang Y, Campbell JM, Poshusta TL, Starker CG, Krug RG, Tan W, Penheiter SG, Ma AC, Leung AY, Fahrenkrug SC, Carlson DF, Voytas DF, Clark KJ, Essner JJ, Ekker SC. In vivo genome editing using a high-efficiency TALEN system. Nature. 2012;491:114–8.
56. Cade L, Reyon D, Hwang WY, Tsai SQ, Patel S, Khayter C, Joung JK, Sander JD, Peterson RT, Yeh JR. Highly efficient generation of heritable zebrafish gene mutations using homo- and heterodimeric TALENs. Nucleic Acids Res. 2012;40:8001–10.
57. Li T, Liu B, Spalding MH, Weeks DP, Yang B. High-efficiency TALEN-based gene editing produces disease-resistant rice. Nat Biotechnol. 2012;30:390–2.
58. Moore FE, Reyon D, Sander JD, Martinez SA, Blackburn JS, Khayter C, Ramirez CL, Joung JK, Langenau DM. Improved somatic mutagenesis in zebrafish using transcription activator-like effector nucleases (TALENs). PLoS One. 2012;7:e37877.
59. Choi SM, Kim Y, Shim JS, Park JT, Wang RH, Leach SD, Liu JO, Deng C, Ye Z, Jang YY. Efficient drug screening and gene correction for treating liver disease using patient-specific stem cells. Hepatology. 2013;57:2458–68.
60. Ma N, Liao B, Zhang H, Wang L, Shan Y, Xue Y, Huang K, Chen S, Zhou X, Chen Y, Pei D, Pan G. Transcription activator-like effector nuclease (TALEN)-mediated gene correction in integration-free β-thalassemia induced pluripotent stem cells. J Biol Chem. 2013;288:34671–9.
61. Sun N, Zhao H. Seamless correction of the sickle cell disease mutation of the HBB gene in human induced pluripotent stem cells using TALENs. Biotechnol Bioeng. 2013;111 (5):1048–53.

62. Li HL, Fujimoto N, Sasakawa N, Shirai S, Ohkame T, Sakuma T, Tanaka M, Amano N, Watanabe A, Sakurai H, Yamamoto T, Yamanaka S, Hotta A. Precise correction of the dystrophin gene in duchenne muscular dystrophy patient induced pluripotent stem cells by TALEN and CRISPR-Cas9. Stem Cell Rep. 2015;4:143–54.
63. Maetzel D, Sarkar S, Wang H, Abi-Mosleh L, Xu P, Cheng AW, Gao Q, Mitalipova M, Jaenisch R. Genetic and chemical correction of cholesterol accumulation and impaired autophagy in hepatic and neural cells derived from Niemann-Pick Type C patient-specific iPS cells. Stem Cell Rep. 2014;2:866–80.
64. Ding Q, Lee YK, Schaefer EA, Peters DT, Veres A, Kim K, Kuperwasser N, Motola DL, Meissner TB, Hendriks WT, Trevisan M, Gupta RM, Moisan A, E Banks, Friesen M, Schinzel RT, Xia F, Tang A, Xia Y, Figueroa E, Wann A, Ahfeldt T, Daheron L, Zhang F, Rubin LL, Peng LF, Chung RT, Musunuru K, Cowan CA. A TALEN genome-editing system for generating human stem cell-based disease models. Cell Stem Cell. 2013;12:238–51.
65. Park CY, Kim J, Kweon J, Son JS, Lee JS, Yoo JE, Cho SR, Kim JH, Kim JS, Kim DW. Targeted inversion and reversion of the blood coagulation factor 8 gene in human iPS cells using TALENs. Proc Natl Acad Sci U S A. 2014;111:9253–8.
66. Chen W, Liu J, Zhang L, Xu H, Guo X, Deng S, Liu L, Yu D, Chen Y, Li Z. Generation of the SCN1A epilepsy mutation in hiPS cells using the TALEN technique. Sci Rep. 2014;4:5404.
67. Pennisi E. The CRISPR craze. Science. 2013;341:833–6.
68. Ishino Y, Shinagawa H, Makino K, Amemura M, Nakata A. Nucleotide sequence of the iap gene, responsible for alkaline phosphatase isozyme conversion in Escherichia coli, and identification of the gene product. J Bacteriol. 1987;169:5429–33.
69. Mojica FJ, Díez-Villaseñor C, García-Martínez J, Soria E. Intervening sequences of regularly spaced prokaryotic repeats derive from foreign genetic elements. J Mol Evol. 2005;60:174–82.
70. Pourcel C, Salvignol G, Vergnaud G. CRISPR elements in Yersinia pestis acquire new repeats by preferential uptake of bacteriophage DNA, and provide additional tools for evolutionary studies. Microbiology. 2005;151:653–63.
71. Barrangou R, Fremaux C, Deveau H, Richards M, Boyaval P, Moineau S, Romero DA, Horvath P. CRISPR provides acquired resistance against viruses in prokaryotes. Science. 2007;315:1709–12.
72. Doudna JA, Charpentier E. Genome editing. The new frontier of genome engineering with CRISPR-Cas9. Science. 2014;346:1258096.
73. Hsu PD, Lander ES, Zhang F. Development and applications of CRISPR-Cas9 for genome engineering. Cell. 2014;157:1262–78.
74. Deltcheva E, Chylinski K, Sharma CM, Gonzales K, Chao Y, Pirzada ZA, Eckert MR, Vogel J, Charpentier E. CRISPR RNA maturation by trans-encoded small RNA and host factor RNase III. Nature. 2011;471:602–7.
75. Deveau H, Barrangou R, Garneau JE, Labonté J, Fremaux C, Boyaval P, Romero DA, Horvath P, Moineau S. Phage response to CRISPR-encoded resistance in Streptococcus thermophilus. J Bacteriol. 2008;190:1390–400.
76. Anders C, Niewoehner O, Duerst A, Jinek M. Structural basis of PAM-dependent target DNA recognition by the Cas9 endonuclease. Nature. 2014;513:569–73.
77. Jinek M, Chylinski K, Fonfara I, Hauer M, Doudna JA, Charpentier E. A programmable dual-RNA-guided DNA endonuclease in adaptive bacterial immunity. Science. 2012;337:816–21.
78. Cong L, Ran FA, Cox D, Lin S, Barretto R, Habib N, Hsu PD, Wu X, Jiang W, Marraffini LA, Zhang F. Multiplex genome engineering using CRISPR/Cas systems. Science. 2013;339:819–23.
79. Mali P, Yang L, Esvelt KM, Aach J, Guell M, DiCarlo JE, Norville JE, Church GM. - RNA-guided human genome engineering via Cas9. Science. 2013;339:823–6.
80. Shalem O, Sanjana NE, Hartenian E, Shi X, Scott DA, Mikkelson T, Heckl D, Ebert BL, Root DE, Doench JG, Zhang F. Genome-scale CRISPR-Cas9 knockout screening in human cells. Science. 2013;343(6166):84–7.

81. Wang T, Wei JJ, Sabatini DM, Lander ES. Genetic screens in human cells using the CRISPR/Cas9 system. Science. 2013;343(6166):80–4.
82. Ding Q, Regan SN, Xia Y, Oostrom LA, Cowan CA, Musunuru K. Enhanced efficiency of human pluripotent stem cell genome editing through replacing TALENs with CRISPRs. Cell Stem Cell. 2013;12:393–4.
83. Smith C, Abalde-Atristain L, He C, Brodsky BR, Braunstein EM, Chaudhari P, Jang YY, Cheng L, Ye Z. Efficient and allele-specific genome editing of disease loci in human iPSCs. Mol Ther. 2015;23:570–7.
84. Yang L, Guell M, Byrne S, Yang JL, De Los Angeles A, Mali P, Aach J, Kim-Kiselak C, Briggs AW, Rios X, Huang PY, Daley G, Church G. Optimization of scarless human stem cell genome editing. Nucleic Acids Res. 2013;41:9049–61.
85. Hou Z, Zhang Y, Propson NE, Howden SE, Chu LF, Sontheimer EJ, Thomson JA. Efficient genome engineering in human pluripotent stem cells using Cas9 from Neisseria meningitidis. Proc Natl Acad Sci U S A. 2013;110:15644–9.
86. Zetsche B, Gootenberg JS, Abudayyeh OO, Slaymaker IM, Makarova KS, Essletzbichler P, Volz SE, Joung J, van der Oost J, Regev A, Koonin EV, Zhang F. Cpf1 Is a Single RNA-Guided Endonuclease of a Class 2 CRISPR-Cas System. Cell. 2015;163(3):759–71.
87. Choi PS, Meyerson M. Targeted genomic rearrangements using CRISPR/Cas technology. Nat Commun. 2014;5:3728.
88. Ye L, Wang J, Beyer AI, Teque F, Cradick TJ, Qi Z, Chang JC, Bao G, Muench MO, Yu J, Levy JA, Kan YW. Seamless modification of wild-type induced pluripotent stem cells to the natural CCR5Δ32 mutation confers resistance to HIV infection. Proc Natl Acad Sci U S A. 2014;111:9591–6.
89. Byrne SM, Ortiz L, Mali P, Aach J, Church GM. Multi-kilobase homozygous targeted gene replacement in human induced pluripotent stem cells. Nucleic Acids Res. 2015;43:e21.
90. Xie F, Ye L, Chang JC, Beyer AI, Wang J, Muench MO, Kan YW. Seamless gene correction of β-thalassemia mutations in patient-specific iPSCs using CRISPR/Cas9 and piggyBac. Genome Res. 2014.
91. Huang X, Wang Y, Yan W, Smith C, Ye Z, Wang J, Gao Y, Mendelsohn L, Cheng L. Production of gene-corrected adult beta globin protein in human erythrocytes differentiated from patient iPSCs after genome editing of the sickle point mutation. Stem Cells. 2015;33:1470–9.
92. Horii T, Tamura D, Morita S, Kimura M, Hatada I. Generation of an ICF syndrome model by efficient genome editing of human induced pluripotent stem cells using the CRISPR system. Int J Mol Sci. 2013;14:19774–81.
93. Kearns NA, Genga RM, Enuameh MS, Garber M, Wolfe SA, Maehr R. Cas9 effector-mediated regulation of transcription and differentiation in human pluripotent stem cells. Development. 2014;141:219–23.
94. Larson MH, Gilbert LA, Wang X, Lim WA, Weissman JS, Qi LS. CRISPR interference (CRISPRi) for sequence-specific control of gene expression. Nat Protoc. 2013;8:2180–96.
95. Mali P, Esvelt KM, Church GM. Cas9 as a versatile tool for engineering biology. Nat Methods. 2013;10:957–63.
96. Mali P, Aach J, Stranges PB, Esvelt KM, Moosburner M, Kosuri S, Yang L, Church GM. CAS9 transcriptional activators for target specificity screening and paired nickases for cooperative genome engineering. Nat Biotechnol. 2013;31:833–8.
97. Perez-Pinera P, Kocak DD, Vockley CM, Adler AF, Kabadi AM, Polstein LR, Thakore PI, Glass KA, Ousterout DG, Leong KW, Guilak F, Crawford GE, Reddy TE, Gersbach CA. - RNA-guided gene activation by CRISPR-Cas9-based transcription factors. Nat Methods. 2013;10:973–6.
98. Qi LS, Larson MH, Gilbert LA, Doudna JA, Weissman JS, Arkin AP, Lim WA. Repurposing CRISPR as an RNA-guided platform for sequence-specific control of gene expression. Cell. 2013;152:1173–83.

99. Gilbert LA, Horlbeck MA, Adamson B, Villalta JE, Chen Y, Whitehead EH, Guimaraes C, Panning B, Ploegh HL, Bassik MC, Qi LS, Kampmann M, Weissman JS. Genome-scale CRISPR-mediated control of gene repression and activation. Cell. 2014;159:647–61.
100. Hilton IB, D'Ippolito AM, Vockley CM, Thakore PI, Crawford GE, Reddy TE, Gersbach CA. Epigenome editing by a CRISPR-Cas9-based acetyltransferase activates genes from promoters and enhancers. Nat Biotechnol. 2015;33:510–7.
101. Konermann S, Brigham MD, Trevino AE, Joung J, Abudayyeh OO, Barcena C, Hsu PD, Habib N, Gootenberg JS, Nishimasu H, Nureki O, Zhang F. Genome-scale transcriptional activation by an engineered CRISPR-Cas9 complex. Nature. 2015;517:583–8.
102. Zalatan JG, Lee ME, Almeida R, Gilbert LA, Whitehead EH, La Russa M, Tsai JC, Weissman JS, Dueber JE, Qi LS, Lim WA. Engineering complex synthetic transcriptional programs with CRISPR RNA scaffolds. Cell. 2015;160:339–50.
103. Pattanayak V, Ramirez CL, Joung JK, Liu DR. Revealing off-target cleavage specificities of zinc-finger nucleases by in vitro selection. Nat Methods. 2011;8:765–70.
104. Fu Y, Foden JA, Khayter C, Maeder ML, Reyon D, Joung JK, Sander JD. High-frequency off-target mutagenesis induced by CRISPR-Cas nucleases in human cells. Nat Biotechnol. 2013;31:822–6.
105. Pattanayak V, Lin S, Guilinger JP, Ma E, Doudna JA, Liu DR. High-throughput profiling of off-target DNA cleavage reveals RNA-programmed Cas9 nuclease specificity. Nat Biotechnol. 2013;31:839–43.
106. Cradick TJ, Fine EJ, Antico CJ, Bao G. CRISPR/Cas9 systems targeting β-globin and CCR5 genes have substantial off-target activity. Nucleic Acids Res. 2013;41:9584–92.
107. Hsu PD, Scott DA, Weinstein JA, Ran FA, Konermann S, Agarwala V, Li Y, Fine EJ, Wu X, Shalem O, Cradick TJ, Marraffini LA, Bao G, Zhang F. DNA targeting specificity of RNA-guided Cas9 nucleases. Nat Biotechnol. 2013;31:827–32.
108. Smith C, Gore A, Yan W, Abalde-Atristain L, Li Z, He C, Wang Y, Brodsky RA, Zhang K, Cheng L, Ye Z. Whole-genome sequencing analysis reveals high specificity of CRISPR/Cas9 and TALEN-based genome editing in human iPSCs. Cell Stem Cell. 2014;15:12–3.
109. Veres A, Gosis BS, Ding Q, Collins R, Ragavendran A, Brand H, Erdin S, Talkowski ME, Musunuru K. Low incidence of off-target mutations in individual CRISPR-Cas9 and TALEN targeted human stem cell clones detected by whole-genome sequencing. Cell Stem Cell. 2014;15:27–30.
110. Suzuki K, Yu C, Qu J, Li M, Yao X, Yuan T, Goebl A, Tang S, Ren R, Aizawa E, Zhang F, Xu X, Soligalla RD, Chen F, Kim J, Kim NY, Liao HK, Benner C, Esteban CR, Jin Y, Liu GH, Li Y, Izpisua Belmonte JC. Targeted gene correction minimally impacts whole-genome mutational load in human-disease-specific induced pluripotent stem cell clones. Cell Stem Cell. 2014;15:31–6.
111. Fu Y, Sander JD, Reyon D, Cascio VM, Joung JK. Improving CRISPR-Cas nuclease specificity using truncated guide RNAs. Nat Biotechnol. 2014;32:279–84.
112. Ran FA, Hsu PD, Lin CY, Gootenberg JS, Konermann S, Trevino AE, Scott DA, Inoue A, Matoba S, Zhang Y, Zhang F. Double nicking by RNA-guided CRISPR Cas9 for enhanced genome editing specificity. Cell. 2013;154:1380–9.
113. Shen B, Zhang W, Zhang J, Zhou J, Wang J, Chen L, Wang L, Hodgkins A, Iyer V, Huang X, Skarnes WC. Efficient genome modification by CRISPR-Cas9 nickase with minimal off-target effects. Nat Methods. 2014;11:399–402.
114. Tsai SQ, Wyvekens N, Khayter C, Foden JA, Thapar V, Reyon D, Goodwin MJ, Aryee MJ, Joung JK. Dimeric CRISPR RNA-guided FokI nucleases for highly specific genome editing. Nat Biotechnol. 2014;32:569–76.
115. Frazer KA, Ballinger DG, Cox DR, Hinds DA, Stuve LL, Gibbs RA, Belmont JW, Boudreau A, Hardenbol P, Leal SM, Pasternak S, Wheeler DA, Willis TD, Yu F, Yang H, Zeng C, Gao Y, Hu H, Hu W, Li C, Lin W, Liu S, Pan H, Tang X, Wang J, Wang W, Yu J, Zhang B, Zhang Q, Zhao H, Zhou J, Gabriel SB, Barry R, Blumenstiel B, Camargo A, Defelice M, Faggart M, Goyette M, Gupta S, Moore J, Nguyen H, Onofrio RC, Parkin M,

Roy J, Stahl E, Winchester E, Ziaugra L, Altshuler D, Shen Y, Yao Z, Huang W, Chu X, He Y, Jin L, Liu Y, Sun W, Wang H, Wang Y, Xiong X, Xu L, Waye MM, Tsui SK, Xue H, Wong JT, Galver LM, Fan JB, Gunderson K, Murray SS, Oliphant AR, Chee MS, Montpetit A, Chagnon F, Ferretti V, Leboeuf M, Olivier JF, Phillips MS, Roumy S, Sallée C, Verner A, Hudson TJ, Kwok PY, Cai D, Koboldt DC, Miller RD, Pawlikowska L, Taillon-Miller P, Xiao M, Tsui LC, Mak W, Song YQ, Tam PK, Nakamura Y, Kawaguchi T, Kitamoto T, Morizono T, Nagashima A, Ohnishi Y, Sekine A, Tanaka T, Tsunoda T, Deloukas P, Bird CP, Delgado M, Dermitzakis ET, Gwilliam R, Hunt S, Morrison J, Powell D, Stranger BE, Whittaker P, Bentley DR, Daly MJ, de Bakker PI, Barrett J, Chretien YR, Maller J, McCarroll S, Patterson N, Pe'er I, Price A, Purcell S, Richter DJ, Sabeti P, Saxena R, Schaffner SF, Sham PC, Varilly P, Stein LD, Krishnan L, Smith AV, Tello-Ruiz MK, Thorisson GA, Chakravarti A, Chen PE, Cutler DJ, Kashuk CS, Lin S, Abecasis GR, Guan W, Li Y, Munro HM, Qin ZS, Thomas DJ, McVean G, Auton A, Bottolo L, Cardin N, Eyheramendy S, Freeman C, Marchini J, Myers S, Spencer C, Stephens M, Donnelly P, Cardon LR, Clarke G, Evans DM, Morris AP, Weir BS, Mullikin JC, Sherry ST, Feolo M, Skol A, Zhang H, Matsuda I, Fukushima Y, Macer DR, Suda E, Rotimi CN, Adebamowo CA, Ajayi I, Aniagwu T, Marshall PA, Nkwodimmah C, Royal CD, Leppert MF, Dixon M, Peiffer A, Qiu R, Kent A, Kato K, Niikawa N, Adewole IF, Knoppers BM, Foster MW, Clayton EW, Watkin J, Muzny D, Nazareth L, Sodergren E, Weinstock GM, Yakub I, Birren BW, Wilson RK, Fulton LL, Rogers J, Burton J, Carter NP, Clee CM, Griffiths M, Jones MC, McLay K, Plumb RW, Ross MT, Sims SK, Willey DL, Chen Z, Han H, Kang L, Godbout M, Wallenburg JC, L'Archevêque P, Bellemare G, Saeki K, An D, Fu H, Li Q, Wang Z, Wang R, Holden AL, Brooks LD, McEwen JE, Guyer MS, Wang VO, Peterson JL, Shi M, Spiegel J, Sung LM, Zacharia LF, Collins FS, Kennedy K, Jamieson R, Stewart J, Consortium IH. A second generation human haplotype map of over 3.1 million SNPs. Nature. 2007;449:851–61.

116. Yang L, Grishin D, Wang G, Aach J, Zhang CZ, Chari R, Homsy J, Cai X, Zhao Y, Fan JB, Seidman C, Seidman J, Pu W, Church G. Targeted and genome-wide sequencing reveal single nucleotide variations impacting specificity of Cas9 in human stem cells. Nat Commun. 2014;5:5507.
117. Kim S, Kim D, Cho SW, Kim J, Kim JS. Highly efficient RNA-guided genome editing in human cells via delivery of purified Cas9 ribonucleoproteins. Genome Res. 2014;24:1012–9.
118. Schumann K, Lin S, Boyer E, Simeonov DR, Subramaniam M, Gate RE, Haliburton GE, Ye CJ, Bluestone JA, Doudna JA, Marson A. Generation of knock-in primary human T cells using Cas9 ribonucleoproteins. Proc Natl Acad Sci U S A. 2015;112:10437–42.
119. Maruyama T, Dougan SK, Truttmann MC, Bilate AM, Ingram JR, Ploegh HL. Increasing the efficiency of precise genome editing with CRISPR-Cas9 by inhibition of nonhomologous end joining. Nat Biotechnol. 2015;33:538–42.
120. Yu C, Liu Y, Ma T, Liu K, Xu S, Zhang Y, Liu H, La Russa M, Xie M, Ding S, Qi LS. Small molecules enhance CRISPR genome editing in pluripotent stem cells. Cell Stem Cell. 2015;16:142–7.
121. Chu VT, Weber T, Wefers B, Wurst W, Sander S, Rajewsky K, Kühn R. Increasing the efficiency of homology-directed repair for CRISPR-Cas9-induced precise gene editing in mammalian cells. Nat Biotechnol. 2015;33:543–8.

Chapter 4
Pluripotent Stem Cells for Kidney Diseases

Navin R. Gupta and Albert Q. Lam

4.1 Introduction

There is a growing need for innovative approaches to the treatment of chronic kidney disease (CKD), as end-stage renal disease (ESRD) has reached epidemic proportions. In the United States alone, more than 600,000 individuals require renal replacement therapy. Annual Medicare expenditures for treatment of ESRD patients exceeded $500 billion as early as 2012 [1]. Meanwhile, current projections indicate that the US population of patients with ESRD may reach more than two million by 2030 [2]. Currently, approximately 70 % of patients receive dialysis-based therapy while 30 % have a functioning renal transplant. Although both treatment modalities prolong survival, each has significant limitations.

Dialysis imperfectly filters blood. Uremic retention products are known to induce premature atherosclerosis [3] and retained beta-2 microglobulin has been linked to the development of amyloidosis [4]. For dialysis patients, the relative risk of mortality has been reported to be as high as 8.2, compared to matched individuals in the general population [5]. Additionally, dialysis does not recapitulate the endocrine functions of the kidney, necessitating erythropoietin and activated vitamin D supplementation. Lastly, dialysis therapy greatly reduces the health-related quality of life of patients of all ages, both genders, and multiple ethnicities [6].

N.R. Gupta, M.D.
Division of Renal Medicine, Department of Medicine, Brigham and Women's Hospital, Harvard Medical School, Boston, MA, USA
e-mail: ngupta12@partners.org

A.Q. Lam, M.D. (✉)
Division of Renal Medicine, Department of Medicine, Brigham and Women's Hospital, Harvard Medical School, Boston, MA, USA

Harvard Stem Cell Institute, Cambridge, MA, USA
e-mail: aqlam@partners.org

E.M. Abdelalim (ed.), *Recent Advances in Stem Cells*, Stem Cell Biology and Regenerative Medicine, DOI 10.1007/978-3-319-33270-3_4

Transplantation, although having both a survival and cost benefit compared to dialysis, suffers from the paucity of transplantable organs. The limited kidney supply, coupled with increasing demand, has resulted in an average transplant-list wait time of >3.8 years for adults in the USA. While 12 people die each day while waiting for a kidney transplant, every 14 min a patient is added to the kidney transplant list (OPTN/UNOS 2015). Despite the development of potent immunosuppressive agents, kidney transplant recipients have a nearly 10 % risk of acute rejection in the first year after transplantation [7]. Additionally, the majority of those patients who receive a kidney transplant require lifelong immunosuppression, which is associated with increased infection risk, morbidity, and mortality.

Given these limitations, stem cell-based regenerative medicine represents an innovative approach to the treatment of CKD and ESRD. By virtue of their intrinsic properties of self-renewal and ability to differentiate into cells of all three germ layers, pluripotent stem cells (PSCs) provide an optimal and scalable cell source for tissue and organ regeneration [8]. Induced pluripotent stem cells (iPSCs) have the added advantage of being theoretically immunocompatible with the host from which they were derived. The implications are that patient-specific, functional kidney tissue may one day be possible.

4.2 Pluripotent Stem Cells

PSCs represent populations of early embryonic progenitor cells, which are believed to correspond to the blastocyst or epiblast stage of mammalian embryonic development [9]. These early cell types arise 5–9 days following human conception and are defined by two intrinsic properties: self-renewal and pluripotency. PSCs have the ability to self-renew theoretically indefinitely in culture, without transformation or differentiation. In addition, PSCs have the capacity to give rise to all cell types derived from the three embryonic germ layers, namely the mesoderm, endoderm, and ectoderm [10]. Perhaps the greatest demonstration for both the differentiation capacity and the ability to generate complex functional tissue from PSCs is cloned mice developed from tetraploid complementation methods [11, 12].

PSCs comprise embryonic stem cells (ESCs) and iPSCs. ESCs are derived from the isolation and culture of cells from the inner cell mass of the embryonic blastocyst [13–15]. In contrast, iPSCs are derived by the retroviral transduction of four key transcription factors (Oct4, Sox2, Klf4, and c-Myc) into adult skin fibroblasts, which directly reprograms them into cells that appear morphologically and behave almost identically to ESCs (Fig. 4.1) [16, 17].

While human ESCs still remain the gold standard for human PSCs and differences do exist between ESCs and iPSCs, human iPSCs have a number of distinct advantages. First, unlike ESCs, iPSC derivation does not involve the use of human embryos, a limitation that has previously led to ethical concerns over the use of human ESCs [18]. Protocols now exist to derive human iPSCs from a variety of different somatic cell types, including peripheral blood mononuclear cells,

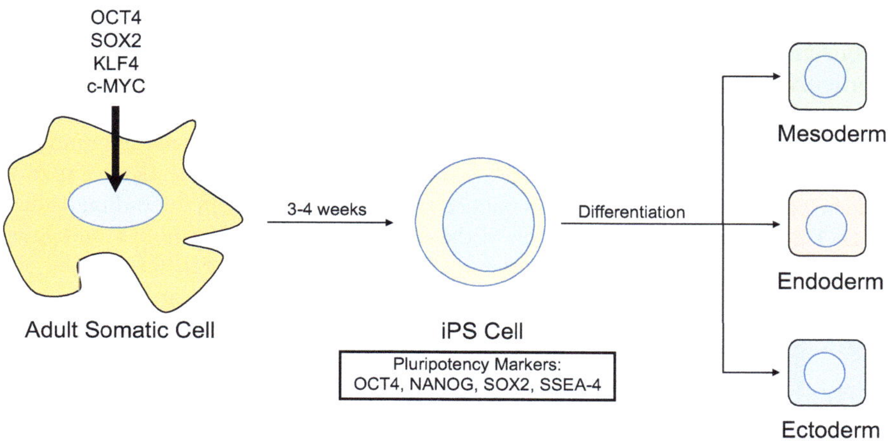

Fig. 4.1 Reprogramming adult somatic cells into induced pluripotent stem (iPS) cells. The retroviral transduction of four pluripotency transcription factors (Oct4, Sox2, c-Myc, and Klf4) converts somatic cells into iPSCs, which are capable of differentiating into cells of the three germ layers of the embryo (mesoderm, ectoderm, endoderm)

keratinocytes, hepatocytes, neural stem cells, and kidney mesangial and tubular epithelial cells using both viral and nonviral reprogramming methods [19–25]. Secondly, because human iPSCs can be generated from essentially any human individual—adult or child, healthy or diseased—and retain the individual's genotype, they represent a starting substrate to generate tissue that is theoretically immunocompatible with the individual from which the iPSCs were originally derived. Thirdly, human iPSCs, which can be generated from patients with specific diseases, can be used to develop in vitro models to better study disease pathogenesis. For diseases that are particularly rare or do not have relevant animal models, iPSCs offer a novel strategy to study pathogenetic mechanisms.

4.3 PSC Differentiation Methods

PSCs can be differentiated into a wide variety of differentiated cell types from multiple organs, including the heart, lungs, liver, pancreas, intestines, kidneys, and nervous system [26]. The withdrawal of growth factors that are required for the maintenance of pluripotency in PSCs results in spontaneous and stochastic differentiation. In the absence of specific exogenous growth factors or chemicals to influence cell fate, PSCs undergo stochastic differentiation into embryoid bodies (EBs) in vitro and teratomas in vivo [15–17]. Both EBs and teratomas are heterogeneous tissues that contain the three embryonic germ layers, confirming pluripotency. However, the efficiency of differentiation into any one particular cell type is low. The efficient generation of specific differentiated cell types with greater purity requires a more directed approach to force PSCs to adopt a particular cell fate. Directed differentiation refers to the process by which PSCs are sequentially treated with growth factors and chemicals to efficiently induce a particular cell or tissue type. Most often, directed differentiation protocols use embryonic organ development as a paradigm for differentiation, subdividing the process into a series of discrete intermediate stages that can be chemically induced and monitored by the expression of key stage-specific markers [26]. Differentiation can be carried out in two-dimensional (2D) monolayer culture, in three-dimensional (3D) EB culture, or a combination of these two approaches. While 2D monolayer culture offers the advantages of better control and monitoring of differentiation, the successful generation of certain organized tissue structures and architecture may require 3D culture environments for realization.

4.4 Mammalian Nephrogenesis

Current strategies to direct the differentiation of PSCs into cells of the kidney lineage have been based on vertebrate animal kidney development as a model. The kidneys are derived from the mesoderm germ layer, specifically from the intermediate mesoderm (IM). During kidney organogenesis, the IM sequentially gives rise to the pronephros, mesonephros, and metanephros (Fig. 4.2). In humans, the pronephros is nonfunctional and regresses by the fourth week of gestation, but for certain primitive jawless fish such as the lamprey and hagfish, it is the primary kidney. The mesonephros forms just prior to degeneration of the pronephros in humans and serves as the primary excretory organ from the fourth to the eighth week of gestation. In females, the mesonephros degenerates, whereas in males it gives rise to portions of the reproductive organs. The metanephros, which begins to form caudal to the mesonephros in the fifth week of gestation, becomes the definitive adult kidney in humans.

The metanephric kidney forms through the reciprocally inductive interactions between two distinct IM tissues, the metanephric mesenchyme (MM) and ureteric bud (UB). The MM arises from the posterior IM and contains a population of multipotent nephron progenitor cells (NPCs) that expresses the transcription factors Six2, Cited1, Pax2, Sall1, and WT1 [27–29]. These Six2+ NPCs are present in the MM that surrounds each UB tip (cap mesenchyme) and, upon receiving inductive Wnt signals from the UB, will undergo mesenchymal-to-epithelial transition and give rise to nearly all the epithelial cells of the nephron except for those of the collecting duct [27, 28]. The UB develops as an epithelial outpouching from the caudal region of the nephric (or Wolffian) duct and, upon receiving inductive signals from the MM, undergoes iterative branching to form the collecting system. Nephrogenesis in humans is completed between 32 and 36 weeks of gestation and results in the formation of approximately one million nephrons in each kidney. After birth, no new nephrons are formed, even under circumstances of kidney injury and repair.

Recent work from Taguchi and colleagues has provided important insight into the embryonic origins of the NPCs in the MM [29]. Employing lineage tracing

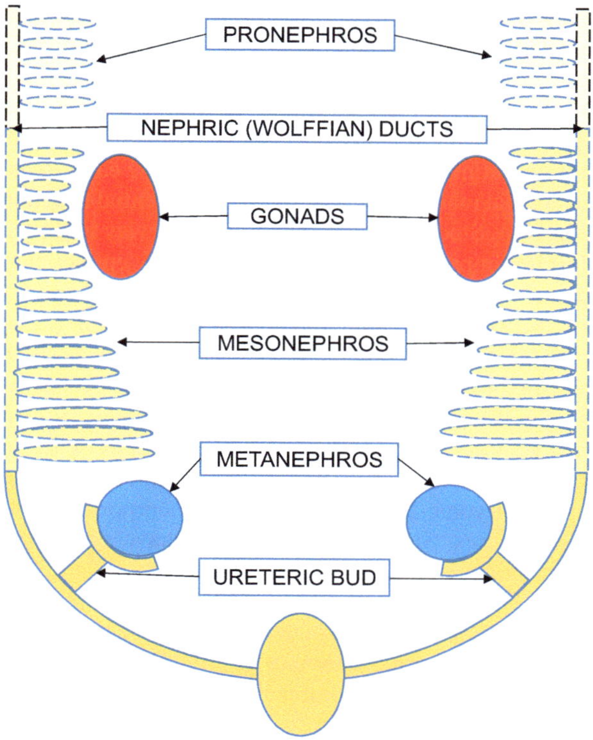

Fig. 4.2 Stages of mammalian kidney development. The pronephros is the initial nephric stage in mammals and degenerates by the fourth week of embryonic life in humans. From the fourth to the eighth week of human embryogenesis, the mesonephros is the primary excretory organ. Thereafter, the developing metanephros gives rise to the mature kidney in humans

techniques in mice, the authors showed that the embryonic origin of NPCs could be traced back to a population of T+ cells in the primitive streak that persists to give rise to T + Tbx6+ posterior nascent mesoderm and then WT1 + Osr1+ posterior IM. In contrast, the UB originates from anterior IM, which is incapable of giving rise to MM. Thus, careful consideration of these diverging developmental pathways is critical for the efficient differentiation of PSCs into cells of these two different lineages.

4.5 Differentiation of Mouse PSCs to Kidney Lineage Cells

Early studies attempting to generate kidney cells from PSCs were performed using mouse ESCs (mESCs). Labeled mESCs microinjected into E12 to E13 mouse metanephroi resulted in the integration of these cells into tubular structures, some of which expressed *Lotus tetragonolobus lectin* (LTL)$^+$ and Na^+/K^+-ATPase$^+$ [30]. EBs generated from the stochastic differentiation of mESCs expressed a number of kidney developmental genes, including *Pax2*, *WT1*, *Lhx1*, *Emx2*, *c-ret*, and *Sall1*. Transplantation of these cells into the mouse retroperitoneum produced teratoma-like growths with regions co-expressing the renal epithelial markers *Dolichos biflorus* agglutinin (DBA) and Pax2 [31]. These early experiments served as proof-of-concept that mammalian PSCs have the potential to generate cells of the kidney lineage in vivo. Stochastic differentiation gave way to directed differentiation in an effort to improve the efficiency of renal epithelial cell induction. Developmental studies identified activin, retinoic acid (RA), and bone morphogenetic proteins (BMPs) as signaling molecules involved in mesoderm and IM differentiation [32]. Utilizing a combination of activin, RA, and BMP7, Kim and Dressler differentiated mouse EBs into cells expressing the IM markers *Pax2*, *WT1*, and *Lhx1* [33]. Vigneau and colleagues treated a *Brachyury* (*T*)-GFP reporter mESC line with activin and generated Brachyury$^+$ cells with 50 % efficiency [34]. In both of the aforementioned studies, transplantation of the differentiated cells into mouse embryonic kidneys resulted in incorporation of the cells into forming tubular structures. Similarly, other studies have shown that activin, RA, and BMPs are potential nephrogenic factors [35–38].

Taguchi and colleagues used a developmental approach, first determining combinations of growth factors and small molecules required to induce differentiation of isolated mouse T$^+$ posterior mesoderm cells into MM cells [29]. Based on these findings, they established multistep protocols to differentiate mESCs and hiPSCs into EBs that expressed multiple markers of NPCs of the MM, including Pax2, Six2, Sall1, and WT1. Co-culture of the EBs containing NPCs with mouse embryonic spinal cord, a tissue known to induce kidney tubulogenesis, resulted in the generation of 3D tubular structures expressing markers of kidney tubules and glomeruli. The protocols for mESCs and hiPSCs were similar, though MM induction required 14 days with hiPSCs compared to 8.5 days with mESCs.

4.6 Differentiation of Human PSCs to Kidney Lineage Cells

The initial approach to kidney differentiation with hPSCs was based on the studies with mPSCs. The work of Batchelder and Lin was the earliest to demonstrate that hESCs could be differentiated into cells expressing developmental kidney markers such as PAX2 and WT1 [39, 40]. Song and colleagues devised a protocol combining EB and monolayer culture methods to generate podocyte-like cells from hiPSCs. Using a combination of activin, BMP7, and RA, the authors generated EBs that incorporated cells bearing the podocyte markers podocin, synaptopodin, and PAX2. Moreover, through a similar but extended protocol, they developed a monolayer culture of these podocyte-like cells that integrated into WT1$^+$

glomerular structures when combined with dissociated-reaggregated E13.5 kidneys [41]. Using a combination of BMP2 and BMP7 in renal epithelial growth medium (REGM), Narayanan and colleagues induced hESCs to differentiate into aquaporin-1 (AQP1)$^+$ proximal tubule-like cells. Flow-sorted AQP1$^+$ cells integrated into tubular compartments of ex vivo newborn mouse kidneys and spontaneously formed cord-like structures when cultured on Matrigel. In addition, AQP1$^+$ cells, increased cAMP production in response to stimulation with parathyroid hormone, demonstrated GGT activity, and produced ammonia [42].

Recent studies have focused on generating populations of kidney progenitor cells, particularly cells of the IM and MM. Mae and colleagues sequentially treated an *OSR1*-GFP reporter hiPSC line with the glycogen synthase kinase-3β inhibitor CHIR99021 (CHIR) and activin followed by BMP7 and generated OSR1+ cells with 90 % efficiency within 11–18 days of differentiation. OSR1-GFP+ cells were capable of differentiating in vitro into cells expressing markers of mature kidneys, adrenal glands, and gonads and could integrate into dissociated-reaggregated E11.5 mouse embryonic kidneys, albeit with low efficiency [43]. The same group of investigators subsequently demonstrated in a follow-up study that substitution of activin and BMP7 with either of the retinoic acid receptor agonists, AM580 and TTNPB, could reduce the time of the original protocol to 6 days [44].

Lam and colleagues sequentially treated hESCs and hiPSCs with CHIR followed by FGF2 and RA and generated PAX2$^+$LHX1$^+$ IM-like cells within 3 days with 70–80 % efficiency [45]. Upon growth factor withdrawal, PAX2$^+$LHX1$^+$ cells stochastically differentiated to form polarized, ciliated, tubular structures that expressed the proximal tubule markers LTL, N-cadherin, and kidney-specific protein. Treatment of PAX2$^+$LHX1$^+$ cells with FGF9 and activin generated cells co-expressing markers of MM including SIX2, SALL1, and WT1. Similar findings were reported by Takasato and colleagues, who treated hESCs with CHIR and FGF9 and induced PAX2$^+$LHX1$^+$ IM cells within 6 days [46]. By maintaining FGF9 treatment of these cells, the authors could generate SIX2$^+$ cells within 14 days with 10–20 % efficiency. Clusters of cells co-expressing PAX2 and E-cadherin were also observed in the same cultures with SIX2$^+$ cells, suggesting that the cultures were heterogeneous and comprised cells of both MM and UB lineages. Mixing these cells with dissociated-reaggregated mouse embryonic kidneys resulted in the incorporation of a small proportion of human cells within mouse tubular structures. Three-dimensional aggregates of SIX2$^+$ cells contained tubular structures expressing markers such as AQP1, AQP2, JAG1, E-cadherin, WT1, and PAX2.

While considerable work has been done to differentiate hPSCs into MM, efforts to differentiate hPSCs into cells of the UB lineage have been limited by comparison. Xia and colleagues treated hESCs and hiPSCs with BMP4 and FGF2, followed by RA, activin, and BMP2 to generate PAX2$^+$, OSR1$^+$, WT1$^+$, LHX1$^+$ IM-like cells that spontaneously upregulated transcripts of the UB markers *HOXB7*, *RET*, and *GFRA1* within 2 days. Upon co-culture with dissociated-reaggregated E11.5 mouse embryonic kidneys, these putative UB progenitor-like cells partially integrated into mouse UB tips and trunks [47].

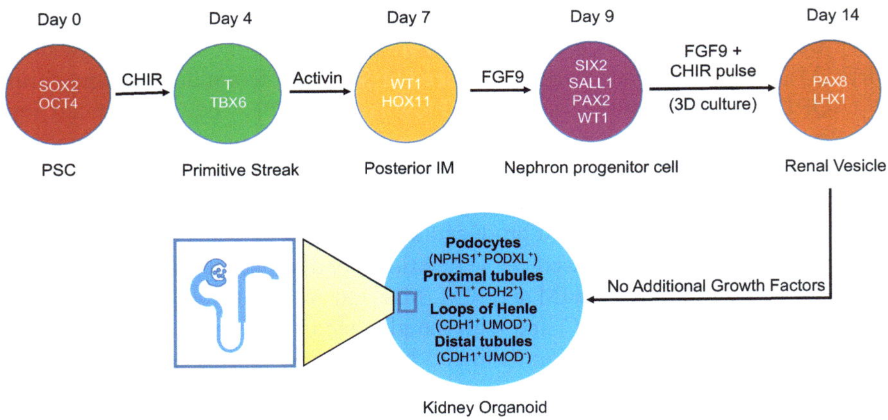

Fig. 4.3 Directed differentiation of hPSCs into 3D kidney organoids. Stepwise induction of hPSCs into late-stage primitive streak (T + TBX6+), posterior intermediate mesoderm (WT1 + HOXD11+), and SIX2 + SALL1 + PAX2 + WT1+ NPCs. NPCs transferred to suspension culture and treated with FGF9 and a transient CHIR pulse self-assemble into 3D organoids that contain multi-segmented, contiguous nephron structures expressing markers of glomerular podocytes, proximal tubules, loops of Henle, and distal tubules

Most recently, two groups demonstrated the ability to differentiate hPSCs into 3D kidney organoids containing complex, multi-segmented nephron-like structures [48, 49]. Takasato and colleagues treated hPSCs with CHIR for 4 days, followed by FGF9 for 3 days, and transferred the cells into 3D suspension culture for up to 20 days to generate kidney organoids. Resultant organoids consisted of nephron-like formations with segmentation into proximal and distal tubules, early loops of Henle, and podocyte-like cells. In addition, organoids contained tubular structures expressing markers of collecting ducts, stromal cells expressing markers of the renal interstitium, and endothelial cells. A pulse of CHIR for 1 h after transferring the cells to suspension culture was optimal for the generation of nephron-like formations. Concurrently, Morizane and colleagues devised a protocol to robustly differentiate hPSCs into $SIX2^{+}SALL1^{+}PAX2^{+}WT1^{+}$ NPCs that could be induced to form nephron organoids in both 2D and 3D culture (Fig. 4.3) [49]. The authors were able to recapitulate the critical stages of MM development by first efficiently differentiating hPSCs into $T^{+}TBX6^{+}$ primitive streak cells with high-dose CHIR for 4 days, inducing $WT1^{+}HOXD11^{+}$ posterior IM cells with activin, then inducing $SIX2^{+}SALL1^{+}PAX2^{+}WT1^{+}$ NPCs with 90 % efficiency using low-dose FGF9. NPCs could be induced with FGF9 and transient CHIR treatment to form $PAX8^{+}$ $LHX1^{+}$ renal vesicles that spontaneously formed nephron-like structures in 2D culture. Transfer of the NPCs into 3D suspension culture resulted in the formation of organoids containing multi-segmented nephron-like formations expressing markers of glomerular podocytes ($NPHS1^{+}PODXL^{+}$), proximal tubules (LTL^{+} $CDH2^{+}$), loops of Henle ($CDH1^{+}UMOD^{+}$), and distal tubules ($CHD1^{+}UMOD^{-}$) in a contiguous arrangement mimicking the in vivo nephron. The authors then

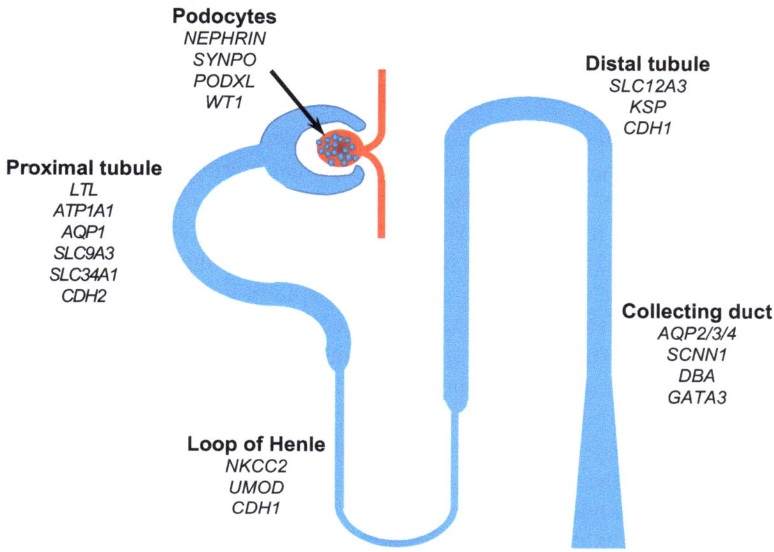

Fig. 4.4 Nephron segment-specific marker expression. Known biomarkers of nephron segments have been used to assess directed differentiation protocols and to determine the efficiency of inducing a cell type of interest. Certain biomarkers are found in multiple distinct nephron segments. It is important to note that traditionally used biomarkers have variable specificity for kidney tissue

demonstrated that these nephron organoids could be applied to study mechanisms of kidney development and drug toxicity.

The establishment of efficient protocols for directing the differentiation of hPSCs into NPCs and kidney organoids marks a significant advance in the ongoing effort to apply human stem cells to the regeneration of kidney tissue, modeling of human kidney disease, and drug testing for therapeutic efficacy and toxicity. However, the development of definitive functional assays and the establishment of reliable genetic markers will be required to verify whether induced hPSC-derived kidney cells and tissues are identical to their in vivo complements (Fig. 4.4).

4.7 Pluripotent Stem Cells for Nephrotoxicity Testing

Toxic effects of drugs and their metabolites often manifest as nephrotoxicity. The kidneys are highly vascular, receiving ~20 % of the cardiac output, and can accumulate toxins in the vascular, interstitial, tubular, and glomerular spaces. A retrospective multinational and multicenter study revealed that 17–26 % of in-hospital AKI was attributed to the administration of a nephrotoxic agent [50]. During drug development, 19 % of failures in Phase III clinical trials are due to nephrotoxicity [51]. The cost to bring a drug to market is currently ~2.6 billion dollars [52]. The availability of high-throughput systems for screening nephrotoxicity during drug development would potentially save considerable time and expenditure.

Recent reports have demonstrated that hPSC-derived kidney cells and tissues may respond to nephrotoxic drugs in a manner that mimics in vivo kidney injury [48, 49, 53]. In the study by Takasato and colleagues, hPSC-derived kidney organoids subjected to the chemotherapeutic agent cisplatin demonstrated histologic evidence of proximal tubular injury as evidenced by the expression of cleaved caspase-3, consistent with known effects of cisplatin-induced AKI [48]. Similar findings were reported by Morizane and colleagues, who subjected nephron organoids to two different nephrotoxic agents. Organoids treated with cisplatin showed upregulation of kidney injury molecule-1 (KIM-1) and γH2AX in injured proximal tubules and a reduction in E-cadherin$^+$ distal tubules, which the authors interpreted as evidence of both proximal and distal tubular toxicity [48]. Treatment of organoids with the antibiotic gentamicin also upregulated KIM-1 in injured proximal tubules without any discernible effect on the distal tubules.

Given that the proximal tubule is a common site of drug-induced nephrotoxicity, Kandasamy and colleagues developed a toxicity assay using hiPSC-derived proximal tubule-like cells. The nephrotoxic response to 30 compounds was determined using a machine learning algorithm called random forest. Human proximal tubular toxicity could be predicted with >87 % accuracy, with hiPSC results congruent with human and animal data [54].

4.8 Pluripotent Stem Cells for Modeling of Kidney Diseases

Patient-derived hiPSCs represent a valuable resource for studying human pathophysiology and the development of novel therapeutics. As hiPSCs carry the genome of the patients from which they are derived, they provide a means of human genetic disease modeling. Additionally, many genetic diseases are rare enough to preclude enrollment in clinical trials. This fact, coupled with the lack of incentive for drug companies to develop pharmaceuticals for the treatment of rare diseases, fuels the hope that hiPSC-based assays can be a scalable and reliable option at low cost. Once established, reliable human disease models may allow for clinical trials-in-a-dish. Human stem cell-based systems may ultimately replace animal testing that is known to be poorly predictive of the human response [55]. To date, human iPSC lines have been generated for autosomal dominant polycystic kidney disease (ADPKD) [47, 53, 56, 57], autosomal recessive polycystic kidney disease (ARPKD) [56], and systemic lupus erythematosus [57, 58].

ADPKD hiPSC lines are particularly noteworthy, owing to the frequency of the disease and uncertainties regarding existing animal models. ADPKD is the most common potentially lethal single gene disorder, affecting 1 in 600–1 in 1000 live births [59]. Approximately 50 % of individuals with ADPKD develop ESRD by age

60. The traditionally used mouse models are homozygous carriers of ADPKD mutations while afflicted humans are heterozygotes, as heterozygote mice manifest only mild cystic disease [60]. Freedman and colleagues established hiPSC lines of three ADPKD and two ARPKD patients via fibroblast reprogramming. ADPKD iPSCs with mutations in the *PKD1* gene, which encodes the protein polycystin-1, exhibited reduced polycystin-2 expression at the primary cilia. Similar results were observed in ADPKD iPSC-derived hepatoblasts, precursors to the biliary cholangiocytes that are the origin of liver cysts in ADPKD patients. The ectopic expression of wild-type polycystin-1 in these hepatoblasts rescued ciliary expression of polycystin-2 [56]. A subsequent study from the same group used gene-editing with the clustered regularly interspaced short palindromic repeats (CRISPR)/Cas9 system to generate knockout *PKD1* or *PKD2* human ESC lines. Two-dimensional kidney organoids derived from these gene-edited hESCs developed cystic structures from kidney tubules, suggesting that this model could potentially serve as a novel means to study cystogenesis in ADPKD [53].

4.9 Pluripotent Stem Cells for Bioengineering Kidney Tissue

The rising prevalence of ESRD, coupled with the shortage of transplantable organs, has led researchers to apply regenerative medicine techniques towards kidney bioengineering. Human iPSCs serve as a theoretically immunocompatible and scalable cell source, with therapeutic applications for both CKD and AKI.

The kidney comprises >50 distinct cell types, arranged in a complex 3D structure that facilitates exocrine, endocrine, and metabolic functions. The primary elements of a bioengineered kidney would include multiple hiPSC-derived cell types and a scaffolding to provide cellular support, segregation, and compartmentalization. Two scaffolding approaches have been undertaken: kidney decellularization and a 3D printed framework.

Decellularized kidney approaches have the benefit of preserving the intricate extracellular matrix (ECM) of distinct kidney compartments, retaining matrix-associated signals and growth factors of specific regions, and conserving the arterial, capillary, and venous vascular tree. Using the detergent sodium dodecyl sulfate (SDS) and the cell membrane toxicant Triton X-100, Nakayama and colleagues decellularized adult rhesus monkey kidney sections. Hematoxylin and eosin (H&E) staining confirmed the removal of cellular material and immunohistochemistry demonstrated the preservation of native ECM [61]. Orlando and colleagues successfully decellularized porcine kidneys and surgically implanted unseeded scaffolds into pigs. Although the decellularized kidneys were easily reperfused, sustained blood pressure, and demonstrated a lack of blood extravasation, the vascular tree was completely thrombosed due to denuded ECM [62]. Song and colleagues seeded decellularized rat kidney scaffolds with rat fetal kidney cells via the ureter and endothelial cells via the renal artery and performed an orthotopic transplantation in a rat. The graft was perfused by the recipient's circulation and produced urine through a ureteral conduit. However, urinary excretion was not substantial and histopathology of the recipient's graft demonstrated vascular thromboses [63]. Similarly, Ross and colleagues seeded murine ESCs into decellularized rat kidneys via the renal artery and ureter. Resultantly, cells lost their pluripotent phenotype and expressed kidney immunohistochemical markers when contacting ECM, while cells not in contact became apoptotic [64]. However, this approach was also limited by small vessel thrombosis. To overcome thrombosis in the small vessel conduits utilized in decellularized scaffolds, Wertheim and colleagues developed a biocompatible polymer that binds denuded ECM. Decellularized rat aortas were lined with poly(1,8-octanediol citrate), functionalized with heparin, and perfused with whole blood. The polymer-ECM reduced platelet adhesion, inhibited whole blood clotting, and supported endothelial cell-adhesion [65]. Given their advantage of maintained architecture, decellularized kidneys represent a valuable resource in the efforts to create a bioengineered kidney. However, it remains to be seen whether proper localization of seeded renal epithelial cell types to their appropriate compartment within the kidney can be achieved. Furthermore, such grafts must also retain significant functionality upon transplantation.

The biologic application of 3D printing has gained both notoriety and credibility with the organ-on-a-chip series, including the lung-on-a-chip, the gut-on-a-chip, the proximal tubule-on-a-chip, and bone marrow-on-a-chip [66–69]. Such devices employ a soft lithography method for the creation of microfluidic chambers, first conceived by Duffy and Whitesides in 1998 [70]. Recent advances in 3D printing have enabled faithful manufacturing of micrometer scale, multicomponent structures. Current precision allows for the biomimicry of multiple physical aspects of native kidneys, such as multicellular architecture, submillimeter tubular diameter, and high surface area to volume ratio. Additionally, applying a perfusate can simulate physiologic levels of shear stress in epithelial and vascular channels. Vascular channels are imperative, as bioengineered tissue structures develop necrotic regions without vasculature within <2 mm of tissue depth [71]. Of note, current commercially available 3D printing resins for both stereolithography and multijet modeling demonstrate poor biocompatibility [72, 73]. To overcome obstacles of resin cytotoxicity and the need for a vascular network in tissue engineering, Kolesky and colleagues used ECM-containing bioink resins to develop a method of printing directly in cells. HUVEC cells, embedded in a Pluronic F127 fugitive hydrogel, were printed in channels and surrounded by gelatin methacrylate (GelMA). Removal of the fugitive ink yielded tubular channels consisting of a confluent monolayer of HUVECs [74].

Fabrication of a bioengineered nephron, the individual functioning unit of the kidney, is a potential intermediate step in the development of a bioengineered kidney. The glomerular, tubular, and collecting duct compartments of the nephron could be modeled separately and connected in series, replete with vasculature, overcoming the compartmentalization difficulties of decellularized kidney methods. Additionally, complex microscale printing provides a means of maximizing absorptive and secretory functions by increased surface area to volume ratio. Homogenous populations of varying types of kidney epithelia may be obtained through cell-sorting of dissociated organoids developed from patient-specific iPSCs. Integration of these cells into 3D printed scaffolds may allow for the generation of an immunocompatible bioengineered nephron, which can be scaled up to restore in vivo kidney filtration.

4.10 Conclusion

Significant advances over the past few years alone have clearly demonstrated that human PSCs represent a powerful tool to study kidney regeneration, disease, and injury. Recently established methods are now capable of directing the differentiation of hESCs and hiPSCs into human kidney organoids in vitro. These kidney organoids can mimic the in vivo pathophysiologic response when subject to nephrotoxic agents, providing novel nephrotoxicity models that may facilitate the identification of lead candidates, reduce developmental costs, and reduce future rates of drug-induced AKI. Patient-derived hiPSCs, bearing naturally occurring human mutations, can recapitulate human disease phenotypes. While disease modeling using hiPSCs may someday supplant animal testing, currently it provides a means of studying rare genetic diseases and allows for clinical trials-in-a-dish. hiPSCs are a theoretically immunocompatible and scalable cell source for kidney regeneration. With the development of advanced bioengineering techniques such as decellularized kidney scaffolds and 3D printing, the integration of stem cell biology with bioengineering may someday contribute to the development of transplantable human kidney tissue.

References

1. Monda KL, et al. Comparative changes in treatment practices and clinical outcomes following implementation of a prospective payment system: the STEPPS study. BMC Nephrol. 2015;16:67.
2. Szczech LA, Lazar IL. Projecting the United States ESRD population: issues regarding treatment of patients with ESRD. Kidney Int Suppl. 2004;90:S3–7.
3. Depner T, Himmelfarb J. Uremic retention solutes: the free and the bound. J Am Soc Nephrol. 2007;18(3):675–6.
4. Floege J, Ketteler M. [beta]2-Microglobulin-derived amyloidosis: an update. Kidney Int. 2001;59(S78):S164–71.
5. Chandrashekar A, Ramakrishnan S, Rangarajan D. Survival analysis of patients on maintenance hemodialysis. Indian J Nephrol. 2014;24(4):206–13.
6. Fukuhara S, et al. Health-related quality of life among dialysis patients on three continents: the Dialysis Outcomes and Practice Patterns Study. Kidney Int. 2003;64(5):1903–10.
7. Stegall MD, Chedid MF, Cornell LD. The role of complement in antibody-mediated rejection in kidney transplantation. Nat Rev Nephrol. 2012;8(11):670–8.

8. Baumann K. Stem cells: multiple routes to pluripotency. Nat Rev Mol Cell Biol. 2015;16(1):1.
9. Lam AQ, Freedman BS, Bonventre JV. Directed differentiation of pluripotent stem cells to kidney cells. Semin Nephrol. 2014;34(4):445–61.
10. Reijo Pera RA, et al. Gene expression profiles of human inner cell mass cells and embryonic stem cells. Differentiation. 2009;78(1):18–23.
11. Boland MJ, et al. Adult mice generated from induced pluripotent stem cells. Nature. 2009;461 (7260):91–4.
12. Zhao XY, et al. iPS cells produce viable mice through tetraploid complementation. Nature. 2009;461(7260):86–90.
13. Martin GR. Isolation of a pluripotent cell line from early mouse embryos cultured in medium conditioned by teratocarcinoma stem cells. Proc Natl Acad Sci U S A. 1981;78(12):7634–8.
14. Evans MJ, Kaufman MH. Establishment in culture of pluripotential cells from mouse embryos. Nature. 1981;292(5819):154–6.
15. Thomson JA, et al. Embryonic stem cell lines derived from human blastocysts. Science. 1998;282(5391):1145–7.
16. Takahashi K, Yamanaka S. Induction of pluripotent stem cells from mouse embryonic and adult fibroblast cultures by defined factors. Cell. 2006;126(4):663–76.
17. Takahashi K, et al. Induction of pluripotent stem cells from adult human fibroblasts by defined factors. Cell. 2007;131(5):861–72.
18. Giacomini M, Baylis F, Robert J. Banking on it: public policy and the ethics of stem cell research and development. Soc Sci Med. 2007;65(7):1490–500.
19. Montserrat N, et al. Generation of induced pluripotent stem cells from human renal proximal tubular cells with only two transcription factors, Oct4 and Sox2. J Biol Chem. 2012;287 (29):24131–8.
20. Song B, et al. Generation of induced pluripotent stem cells from human kidney mesangial cells. J Am Soc Nephrol. 2011;22(7):1213–20.
21. Zhou T, et al. Generation of human induced pluripotent stem cells from urine samples. Nat Protoc. 2012;7(12):2080–9.
22. Seki T, Yuasa S, Fukuda K. Generation of induced pluripotent stem cells from a small amount of human peripheral blood using a combination of activated T cells and Sendai virus. Nat Protoc. 2012;7(4):718–28.
23. Aasen T, et al. Efficient and rapid generation of induced pluripotent stem cells from human keratinocytes. Nat Biotechnol. 2008;26(11):1276–84.
24. Liu H, et al. Generation of endoderm-derived human induced pluripotent stem cells from primary hepatocytes. Hepatology. 2010;51(5):1810–9.
25. Kim JB, et al. Pluripotent stem cells induced from adult neural stem cells by reprogramming with two factors. Nature. 2008;454(7204):646–50.
26. Cohen DE, Melton D. Turning straw into gold: directing cell fate for regenerative medicine. Nat Rev Genet. 2011;12(4):243–52.
27. Kobayashi A, et al. Six2 defines and regulates a multipotent self-renewing nephron progenitor population throughout mammalian kidney development. Cell Stem Cell. 2008;3(2):169–81.
28. Self M, et al. Six2 is required for suppression of nephrogenesis and progenitor renewal in the developing kidney. EMBO J. 2006;25(21):5214–28.
29. Taguchi A, et al. Redefining the in vivo origin of metanephric nephron progenitors enables generation of complex kidney structures from pluripotent stem cells. Cell Stem Cell. 2014;14 (1):53–67.
30. Steenhard BM, et al. Integration of embryonic stem cells in metanephric kidney organ culture. J Am Soc Nephrol. 2005;16(6):1623–31.
31. Yamamoto M, et al. Branching ducts similar to mesonephric ducts or ureteric buds in teratomas originating from mouse embryonic stem cells. Am J Physiol Renal Physiol. 2006;290(1):F52–60.
32. Dressler GR. Advances in early kidney specification, development and patterning. Development. 2009;136(23):3863–74.

33. Kim D, Dressler GR. Nephrogenic factors promote differentiation of mouse embryonic stem cells into renal epithelia. J Am Soc Nephrol. 2005;16(12):3527–34.
34. Vigneau C, et al. Mouse embryonic stem cell-derived embryoid bodies generate progenitors that integrate long term into renal proximal tubules in vivo. J Am Soc Nephrol. 2007;18 (6):1709–20.
35. Bruce SJ, et al. In vitro differentiation of murine embryonic stem cells toward a renal lineage. Differentiation. 2007;75(5):337–49.
36. Morizane R, Monkawa T, Itoh H. Differentiation of murine embryonic stem and induced pluripotent stem cells to renal lineage in vitro. Biochem Biophys Res Commun. 2009;390 (4):1334–9.
37. Nishikawa M, et al. Stepwise renal lineage differentiation of mouse embryonic stem cells tracing in vivo development. Biochem Biophys Res Commun. 2012;417(2):897–902.
38. Morizane R, et al. Kidney specific protein-positive cells derived from embryonic stem cells reproduce tubular structures in vitro and differentiate into renal tubular cells. PLoS One. 2014;8(6):e64843.
39. Batchelder CA, et al. Renal ontogeny in the rhesus monkey (Macaca mulatta) and directed differentiation of human embryonic stem cells towards kidney precursors. Differentiation. 2009;78(1):45–56.
40. Lin SA, et al. Subfractionation of differentiating human embryonic stem cell populations allows the isolation of a mesodermal population enriched for intermediate mesoderm and putative renal progenitors. Stem Cells Dev. 2010;19(10):1637–48.
41. Song B, et al. The directed differentiation of human iPS cells into kidney podocytes. PLoS One. 2012;7(9):e46453.
42. Narayanan K, et al. Human embryonic stem cells differentiate into functional renal proximal tubular-like cells. Kidney Int. 2013;83(4):593–603.
43. Mae S, et al. Monitoring and robust induction of nephrogenic intermediate mesoderm from human pluripotent stem cells. Nat Commun. 2013;4:1367.
44. Araoka T, et al. Efficient and rapid induction of human iPSCs/ESCs into nephrogenic intermediate mesoderm using small molecule-based differentiation methods. PLoS One. 2014;9(1):e84881.
45. Lam AQ, et al. Rapid and efficient differentiation of human pluripotent stem cells into intermediate mesoderm that forms tubules expressing kidney proximal tubular markers. J Am Soc Nephrol. 2014;25(6):1211–25.
46. Takasato M, et al. Directing human embryonic stem cell differentiation towards a renal lineage generates a self-organizing kidney. Nat Cell Biol. 2014;16(1):118–26.
47. Xia Y, et al. Directed differentiation of human pluripotent cells to ureteric bud kidney progenitor-like cells. Nat Cell Biol. 2013;15(12):1507–15.
48. Takasato M, et al. Kidney organoids from human iPS cells contain multiple lineages and model human nephrogenesis. Nature. 2015;526:564–8.
49. Morizane R, et al. Nephron organoids derived from human pluripotent stem cells model kidney development and injury. Nat Biotechnol. 2015;33(11):1193–200.
50. Pazhayattil GS, Shirali AC. Drug-induced impairment of renal function. Int J Nephrol Renov Dis. 2014;7:457–68.
51. Su R, et al. Supervised prediction of drug-induced nephrotoxicity based on interleukin-6 and -8 expression levels. BMC Bioinf. 2014;15 Suppl 16:S16.
52. Bertolini F, Sukhatme VP, Bouche G. Drug repurposing in oncology[mdash]patient and health systems opportunities. Nat Rev Clin Oncol. 2015;12(12):732–42.
53. Freedman BS, et al. Modelling kidney disease with CRISPR-mutant kidney organoids derived from human pluripotent epiblast spheroids. Nat Commun. 2015;6.
54. Kandasamy K, et al. Prediction of drug-induced nephrotoxicity and injury mechanisms with human induced pluripotent stem cell-derived cells and machine learning methods. Sci Rep. 2015;5:12337.

55. Olson H, et al. Concordance of the toxicity of pharmaceuticals in humans and in animals. Regul Toxicol Pharmacol. 2000;32(1):56–67.
56. Freedman BS, et al. Reduced ciliary polycystin-2 in induced pluripotent stem cells from polycystic kidney disease patients with PKD1 mutations. J Am Soc Nephrol. 2013;24 (10):1571–86.
57. Thatava T, et al. Successful disease-specific induced pluripotent stem cell generation from patients with kidney transplantation. Stem Cell Res Ther. 2011;2(6):48.
58. Chen Y, et al. Generation of systemic lupus erythematosus-specific induced pluripotent stem cells from urine. Rheumatol Int. 2013;33(8):2127–34.
59. Iglesias CG, et al. Epidemiology of adult polycystic kidney disease, Olmsted County, Minnesota: 1935–1980. Am J Kidney Dis. 1983;2(6):630–9.
60. Wilson PD. Mouse models of polycystic kidney disease. Curr Top Dev Biol. 2008;84:311–50.
61. Nakayama KH, et al. Decellularized rhesus monkey kidney as a three-dimensional scaffold for renal tissue engineering. Tissue Eng Part A. 2010;16(7):2207–16.
62. Orlando G, et al. Production and implantation of renal extracellular matrix scaffolds from porcine kidneys as a platform for renal bioengineering investigations. Ann Surg. 2012;256 (2):363–70.
63. Song JJ, et al. Regeneration and experimental orthotopic transplantation of a bioengineered kidney. Nat Med. 2013;19(5):646–51.
64. Ross EA, et al. Embryonic stem cells proliferate and differentiate when seeded into kidney scaffolds. J Am Soc Nephrol. 2009;20(11):2338–47.
65. Jiang B, et al. A polymer-extracellular matrix composite with improved thromboresistance and recellularization properties. Acta Biomater. 2015;18:50–8.
66. Huh D, et al. A human disease model of drug toxicity-induced pulmonary edema in a lung-on-a-chip microdevice. Sci Transl Med. 2012;4(159):159ra147.
67. Kim HJ, et al. Human gut-on-a-chip inhabited by microbial flora that experiences intestinal peristalsis-like motions and flow. Lab Chip. 2012;12(12):2165–74.
68. Jang KJ, et al. Human kidney proximal tubule-on-a-chip for drug transport and nephrotoxicity assessment. Integr Biol (Camb). 2013;5(9):1119–29.
69. Torisawa YS, et al. Bone marrow-on-a-chip replicates hematopoietic niche physiology in vitro. Nat Methods. 2014;11(6):663–9.
70. Duffy DC, et al. Rapid prototyping of microfluidic systems in poly(dimethylsiloxane). Anal Chem. 1998;70(23):4974–84.
71. Griffith CK, et al. Diffusion limits of an in vitro thick prevascularized tissue. Tissue Eng. 2005;11(1–2):257–66.
72. Chia HN, Wu BM. Recent advances in 3D printing of biomaterials. J Biol Eng. 2015;9:4.
73. Macdonald NP, et al. Assessment of biocompatibility of 3D printed photopolymers using zebrafish embryo toxicity assays. Lab Chip. 2016;16(2):291–7.
74. Kolesky DB, et al. 3D bioprinting of vascularized, heterogeneous cell-laden tissue constructs. Adv Mater. 2014;26(19):3124–30.

Chapter 5
Pluripotent Stem Cells for Modeling Motor Neuron Diseases

Delphine Bohl

5.1 Introduction

Motoneuron diseases (MNDs) are a group of progressive neurological diseases affecting the neurons that control voluntary muscle activities like walking, breathing, and speaking. They are characterized by a muscular weakness and muscle atrophy that result in paralysis and often death of patients. Both children and adults can be affected. Today there is no effective treatment. Specific supportive cares and symptom relief are the only cures.

MNDs can be classified according to whether affected motoneurons (MNs) are located in the motor cortex (upper MNs) or in the brain stem and/or the spinal cord (lower MNs). Spinal muscular atrophy (SMA), spinal and bulbar muscular atrophy (Kennedy's disease), progressive muscular atrophy, and hereditary motor neuropathies affect lower MNs, while primary lateral sclerosis (PLS), hereditary spastic paraplegia, progressive bulbar and pseudobulbar palsy, and SMA with respiratory distress type I affect lower MNs. In Amyotrophic Lateral Sclerosis (ALS), both upper and lower MNs are targets of the degeneration process. Among these diseases, ALS and SMA type I are the two most common adult and infantile MNDs, respectively. Their prognosis is fatal. In order to study disease pathology and to try to identify molecular and chemical processes leading to specific motoneuronal degeneration in these diseases, various animal models were developed, as well as in vitro cellular approaches. Unfortunately, despite decades of studies,

---

D. Bohl
Inserm U 1127, CNRS UMR 7225, Sorbonne Universités, UPMC Univ Paris 06 UMR S 1127, Institut du Cerveau et de la Moelle épinière, ICM, Paris F-75013, France
e-mail: delphine.bohl@icm-institute.org

E.M. Abdelalim (ed.), *Recent Advances in Stem Cells*, Stem Cell Biology and Regenerative Medicine, DOI 10.1007/978-3-319-33270-3_5

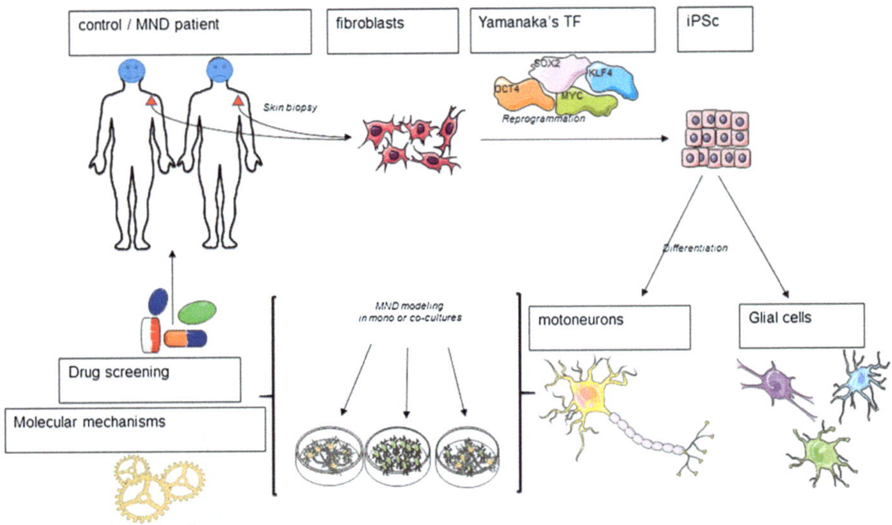

Fig. 5.1 Modeling MND with iPSC. Skin biopsies from control subjects and MND patients are performed and fibroblast cultures are established. Then, reprogrammation of these somatic cells is obtained through the forced expression of the four Yamanaka's transcription factors (TF). iPSC clones are isolated, amplified, and fully characterized at the molecular and functional levels. To compare human MND and control cells (including motoneurons and glial cells) affected in MND, specific protocols have to be applied to ensure that iPS-differentiated cultures can be compared at the phenotypic level. Even if MNs are the primary targets of the neurodegeneration process, glial cells may influence their fate. Disease modeling relies on studies of both cultures of pure MNs or glial cells as well as co-cultures to reveal molecular mechanisms and specific cellular interactions that could be the targets for future drug screenings

hypothesis and results do not lead to effective treatments. One reason may reside in the genotypic and phenotypic differences between human patients and the nonhuman models that were used.

With the recent discovery of the induced pluripotent stem cell (iPSC) technology, new hopes arise to generate new cellular models for MNDs [1, 2]. For neurodegenerative disorders in general, and MNDs in particular, iPSCs offer the unique possibility to have access to human neurons, as there is no possibility to obtain human biopsies of the central nervous system. Until now the only human samples accessible were derived from the blood, muscle biopsies, or brain and spinal cord postmortem tissues which represent the end stage of the disease. In this chapter, I will present the unique human models generated with human iPSC to study SMA and ALS in the perspective to better understand mechanisms leading to MN death and to find new treatments (Fig. 5.1).

5.2 Differentiation of iPSC into Human Motoneurons

In both SMA and ALS, alterations occur at first in MNs but other cells around them, especially glial cells, may be involved in disease progression [3–5]. The development of protocols for efficient and rapid production of either MNs or glial cells is thus extremely important. For glial cells, few protocols exist to generate human astrocytes, oligodendrocytes, or microglia [6–9]. These protocols are quite long and not used for MNDs modeling except for iPSC-derived astrocytes [8] that will be described below. For MNs, many protocols are described in the literature and they are improved very quickly year after year. Their setup benefited from developmental studies and from protocols developed in the past from mouse and human embryonic stem cells (ESCs) [10, 11]. Nevertheless, the majority of the protocols allow the production of spinal MNs (see below). Only one protocol described recently the generation of human iPSC-derived cranial MNs [12] and a study reported the generation of upper MN-like cells (layer 5 cortical neurons) to study specific ALS defects (see below) [13].

5.2.1 *Generation of Spinal Motor Neurons*

Until recently, protocols for the generation of human spinal MNs followed always the same scheme: neuralization of pluripotent stem cells in the presence of retinoic acid for caudalization and a Sonic hedgehog agonist for ventralization [14, 15]. Protocols lasted at least 2 months with the production of MNs positive for the MN-specific transcription factors HB9 and ISLET1 in relatively low proportions (5–40 % of HB9-positive neurons) [14–17]. Despite this successful generation of human spinal MNs with these protocols, a problem emerged for iPSC modeling: the persistence of proliferative neural cells in cultures and their uncontrolled differentiation, leading to the generation of asynchronous cultures with MNs at different stages of maturation, thus preventing reliable comparisons between control and patient cultures.

To solve this problem, laboratories focused either on improvements of protocols or developed tools to purify MNs either by FACS or gradient centrifugation [18, 19]. Several laboratories have now improved protocols and offer the possibility to obtain iPS-differentiated cultures enriched in MNs (30–90 %) within 2–3 weeks [12, 20–23]. Improvement of stem cell neural conversion was reached through the dual SMAD inhibition with molecules able to inhibit transforming growth factor-β (TGF-β) and bone morphogenetic protein (BMP) signaling [24, 25]. Also a crucial timing for initiation of neural patterning was underscored by Qu et al. [22]. Under optimal conditions, human iPSCs treated with Noggin or a substitute, LDN-193189, and SB-431542 led to the formation of more than 90 % of PAX6 neural precursors within a week. For MN generation, Amoroso et al. [20] generated embryoid bodies from human iPSCs and then treated these cell clusters first with both LDN-193189 and SB-431542 and second with both retinoic acid and two ventralizing Smoothened (Smo) agonists. This protocol led to the accelerated generation of MNs within 3 weeks at up to 50 % abundance. To reach 70–90 % of MNs, some studies reported the use of the Wnt agonist Chir-99021 [12, 21, 23]. The activation of Wnt signaling was shown to allow the efficient and accelerated specification of MN progenitors in cooperation with a Sonic Hedgehog agonist and retinoic acid. Moreover, the addition of a gamma-secretase inhibitor, DAPT or Compound E, accelerated the next step in the protocol for the efficient conversion of MN progenitors into postmitotic MNs in less than a week [12, 23]. Taken together, all these studies led to the establishment of more standardized and reproducible methods allowing in 2–3 weeks the production of MNs in high proportions in a synchronous way and without contaminating proliferative cells. These iPSC-derived MNs were proven to be mature. They expressed for example the choline acetyltransferase MN marker, formed neuromuscular junctions in co-culture with myotubes, acquire electrophysiological properties, and integrated into the developing chick spinal cord.

5.2.2 Subtypes of Motoneurons Affected in SMA and ALS

In SMA and ALS, MNs are the first targets of degeneration. However, MNs are not a homogenous group of neurons. There is a high diversity in terms of functional properties and the fate in response to disease differs significantly between MN subtypes. In mammals, MNs are grouped into motor columns: the medial motor column (MMC), the hypaxial motor column (HMC), and the lateral motor columns (LMC) [26]. In ALS and SMA, the LMC MNs including brain stem and limb-innervating MNs, and both the MMC and HMC including axial muscle-innervating MNs, are preferentially affected, respectively. These MN subtypes were shown to express different combination of transcription factors. Among these factors, some distinguish between MMC MNs, which are LHX3-positive, and LMC MNs which are FOXP1-positive [26].

Few reports described the generation of these specific MN subtypes from hESCs or hiPSCs [20, 27, 28]. Patani et al. [28] showed that retinoid-independent motor neurogenesis resulted in the preferential differentiation of LHX3-positive MNs with a MMC identity. Amoroso et al. [20] succeeded to force the generation of FOXP1-positive MNs through a modification of the Sonic Hedgehog and retinoic acid signaling in stem cells. Finally, Adams et al. [27] reprogrammed the production of LMC MNs through misexpression of FOXP1 into neurons. One major limitation that needs now to be addressed is the non-purity of MN subtype cultures. Constructions of viral vectors expressing fluorescent proteins under the control of the LHX3 or FOXP1 promoters would help to reach the objective and this would open new perspectives to better understand the selective death of MN subtypes in SMA and SLA.

5.3 Modeling of Spinal Muscular Atrophy

5.3.1 SMA

SMAs are a group of inherited disorders with a wide spectrum of clinical and genetic phenotypes. Today 33 causative genes have been identified. However, SMA often refers to the most common form caused by mutation or deletion in the survival motor neuron 1 (SMN1) gene leading to reduced levels of ubiquitously expressed full-length SMN protein [29]. SMA is the leading inherited cause of infant mortality and the disease is primarily characterized by progressive degeneration of lower MNs as well as muscle weakness and atrophy that affect mainly proximal muscles. The incidence is of 1 per 6000–10,000 live births. Clinically, SMA disease phenotypes range from severe type I to milder types III and IV on the basis of the age of onset, clinical severity, and the ability to achieve milestones of motor coordination development. In infants with SMA type I (also known as Werdnig–Hoffman disease) disease onset is before 6 months of age and death usually occurs within the first 2 years due to respiratory failure. Today, at least 26 clinical trials have investigated potential treatments and unfortunately all have failed to show any benefit to patients [29].

In cells, the SMN protein has several functions. It is involved in pre-RNA splicing, mRNA transport, and axonal growth. It is a central component of the complex required for assembly of spliceosomal small nuclear ribonucleic particles called snRNPs. Several transgenic mouse models of SMA were created and allowed advances in the understanding of the disease and in particular the pathological changes of the neuromuscular junction preceding MN loss [30, 31]. However, murine models remain different from humans both at the anatomical and the physiological levels and they cannot fully recapitulate human pathologies. This is of particular importance for SMA as humans have a unique genetic situation compared to rodents. They possess a SMN2 paralogous gene which is almost identical to the SMN1 gene but which produces 90 % of a truncated and unstable SMN protein. The remaining 10 % are full-length transcripts. Thus, individuals affected by SMA retain a variable number of SMN2 copies and a direct correlation was shown between this copy number and the severity of the disease. In this context, the generation of human iPSCs from SMA patients with the different severities promises to fill an important niche between studies in rodents and humans in deciphering mechanisms.

5.3.2 Induced Pluripotent Stem Cells (iPSCs) to Model SMA

Human iPSCs models generated to study SMA are listed in Table 5.1. Except one paper describing phenotypes in SMA astrocytes [5], all other reports described the generation of spinal MNs from SMA patients with different types (I–IV)

Table 5.1 Phenotypes in iPSC-derived motoneurons or astrocytes with SMN1 mutations

SMA subtype	Phenotype	Tested drug	Reference
One patient, type I	Reduction in number and size of MNs	Valproic acid	[33]
Two patients, type I	Increase in Fas ligand-mediated apoptosis in MNs	Fas blocking antibodies	[36]
Two patients, type I	Decrease in gem numbers in MNs	–	[18]
	Reduction in number and size of MNs, in their axonal length and in the formation of neuromuscular junctions		
	Gene expression profiling in MNs: defects in cytoskeleton proteins, neuronal development, MN differentiation, and synaptic generation		
	Alteration in the splicing profile of MNs		
Two patients, type I	Deficits in internal calcium signaling mechanisms in astrocytes	Thapsigargin	[5]
One patient, type I	Decrease of SMN protein levels	Splicing modifiers	[75]
One patient, type II			
Three patients, type I	Hyperexcitability of MNs	–	[34]
Two patients, type I	Impairment of neuromuscular junction formation or maturation	Valproic acid	[37]
One patient, type I	Decreased soma size of MNs	Inhibitors of endoplasmic reticulum stress	[35]
One patient, type II	Increased apoptosis in MNs		
	Gene expression profiling in MNs: hyper-activation of the endoplasmic reticulum stress pathway		
Four patients, a consanguineous family with chronic SMA	Significant differences in MN neurite length and number between family members	–	[32]

[18, 32–37]. Validation of iPSC models was performed through analysis of previously described phenotypes considered as hallmarks in SMA animal models and patients. These phenotypes include nuclear gem deficits which are specific protein-nuclear complexes. They form when the SMN protein is present and they are essential for protein splicing.

The paper by Ebert et al. [33] was the first published study describing a phenotype in iPSC-derived cells. They showed nuclear gem defects in iPSCs and a decrease in number and size of iPSC-derived MNs. Other reports validated their different iPSC models and showed nuclear condensation, decreased in MN soma size and number, and Fas ligand-mediated apoptosis. Defects in neurite growth, impairment of neuromuscular junction formation or maturation as well as endoplasmic reticulum stress were also described [18, 32, 35–37]. Interestingly, Boza-Moran et al. generated iPSCs from members of a discordant consanguineous family with chronic SMA (one SMA type IV asymptomatic and two type IIIa sisters).

Significant differences were observed in neurite length and number between family members, but defects were modest compared to previously reported for SMA type I [32]. They also report a progressive decay in SMN protein levels occurred during iPSC differentiation, which recapitulates previous developmental observations. In some reports pharmacological compounds were shown to inhibit some alterations in these iPSC models [33, 35, 36]. Corti et al. [18] also described genetic editing of iPSCs with oligonucleotides to modify SMN2 in order to produce a functional SMN-like protein. MNs derived from genetically corrected SMA-iPSCs showed rescue of disease-specific features. Gene expression profiling analysis showed that SMA MNs had specific alterations in genes encoding proteins involved in cytoskeleton, neuronal development and synaptic generation. Splicing alterations secondary to SMN1 deficiency were also identified and highlighted defects in axon guidance, MN differentiation, DNA linkage, and signal transduction [18]. Further investigations are now necessary to better understand the role of the identified dysregulated genes in SMA pathogenesis.

5.4 Modeling of Amyotrophic Lateral Sclerosis

5.4.1 Amyotrophic Lateral Sclerosis

ALS (also known as Lou Gehrig's disease) is an incurable degenerative MN disorder. It is one of the most devastating neurodegenerative diseases known in adults. The age onset is around 50–60 years. ALS is inexorably worsening, leading progressively and very rapidly to muscle atrophy, paralysis, and death usually by respiratory failure, with a median survival of 3–5 years after diagnosis [38]. Upper and lower MN involvement is variable, and in rare cases cerebellar, extrapyramidal, sensory, and autonomic systems can be affected. Consequently, ALS should not be seen any more as a homogenous neurodegenerative disorder, but rather as a heterogeneous multisystem neurodegenerative disease [38, 39]. The prevalence (3–6 per 100,000) is relatively low compared to other neurodegenerative disorders. However this reflects the short duration of the disease. More than 100,000 patients are affected worldwide. With an incidence of ~2 per 100,000, ALS is today the most common adult onset motor neuron disease [40]. After decades of clinical trials, Riluzole, a glutamate-release inhibitor with neuroprotective properties, is to date the only product that has demonstrated anti-neurodegenerative activity in ALS patients [41, 42]. However, its efficacy is moderate and prolongs mean survival of ALS patients by only a few months.

ALS can be divided into familial forms (F-ALS) which account for ~10 % of cases and ~90 % of sporadic ALS (S-ALS) cases, with no family history. The major genetic causes are of dominant inheritance and gain of functions of mutant proteins were shown for most genes. The four main genes responsible for ALS include mutations in SOD1 (Superoxyde Dismutase 1) (~10 % of F-ALS) [43], TARDBP

(TAR DNA-binding protein 43 (TDP-43)) [44–49], FUS (fused in sarcoma) [50, 51] (~5 % of F-ALS), and the newly discovered intronic hexanucleotide expansions in C9ORF72 (an unknown protein) that is the most common cause of F-ALS (~23–46 %) [52, 53]. Other rare mutations in ANG, VAPB, DAO, OPTN, and UBQLN2 represent <1 % of F-ALS. The remaining forms of ALS may be of genetic, nongenetic, or epigenetic origin. The functional consequences of these different mutations remain to be characterized in relevant cellular and animal models.

Mechanisms leading to the selective death of MNs were first described in animal model systems [54, 55]. They may involve misfolded protein aggregation, depletion of neurotrophic factors, oxidative damage by free radicals, excitotoxic processes related to decreased synaptic reuptake of glutamate, impaired axonal transport, mitochondrial dysfunction, endoplasmic reticulum stress, neurotoxins, viruses, altered astrocyte function, impaired blood–brain barrier, chronic hypoxia, and defective energy metabolism [55]. Several experimental systems have also provided evidence on the involvement of glial cells, and in particular astrocytes, and non-cell autonomous mechanisms in ALS [3, 4].

Most of studies to better understand mechanisms leading to ALS development were performed in mice and rats with various mutations in the SOD1 gene and today these models remain the best nonhuman models compared to animal models based on other mutant genes (TDP-43, FUS) [54]. Unfortunately, despite a large number of positive therapeutic assays in the mutant SOD1 rodent models, translation into human clinical trials was unsuccessful [56]. In the context of ALS, the generation of human iPSCs from patients with various ALS forms and the comparisons between the different ALS MN cultures may help to identify common and divergent affected pathways involved in ALS development in a perspective to identify new therapeutic compounds.

5.4.2 *Induced Pluripotent Stem Cells (iPSCs) to Model ALS*

Today, published studies described the generation of iPSCs from patients with mutations in the four main genes responsible for ALS: C9ORF72 [57–59], SOD1 [20, 21, 60, 61], TDP-43 [62–65], and FUS [66–68]. One paper reported the generation of iPSC with a rare mutation in VAPB (vamp-associated protein B/C) [69] and two papers described patients with S-ALS [13, 70] (Tables 5.2 and 5.3). In the large majority of these papers, iPSCs were differentiated into spinal MNs. In only one paper both spinal MNs and layer 5 cortical neurons were produced and analyzed [13] and one paper studied the phenotype of iPSC-derived astrocytes from mutant TDP-43 patients [8]. There is no report today about the generation of iPSC-derived oligodendrocytes or microglial cells from ALS patients.

To validate these different iPSCs models, analysis of hallmark ALS phenotypes previously reported in animal models and patients was performed. As shown in Table 5.2 first analyzed phenotypes were for most of them related to protein defects

Table 5.2 Phenotypes in iPSC-derived motoneurons with either SOD1, TDP-43, FUS, C9ORF72, VAPB mutations or from sporadic ALS cases

ALS forms	Phenotypes in motor neurons	Tested drug	Reference
Mutant in SOD1			
• SOD1 L144F	Not studied	–	[61]
• SOD1 A4V	Not studied	–	[20]
SOD1 N139K			
SOD1 V148G			
• SOD1 N87S	Not studied	–	[60]
SOD1 S106L			
• SOD1 A4V	Neurofilament aggregation	–	[21]
SOD1 D90A	Neurite degeneration		
Mutant in TDP-43			
• TDP-43 Q343R	TDP-43 cytosolic aggregates	Anacardic acid	[64]
TDP-43 M337V	Reduced neurite length		
TDP-43 G298S	Increased susceptibility to arsenite exposure		
	Gene expression profiling: decrease in expression of genes of cytoskeletal intermediates filaments		
• TDP-43 M337V	Increase in insoluble TDP-43	–	[63]
• TDP-43 M337V	Increase in cytosolic TDP-43	–	[65]
• TDP-43	Formation of cytoplasmic mRNP granules	–	[62]
	Impairment of mRNA axonal transport		
Mutant in FUS			
• FUS R521C	Cytoplasmic FUS accumulation	–	[66]
R495QfsX527			
• FUS R521C	Cytoplasmic FUS accumulation	–	[67]
FUS R514S	FUS recruitment into stress granules		
FUS P525L			
• FUS P525L	Cytoplasmic FUS aggregates	–	[68]
Expansions in C9ORF72			
• GGGGCC expansions	RNA foci, RNA translation products	ASOS	[57]
• GGGGCC expansions	Increased susceptibility to glutamate excitotoxicity	ASOS	[59]
• GGGGCC expansions	RNA foci	–	[58]
	Reduced electrical excitability		
	Increased number of P bodies		
VAPB			
• P56S	Reduction of VAPB protein levels	–	[69]
	No cytoplasmic aggregates		

(continued)

Table 5.2 (continued)

ALS forms	Phenotypes in motor neurons	Tested drug	Reference
Sporadic cases			
• **2 SLA-S** (no mutation found in SOD-1, TARDBP, C9ORF72)	Gene expression profiling supports impairment of intracellular trafficking, intercellular signaling, oxidative phosphorylation, neurotrophic factor function	–	[70]
	Mitochondrial dysfunction		

Table 5.3 Common molecular mechanisms of ALS pathogenesis in iPS-derived mutant motoneurons

ALS forms	Phenotype in motoneurons	Tested drug	References
SOD1 A4V	TDP-43 intranuclear aggregates in 3/16 sALS	Cardiac glycosides	[13]
SOD1 N139K			
TDP-43 A315T			
FUS G566A			
Sporadic (16 cases)			
SOD1 A4V	Hyperexcitability	Retigabine	[73]
FUS H517Q			
C9ORF72 $(G^4C^2)^N$			
TDP-43 M337V	Initial hyperexcitability followed by progressive loss of action potential input and synaptic activity	–	[72]
C9ORF72 $(G^4C^2)^N$			
SOD1 A4V	In SOD1 MNs: mitochondrial defects, ER stress	–	[71]
C9ORF72 $(G^4C^2)^N$	Gene expression profiling		
	In SOD-1: increased oxidative stress, reduced mitochondrial function, altered subcellular transport, activation of the ER stress, and UPR response pathways		
	In C9ORF72: conservation of a subset of these changes		

into MNs. Such defects had been previously described in human postmortem tissues. Aberrant TDP-43 protein aggregation or nuclear exclusion in patients with mutant TDP-43 and in sporadic cases [13, 64, 65], cytoplasmic FUS accumulation in patients with FUS mutations [66–68], RNA foci formation and P-bodies increases in patients with C9ORF72 expansions [57–59], and neurofilaments aggregation in mutant SOD1 patients [21] were described. Other studies described neurite defects in mutant SOD1 and TDP-43 patients [21, 64], as well as mitochondrial defects and reticulum endoplasmic stress in a mutant SOD1 patient [71]. Gene expression profiles identified affected pathways in mutant MNs, suggesting impairment of intracellular trafficking, intercellular signaling, neurotrophic functions, or mitochondrial dysfunction in patients with mutations in TDP-43 [64], SOD1, C9ORF72 [71] and in S-ALS patients [70]. Pharmacological compounds, siRNA, and antisense oligonucleotides (ASOS) were shown to inhibit some alterations in these iPSCs models [13, 57, 59, 64, 65, 71].

Only one report described the generation of iPSC-derived astrocytes [8] from mutant TDP-43 patients. In contrast to previous results showing the toxic contribution of human mutant SOD1 and sporadic astrocytes (not derived from iPSCs) to MN death [4], mutant TDP-43 iPSC-derived astrocytes did not affect MN survival. This result questions on the exact contribution of mutant astrocytes carrying different ALS mutations on MNs and more studies are now necessary to understand the exact role of MN neighboring cells in ALS development.

To advance further in the modeling with human iPSC, and as the ALS syndrome may be viewed more like a spectrum of diseases, comparisons of phenotypes of MNs with different ALS forms may identify common and divergent pathways that may be affected and this may help to identify new approaches to develop personalized therapies. Table 5.3 lists the only four reports which compare MNs from different ALS patients [13, 71–73]. Burkhardt et al. [13] focused on nuclear TDP-43 aggregates and compared the phenotypes in iPSC-derived MNs of a large cohort of patients including 16 S-ALS patients and 8 patients with mutations in SOD1, TDP-43, and FUS. Interestingly and surprisingly, only three S-ALS patients had TDP-43 aggregates in both upper and lower MNs, bringing out heterogeneity among ALS patients. Two reports focused on electrophysiological properties of ALS MNs. The studies on SOD1 mutant mice strongly suggested that early on the morphogenesis of MNs is impaired and that it entails the electrophysiological characteristics of the MNs. While Wainger et al. [73] suggested that hyperexcitability in ALS MNs was recapitulated in patients with SOD1, C9ORF72, and FUS mutations, Devlin et al. described an initial hyperexcitability in C9ORF72 and TDP-43 patients followed by a progressive loss with time of action potential input and synaptic activity [72]. In both studies, MNs cultures were not pure and a role of astrocytes on the deleterious effect observed by Devlin et al. is currently suggested. Consequently, future experiments with pure cultures of MNs are now required, as well as analysis of MNs of sporadic cases to compare the various ALS forms. Finally, comparison of gene expression profiling between one patient with a SOD1 mutation and one patient with a C9ORF72 expansion allowed to highlight that both ALS cases shared only a subset of transcriptional changes [71], showing one more time that ALS should be seen as a group of diseases. Nevertheless, common identified pathways need now to be investigated in detail to define if they could represent therapeutic targets.

5.5 Conclusion: The Perspective for Drug Discovery

Eight years after the description of the iPSC technology, researchers have to their availability a great number of new human cellular models. They also have efficient protocols to produce the main cell type affected in MNDs, the MNs. Despite these very rapid advances in the field, much remains to be done. As said above, the large majority of the studies focused on spinal MNs that were produced with different protocols. Consequently cell yields were different and cultures were, in most reports, not completely pure. As non-cell autonomous mechanisms may be involved in MN death, researchers still have to pay attention to "contaminating" cell types present in cultures of MNs and thus to conclusions and interpretations. More developments are also necessary in order to be able to analyze more precisely the different MN subtypes as well as the other MN types affected in ALS, the upper MNs.

Nevertheless, we have now the proof-of-concept that SMA and ALS phenotypic hallmarks are recapitulated in human iPS-derived MNs. Comparisons between various forms of the diseases are in progress [13, 32, 71–73] and need now to be reproduced to clarify which affected pathways may be the best targets. Some drugs were tested with success in the human iPSC models but there is no definitive proof yet that drugs could be efficient in patients. Nevertheless, recent studies suggest that human iPSC MNs could help to validate compound efficacy for human trials [35, 74, 75]. In the SMA field, based on an approach of SMN-dependant therapy, PTC Therapeutics and Roche Pharmaceutical Research showed spectacular effects of SMN2 splicing modifiers on SMN protein levels in SMA iPSC-derived MNs and a mouse model [75]. A phase 1 clinical trial is in progress. On the other hand and to develop SMN-independent therapies, Ng et al. tested different endoplasmic reticulum stress inhibitors on iPSC-derived MNs. Guanabenz was shown to be the most effective inhibitor in vitro on human iPSC-derived MNs and in SMA mice it was also the one which preserved MN number and size. Interestingly, 4-phenylbutyrate which has been tested in clinical trials on SMA patients and that failed in phase II, had no efficacy on human MNs in vitro [35]. In the ALS field, Yang et al. combined rodent and human stem cell-derived MNs to screen for molecules able to increase ALS MN survival. They identified kenpaullone as the best candidate and compared its effects on human iPSC-derived MNs with effects of two molecules that failed in human clinical trials, olesoxime and dexpramipexole. They showed that these two molecules were barely effective in rescuing MNs from death [74]. Taken together, these studies are proof of principle that a screening approach with human iPSC-derived MNs might predict efficacies of new drugs and it seems clear that this technology could become a useful and relevant tool to accelerate drug discovery.

References

1. Faravelli I, et al. Motor neuron derivation from human embryonic and induced pluripotent stem cells: experimental approaches and clinical perspectives. Stem Cell Res Ther. 2014;5 (4):87.
2. Winner B, et al. Human-induced pluripotent stem cells pave the road for a better understanding of motor neuron disease. Hum Mol Genet. 2014;23(R1):R27–34.
3. Boillee S, Vande Velde C, Cleveland DW. ALS: a disease of motor neurons and their nonneuronal neighbors. Neuron. 2006;52(1):39–59.
4. Haidet-Phillips AM, et al. Astrocytes from familial and sporadic ALS patients are toxic to motor neurons. Nat Biotechnol. 2011;29(9):824–8.
5. McGivern JV, et al. Spinal muscular atrophy astrocytes exhibit abnormal calcium regulation and reduced growth factor production. Glia. 2013;61(9):1418–28.
6. Almeida S, et al. Modeling key pathological features of frontotemporal dementia with C9ORF72 repeat expansion in iPSC-derived human neurons. Acta Neuropathol. 2013;126 (3):385–99.
7. Ogawa S, et al. Induction of oligodendrocyte differentiation from adult human fibroblast-derived induced pluripotent stem cells. In Vitro Cell Dev Biol Anim. 2011;47(7):464–9.
8. Serio A, et al. Astrocyte pathology and the absence of non-cell autonomy in an induced pluripotent stem cell model of TDP-43 proteinopathy. Proc Natl Acad Sci U S A. 2013;110 (12):4697–702.
9. Wang S, et al. Human iPSC-derived oligodendrocyte progenitor cells can myelinate and rescue a mouse model of congenital hypomyelination. Cell Stem Cell. 2013;12(2):252–64.
10. Chipman PH, Toma JS, Rafuse VF. Generation of motor neurons from pluripotent stem cells. Prog Brain Res. 2012;201:313–31.
11. Davis-Dusenbery BN, et al. How to make spinal motor neurons. Development. 2014;141 (3):491–501.
12. Maury Y, et al. Combinatorial analysis of developmental cues efficiently converts human pluripotent stem cells into multiple neuronal subtypes. Nat Biotechnol. 2015;33(1):89–96.
13. Burkhardt MF, et al. A cellular model for sporadic ALS using patient-derived induced pluripotent stem cells. Mol Cell Neurosci. 2013;56:355–64.
14. Hu BY, Zhang SC. Differentiation of spinal motor neurons from pluripotent human stem cells. Nat Protoc. 2009;4(9):1295–304.
15. Lopez-Gonzalez R, Velasco I. Therapeutic potential of motor neurons differentiated from embryonic stem cells and induced pluripotent stem cells. Arch Med Res. 2012;43(1):1–10.
16. Hu BY, et al. Neural differentiation of human induced pluripotent stem cells follows developmental principles but with variable potency. Proc Natl Acad Sci U S A. 2010;107 (9):4335–40.
17. Jha BS, Rao M, Malik N. Motor neuron differentiation from pluripotent stem cells and other intermediate proliferative precursors that can be discriminated by lineage specific reporters. Stem Cell Rev. 2015;11(1):194–204.
18. Corti S, et al. Genetic correction of human induced pluripotent stem cells from patients with spinal muscular atrophy. Sci Transl Med. 2012;4(165):165ra162.
19. Toli D, et al. Modeling amyotrophic lateral sclerosis in pure human iPSc-derived motor neurons isolated by a novel FACS double selection technique. Neurobiol Dis. 2015;82:269–80.
20. Amoroso MW, et al. Accelerated high-yield generation of limb-innervating motor neurons from human stem cells. J Neurosci. 2013;33(2):574–86.
21. Chen H, et al. Modeling ALS with iPSCs reveals that mutant SOD1 misregulates neurofilament balance in motor neurons. Cell Stem Cell. 2014;14(6):796–809.
22. Qu Q, et al. High-efficiency motor neuron differentiation from human pluripotent stem cells and the function of Islet-1. Nat Commun. 2014;5:3449.
23. Du ZW, et al. Generation and expansion of highly pure motor neuron progenitors from human pluripotent stem cells. Nat Commun. 2015;6:6626.

24. Chambers SM, et al. Highly efficient neural conversion of human ES and iPS cells by dual inhibition of SMAD signaling. Nat Biotechnol. 2009;27(3):275–80.
25. Kim DS, et al. Robust enhancement of neural differentiation from human ES and iPS cells regardless of their innate difference in differentiation propensity. Stem Cell Rev. 2010;6 (2):270–81.
26. Kanning KC, Kaplan A, Henderson CE. Motor neuron diversity in development and disease. Annu Rev Neurosci. 2010;33:409–40.
27. Adams KL, et al. Foxp1-mediated programming of limb-innervating motor neurons from mouse and human embryonic stem cells. Nat Commun. 2015;6:6778.
28. Patani R, et al. Retinoid-independent motor neurogenesis from human embryonic stem cells reveals a medial columnar ground state. Nat Commun. 2011;2:214.
29. Farrar MA, Kiernan MC. The genetics of spinal muscular atrophy: progress and challenges. Neurotherapeutics. 2015;12(2):290–302.
30. Kong L, et al. Impaired synaptic vesicle release and immaturity of neuromuscular junctions in spinal muscular atrophy mice. J Neurosci. 2009;29(3):842–51.
31. Thomson SR, et al. Morphological characteristics of motor neurons do not determine their relative susceptibility to degeneration in a mouse model of severe spinal muscular atrophy. PLoS One. 2012;7(12):e52605.
32. Boza-Moran MG, et al. Decay in survival motor neuron and plastin 3 levels during differentiation of iPSC-derived human motor neurons. Sci Rep. 2015;5:11696.
33. Ebert AD, et al. Induced pluripotent stem cells from a spinal muscular atrophy patient. Nature. 2009;457(7227):277–80.
34. Liu H, et al. Spinal muscular atrophy patient-derived motor neurons exhibit hyperexcitability. Sci Rep. 2015;5:12189.
35. Ng SY, et al. Genome-wide RNA-seq of human motor neurons implicates selective ER stress activation in spinal muscular atrophy. Cell Stem Cell. 2015;17(5):569–84.
36. Sareen D, et al. Inhibition of apoptosis blocks human motor neuron cell death in a stem cell model of spinal muscular atrophy. PLoS One. 2012;7(6):e39113.
37. Yoshida M, et al. Modeling the early phenotype at the neuromuscular junction of spinal muscular atrophy using patient-derived iPSCs. Stem Cell Rep. 2015;4(4):561–8.
38. Swinnen B, Robberecht W. The phenotypic variability of amyotrophic lateral sclerosis. Nat Rev Neurol. 2014;10(11):661–70.
39. Millecamps S, et al. SOD1, ANG, VAPB, TARDBP, and FUS mutations in familial amyotrophic lateral sclerosis: genotype-phenotype correlations. J Med Genet. 2010;47 (8):554–60.
40. Robberecht W, Philips T. The changing scene of amyotrophic lateral sclerosis. Nat Rev Neurosci. 2013;14(4):248–64.
41. Bensimon G, Lacomblez L, Meininger V. A controlled trial of riluzole in amyotrophic lateral sclerosis. ALS/Riluzole Study Group. N Engl J Med. 1994;330(9):585–91.
42. Lacomblez L, et al. Dose-ranging study of riluzole in amyotrophic lateral sclerosis. Amyotrophic Lateral Sclerosis/Riluzole Study Group II. Lancet. 1996;347(9013):1425–31.
43. Rosen DR, et al. Mutations in Cu/Zn superoxide dismutase gene are associated with familial amyotrophic lateral sclerosis. Nature. 1993;362(6415):59–62.
44. Gitcho MA, et al. TDP-43 A315T mutation in familial motor neuron disease. Ann Neurol. 2008;63(4):535–8.
45. Kabashi E, et al. TARDBP mutations in individuals with sporadic and familial amyotrophic lateral sclerosis. Nat Genet. 2008;40(5):572–4.
46. Kuhnlein P, et al. Two German kindreds with familial amyotrophic lateral sclerosis due to TARDBP mutations. Arch Neurol. 2008;65(9):1185–9.
47. Rutherford NJ, et al. Novel mutations in TARDBP (TDP-43) in patients with familial amyotrophic lateral sclerosis. PLoS Genet. 2008;4(9):e1000193.
48. Sreedharan J, et al. TDP-43 mutations in familial and sporadic amyotrophic lateral sclerosis. Science. 2008;319(5870):1668–72.

49. Van Deerlin VM, et al. TARDBP mutations in amyotrophic lateral sclerosis with TDP-43 neuropathology: a genetic and histopathological analysis. Lancet Neurol. 2008;7(5):409–16.
50. Kwiatkowski Jr TJ, et al. Mutations in the FUS/TLS gene on chromosome 16 cause familial amyotrophic lateral sclerosis. Science. 2009;323(5918):1205–8.
51. Vance C, et al. Mutations in FUS, an RNA processing protein, cause familial amyotrophic lateral sclerosis type 6. Science. 2009;323(5918):1208–11.
52. DeJesus-Hernandez M, et al. Expanded GGGGCC hexanucleotide repeat in noncoding region of C9ORF72 causes chromosome 9p-linked FTD and ALS. Neuron. 2011;72(2):245–56.
53. Renton AE, et al. A hexanucleotide repeat expansion in C9ORF72 is the cause of chromosome 9p21-linked ALS-FTD. Neuron. 2011;72(2):257–68.
54. Philips T, Rothstein JD. Rodent models of amyotrophic lateral sclerosis. Curr Protoc Pharmacol 2015;69:5.67.1–21.
55. Valetdinova KR, Medvedev SP, Zakian SM. Model systems of motor neuron diseases as a platform for studying pathogenic mechanisms and searching for therapeutic agents. Acta Naturae. 2015;7(1):19–36.
56. Mitsumoto H, Brooks BR, Silani V. Clinical trials in amyotrophic lateral sclerosis: why so many negative trials and how can trials be improved? Lancet Neurol. 2014;13(11):1127–38.
57. Donnelly CJ, et al. RNA toxicity from the ALS/FTD C9ORF72 expansion is mitigated by antisense intervention. Neuron. 2013;80(2):415–28.
58. Haeusler AR, et al. C9orf72 nucleotide repeat structures initiate molecular cascades of disease. Nature. 2014;507(7491):195–200.
59. Sareen D, et al. Targeting RNA foci in iPSC-derived motor neurons from ALS patients with a C9ORF72 repeat expansion. Sci Transl Med. 2013;5(208):208ra149.
60. Chestkov IV, et al. Patient-specific induced pluripotent stem cells for SOD1-associated amyotrophic lateral sclerosis pathogenesis studies. Acta Naturae. 2014;6(1):54–60.
61. Dimos JT, et al. Induced pluripotent stem cells generated from patients with ALS can be differentiated into motor neurons. Science. 2008;321(5893):1218–21.
62. Alami NH, et al. Axonal transport of TDP-43 mRNA granules is impaired by ALS-causing mutations. Neuron. 2014;81(3):536–43.
63. Bilican B, et al. Mutant induced pluripotent stem cell lines recapitulate aspects of TDP-43 proteinopathies and reveal cell-specific vulnerability. Proc Natl Acad Sci U S A. 2012;109 (15):5803–8.
64. Egawa N, et al. Drug screening for ALS using patient-specific induced pluripotent stem cells. Sci Transl Med. 2012;4(145):145.
65. Nishimura AL, et al. Allele-specific knockdown of ALS-associated mutant TDP-43 in neural stem cells derived from induced pluripotent stem cells. PLoS One. 2014;9(3):e91269.
66. Japtok J, et al. Stepwise acquirement of hallmark neuropathology in FUS-ALS iPSC models depends on mutation type and neuronal aging. Neurobiol Dis. 2015;82:420–9.
67. Lenzi J, et al. ALS mutant FUS proteins are recruited into stress granules in induced pluripotent stem cell-derived motoneurons. Dis Model Mech. 2015;8(7):755–66.
68. Liu X, et al. The fused in sarcoma protein forms cytoplasmic aggregates in motor neurons derived from integration-free induced pluripotent stem cells generated from a patient with familial amyotrophic lateral sclerosis carrying the FUS-P525L mutation. Neurogenetics. 2015;16(3):223–31.
69. Mitne-Neto M, et al. Downregulation of VAPB expression in motor neurons derived from induced pluripotent stem cells of ALS8 patients. Hum Mol Genet. 2011;20(18):3642–52.
70. Alves CJ, et al. Gene expression profiling for human iPS-derived motor neurons from sporadic ALS patients reveals a strong association between mitochondrial functions and neurodegeneration. Front Cell Neurosci. 2015;9:289.
71. Kiskinis E, et al. Pathways disrupted in human ALS motor neurons identified through genetic correction of mutant SOD1. Cell Stem Cell. 2014;14(6):781–95.
72. Devlin AC, et al. Human iPSC-derived motoneurons harbouring TARDBP or C9ORF72 ALS mutations are dysfunctional despite maintaining viability. Nat Commun. 2015;6:5999.

73. Wainger BJ, et al. Intrinsic membrane hyperexcitability of amyotrophic lateral sclerosis patient-derived motor neurons. Cell Rep. 2014;7(1):1–11.
74. Yang YM, et al. A small molecule screen in stem-cell-derived motor neurons identifies a kinase inhibitor as a candidate therapeutic for ALS. Cell Stem Cell. 2013;12(6):713–26.
75. Naryshkin NA, et al. Motor neuron disease. SMN2 splicing modifiers improve motor function and longevity in mice with spinal muscular atrophy. Science. 2014;345(6197):688–93.

Chapter 6
Pluripotent Stem Cell-Derived Pancreatic β Cells: From In Vitro Maturation to Clinical Application

Essam M. Abdelalim and Mohamed M. Emara

6.1 Introduction

Embryonic development is initiated by the formation of a small hollow sphere known as blastocyst. This structure possesses an outer layer of cells (trophoblast) and a cluster of inner cells called inner cell mass (ICM). Although the ICM is small in size, it has a great potential in development, because this group of cells is capable to differentiate into the three germ layers derived tissues (ectoderm, mesoderm, and endoderm) that eventually give raise to an embryo in a predominant phenomenon known as pluripotency. Pluripotent stem cells (PSCs) are characterized by a unique ability to self-renew or differentiate into various types of cells [1, 2]. The most important types of PSCs are embryonic stem cells (ESCs), which are isolated from the ICM [1], and induced PSC (iPSCs) that are generated from somatic cells in vitro, such as skin fibroblast, keratinocytes, and blood cells (Fig. 6.1) [2, 3]. In iPSC technology, somatic cells are reprogrammed to become pluripotent by insertion of three or four transcription factors, which are known to be essential for ESC pluripotency, including OCT4, C-MYC, SOX2, KLF4, SOX2, NANOG, and LIN28 [2, 4]. ESCs and iPSCs have similar characteristics and have a great ability to propagate indefinitely in vitro with maintaining the genome integrity [5, 6], therefore, they hold great promises in cell replacement therapies for different critical diseases such as diabetes.

Diabetes mellitus (DM) is a common disease, which is characterized by imbalance between insulin production, insulin need, and the body's ability to utilize the available insulin. This imbalance is resulted due to array of dysfunctions, ranging from inefficiency of β cells in the pancreas to produce insulin, defective insulin

E.M. Abdelalim, Ph.D. (✉) • M.M. Emara
Qatar Biomedical Research Institute, Hamad Bin Khalifa University (HBKU),
Qatar Foundation, Education City, Doha 5825, Qatar
e-mail: emohamed@qf.org.qa

E.M. Abdelalim (ed.), *Recent Advances in Stem Cells*, Stem Cell Biology and Regenerative Medicine, DOI 10.1007/978-3-319-33270-3_6

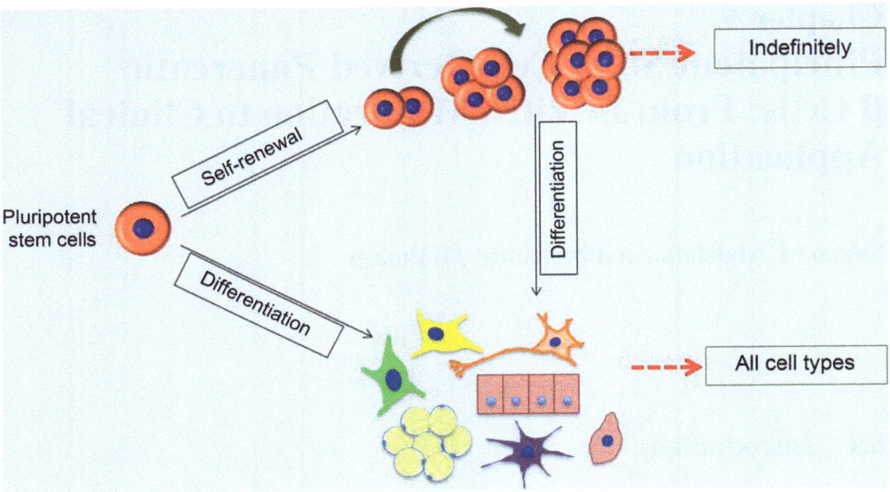

Fig. 6.1 Schematic showing the unique characteristics of pluripotent stem cells (PSCs). PSCs can be propagated and maintained indefinitely in vitro under strict culture conditions. Also, they have the ability to differentiate into all types of cell body including all germ layers (ectoderm, mesoderm, and endoderm)

receptors in specific body tissues that mediate insulin action, or production of defective insulin hormone. Insulin is a peptide hormone that regulates glucose uptake in body tissues; therefore inadequate insulin secretion and/or tissue-specific insulin resistance leads to the accumulation of glucose in the blood stream in levels above normal fasting glucose levels developing a condition known as hyperglycemia. DM is classified mainly into two well-characterized types, type 1 (T1D) and type 2 (T2D). T1D is characterized by a total lack of insulin production resulting from the destruction of insulin-secreting β cells in pancreatic islets by autoimmune attack [7]. This autoimmune process predominantly was found to be due to a combination of genetic and environmental factors that might be developed during childhood over several years before the disease diagnosis. Since the lack of insulin production is the sole cause of T1D and this type usually appears in young age so T1D was known as insulin-dependent diabetes and/or juvenile diabetes. Similarly the development of T2D involves both genetic and acquired environmental factors. Among these environmental factors obesity stands out as one of the most important components that is linked to T2D [8, 9]. T2D represents ~90 % of patients suffering from diabetes worldwide; therefore, it is considered the main type. T2D are characterized by insulin resistance in insulin target tissues (muscle, liver, and fat) and/or inadequate insulin secretion from the insulin-secreting β cells in the pancreatic islets [10]. It has been recently reported that obesity induces a specific type of stress that suppresses signals to insulin receptors and thus forces tissues of the body to become resistant to normal or even high levels of insulin [8, 9]. Tissue-specific insulin resistance leads to hyperglycemia, which stimulates β cells in the pancreas to secrete more insulin to compensate high glucose levels in the blood. Insulin-secreting β cells gradually lose their ability to produce sufficient amounts of insulin needed for the body. Therefore T1D and T2D patients suffer from inadequate insulin secretion and damage of insulin-secreting β cells by distinct mechanisms [11, 12]. Other form of diabetes called "monogenic," including maturity-onset diabetes of the young (MODY) [13] and neonatal diabetes mellitus (NDM) [14], which are rare disorders. These forms occur as a result of mutation(s) in a single gene that is involved in the development of insulin-secreting β cells and/or functionality of β cells (decreased glucose response of beta cells, induced cell death of β cells, or loss of membrane depolarization) [14].

Recently pancreatic β cells derived from PSCs are recognized as one of the potential sources for cell-based therapy as well as disease modeling for diabetes. This makes them a great tool in medicine that shows great promises to save millions of diabetic patients in the years to come. Human iPSCs (hiPSCs) generated from individuals suffering from the same type of diabetes and show similar clinical manifestations may offer valuable information about certain predisposing genes in diabetes and therefore allow a rational design of personalized therapies. Therefore, in this chapter we give orientations to various aspects of ESCs and iPSCs differentiation into pancreatic β cells and discuss the possibility of using PSC-derived β cells as a tool for in vitro disease modeling and cell-based therapy for diabetes.

6.2 Differentiation of Pluripotent Stem Cells into Pancreatic β Cells

During embryonic development undifferentiated and unspecialized PSCs have a unique power to generate several different kinds of cells, that buildup the human body, through a process known as differentiation. Differentiation is a stepwise process that starts with specific cell lineage determination and ends by irreversible terminal differentiation to a specific cell type. This sophisticated process defines a delicate balanced network of genes that are expressed under the control of complex regulatory signal transduction pathways and synergistically work together to create a molecular signature for each specific cell type [15, 16].

Human ESCs (hESCs) and hiPSCs are PSCs that are identical in their characteristics and properties and fulfill the same differentiation capacity to generate various cell types. This encourages several researchers to establish in vitro protocols that mimic the differentiation process during embryonic development [2, 17, 18]. Among these differentiation trials, differentiation of ESCs and/or iPSCs into insulin-secreting β cells has been extensively studied, because of the importance of these cells in diabetes research [19–24]. Successful generation of insulin-secreting β cells from specific patient with a known form of diabetes will allow modeling

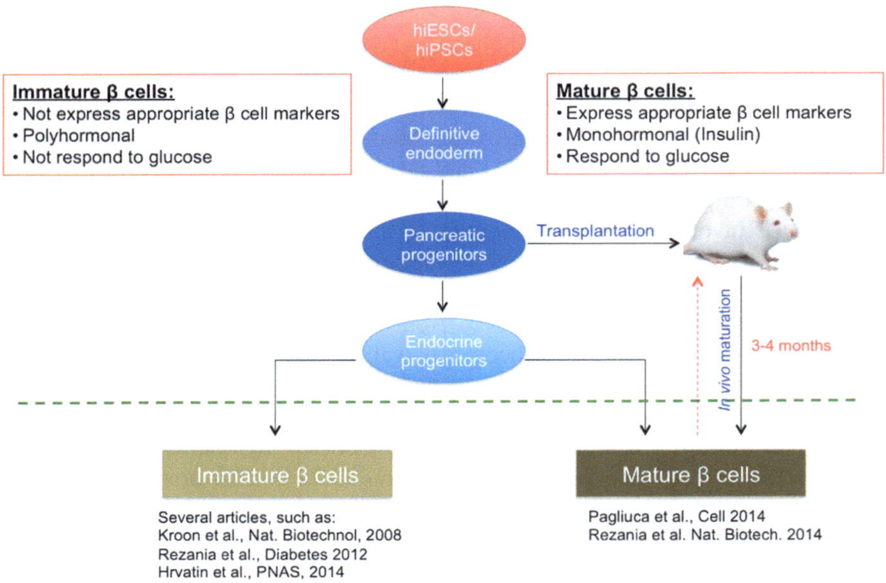

Fig. 6.2 Schematic representation showing the differentiation of pluripotent stem cells into mature pancreatic β cells. Several reports showed the differentiation of hESCs and hiPSCs into pancreatic β cells, which are not fully functional in vitro. However, transplanting the differentiated cells at the stage of pancreatic progenitors into mice leads to their maturation in vivo. Two recent studies showed the ability of PSCs to differentiate into fully functional pancreatic β cells

diabetes and studying the disease pathogenesis in vitro. Furthermore, functional β cells generation may be a tool to cure diabetes through cell-based therapy.

There are several factors that tightly regulate pancreatic development and β cell differentiation ranging from the expression of specific genes to the regulation of signaling pathways. For instance Wnt signaling [25–27] and nodal/activin signaling [28–30] have been reported to play an essential role in proper germ layer formation during development. Therefore, the differentiation of PSCs (hiPSCs and hESCs) into insulin-secreting β cells in vitro is performed in an optimized culture conditions that harbor all the components needed for initiating the gene expression of main transcription factors, which are essentially involved in pancreatic development. Such strictly and controlled culture conditions is considered one of the most critical factors that support the generation of functional pancreatic insulin-secreting β cells from PSCs. Initially, a stepwise protocol that induces embryonic signal transduction pathways was widely used to differentiate hESCs into insulin-secreting β cells [31]. This protocol guides PSCs into sequential differentiation of PSCs into definitive endoderm (DE), pancreatic progenitors (PP), pancreatic endocrine (PE) progenitors, and finally pancreatic β cells (Fig. 6.2).

Although the multistep differentiation protocol was widely used to differentiate pancreatic β cells from PSCs [19–21, 32, 33], the efficiency of differentiation varies between different hPSC lines [34, 35]. It is possible that this discrepancy in pancreatic β cell differentiation is due to the use of different cell lines. Indeed, several studies reported the generation of pancreatic β cells from ESCs [21, 24, 32, 33, 36] and iPSCs [19–24]. However, there was limited capacity to generate pancreatic β cells from PSCs that are capable to secrete adequate insulin levels under different growth factors and conditions [32, 36, 37]. To overcome this problem several trials have been done to modify culture conditions in a way to enhance PSCs differentiation to functional cells that are capable of insulin secretion [32, 36, 38, 39]. A number of studies focused on the modifications of the two-dimensional monolayer cultures [32, 33, 36, 38, 40, 41] by exposing PSCs to distinct signaling factors, that regulate specific signaling pathways, to mediate β cells differentiation. For example, transforming growth factor β (TGFβ) signaling was shown to be required for appropriate β cell differentiation and thus increases the number of insulin-secreting cells to about 25 % [42]. This in vitro modifications approach gathered sound evidence that indicate the vital role of specific pathways in β cell differentiation enhancement. Also, several studies have used xeno-free culture system to generate pancreatic β cells from PSCs in vitro [43–46].

Another approach that has been applied to enhance β cell differentiation was the use of the three-dimensional culture conditions to form multicellular aggregates known as embryoid bodies (EBs) [42, 47]. The three-dimensional approach helps to enhance cell–cell and/or cell–extracellular matrices interactions, which has been found to play an important role in β cell proliferation and function [48–50]. It is possible that EBs formation enhances the interactions between insulin-secreting cells by intercellular electric coupling, which in turn have a direct effect on enhancing the kinetics of insulin production [51]. Yet the efficiency of β cell differentiation in the modified three-dimensional EBs cultures was similar to that of the two-dimensional monolayer one [42]. Notably, all these efforts to critically refine β cell differentiation succeeded to enhance the maturation of insulin-secreting cells generated from hESCs, only, when those cells were transplanted into animals. In engrafted mice, hESCS-derived β cells were capable to respond efficiently and secret insulin in response to glucose [38]. This indicate that there are some specific signals and transcription factors that are still missing during the in vitro differentiation process and are essential for the completion of β cell maturation. Recently, Pagliuca and colleagues were able to identify those factors and thus increase the efficiency of hPSCs to generate mature and functional pancreatic β cells in vitro and in vivo [24]. In this study, the generated pancreatic β cells were produced in massive scale, were significantly similar in character and function to normal human β cells, and were able to restore glucose levels in diabetic mice. Such successful attempt to generate mature and functional pancreatic β cells is considered a big leap towards a potential cell therapy treatment for diabetes.

6.2.1 Differentiation into Definitive Endoderm

At the late blastocyst stage, ICM segregates into two distinct lineages, primitive endoderm (PE) and epiblast. The PE forms the extraembryonic tissues, which surround the embryo, whereas the epiblast gives rise to the three primary germ layers. The innermost layer of the three germ layers derived tissues is the endoderm, which is also called definitive endoderm (DE). DE is different than PE as it setup a landmark for the development of many important tissues and organs of the respiratory and digestive tracts including lung, liver, gall bladder, and pancreas [52]. Importantly, several studies had demonstrated the formation of a transit germ layer known as mesendoderm during the development of a number of animal models such as zebrafish and mouse. This transitional germ layer has the capacity to differentiate into either mesoderm or DE, hence the name [53–56]. Thus the formation of DE is considered a main initial step in its subsequent lineage specification and differentiation processes for the generation of desired organs in vivo. Likewise, in vitro differentiation of PSCs to generate cells belonging to the endodermal lineage depends to a large great extent on the successful stimulation of DE as a leading step during this multistep event (Fig. 6.2).

It has been shown that DE differentiation is recognized by the expression of specific markers [57–60]. Several DE markers have been discovered, of which SOX17, FOXA2, CXCR4, and GSC stand out as the most common and well-known markers that discriminate DE from other tissues during development. During hESCs differentiation to DE, 60–80 % of the cells express an array of DE markers, however the PE marker, SOX7, was not detected in those cells [21, 31, 32, 38, 61, 62]. Interestingly, Sox17 alone was found to be enough to distinguish DE from the other germ layers [63]. However, at the late blastocyst stage, Sox17 expression was found to co-localize and coincide well with the expression of the PE marker Gata6 [64, 65], indicating that Sox17 cannot act as a single marker to distinguish DE from PE. Altogether, it is not surprising that all those markers could be used as molecular signature to purify and/or isolate DE from mouse ESCs (mESCs) as well as hESCs [60].

It has been previously reported that there are several signals orchestrating the differentiation of DE early during development [57, 58]. The first step in DE differentiation is the formation of the primitive streak (PS), which is induced by Nodal/Activin A signaling. Nodal is a ligand that is activated by Activin A, one of the members of TGFβ super family for growth and differentiation, to stimulate a cascade of signaling events that regulates DE development [66]. It has been previously shown that Nodal is the master regulator that induces DE [67]. Notably, the crucial role of Nodal in the generation of DE and its subsequent derivatives comes from the findings that demonstrated the absence of PS formation in Nodal−/− mutant mouse embryo [28, 68]. This was further confirmed by the overexpression of Nodal in mES cell lines, which upregulates the expression of ectoderm and DE markers [69]. Similarly WNT signaling pathway plays an important role in embryonic DE differentiation. Like Nodal−/− mutant mouse embryo, it has been shown that PS is not formed in mouse embryos lacking WNT pathway [26, 70]. This clear involvement of specific signaling pathways in the DE development encourages many researchers to develop a mimic DE differentiation system in vitro.

DE differentiation in vitro, from mESCs, hESCs, hiPSCs, is properly initiated by various number of signaling pathways [21, 31, 36, 71–73], where Nodal/Activin pathway stands out as the most prominent one. The differentiation of DE in vitro was demonstrated by treating ESCs, in adherent [31, 56, 74, 75] or EBs suspension cultures [57, 76], with Activin A, to activate Nodal signaling. Importantly, such activation is found to be dependent on the concentration of Activin A as it appears to be crucial on cell fate determination. High concentrations (50–100 ng/mL) of Activin A efficiently induces Nodal signaling, which in turn leads to DE differentiation, whereas the mesoderm differentiation is initiated with the low concentrations of Activin A (1–3 ng/mL) [47, 57, 77, 78]. Although Activin A was shown to be vital for driving DE formation in both mESCs and hESCs, DE induction by Activin A was significantly efficient in hESCs adherent cultures as compared to that of mESCs [31, 74]. Altogether, these findings suggest the essential role of Activin A in DE induction, which may reflect its widespread use in a number of pancreatic or hepatic differentiation protocols [36, 38, 61, 79, 80].

Remarkably, this significant effect of Activin A is boosted by its combination with other factors that have been shown to play an important role in DE differentiation. The association of Activin A and bone morphogenetic protein (BMP), another member of TGFβ family, leads to a synergistic promotion of DE differentiation in hESCs as measured by the co-expression of the DE specific markers, FOXA2 and SOX17 [80, 81]. Consistent with above findings, the association of Activin A with one of its family members, GDF8 (myostatin), effectively stimulates the differentiation of ESCs into SOX17-expressing DE cells [82]. Thus, the synergistic action of Activin and other TGFβ family members is critical for proper generation of DE. Beside TGFβ family members, the association of WNT signaling activators, such as WNT3A, CHIR9902, or GSK3β inhibitor, with Activin A enhanced DE induction [74]. Notably, CHIR99021 [41] and GSK3β inhibitor [83] were more potent in promoting SOX17- and FOXA2-positive endodermal cells as compared to WNT3A. Given these results, it is perhaps not surprising that many investigators have used Activin A and WNT activators as a standard combination in their DE induction protocols to eventually generate hepatic or pancreatic lineages from different cell lines including iPSCs [27, 31, 38, 42, 61, 62, 72]. However, recently, these combination experiments with Activin A were expanded to include sodium butyrate [32] or PI3K pathway antagonists [21, 71]. Interestingly, the efficiency of hESCs differentiation to the DE lineage significantly increases to reach approximately 90 % after cells were treated with a mixed combination of activin A, CHIR99021, and wortmannin (PI3K inhibitor) [84], indicating the vital role played by several signaling pathways, by either activation or inhibition, in DE differentiation. Although this crucial role was demonstrated by Activin A and its associated factors in DE differentiation, the addition of small molecules such as IDE1 and IDE2 was found to mimic Activin A and stimulate the differentiation of 80 % of hESCs into the DE lineage [85]. This is significantly higher number of differentiated cells as compared to the ones generated using Activin A alone. Therefore, it is possible to predict the wide use of chemical compounds instead of recombinant proteins in the future DE differentiation experiments.

Finally, the efficiently generated DE is anticipated to further differentiate into its final endodermal derivatives such as liver and pancreas progeny cells. Thus, to stimulate pancreatic lineage differentiation, in vitro, the hepatic lineage has to be blocked. To induce this specific lineage inhibition, several types of growth factors such as SU5402 (FGF receptor antagonist) and Noggin (BMP antagonist) [61] have been identified and found to switch off the direction to hepatic generation in treated cells. This is considered a critical step towards engaging DE towards the differentiation into pancreatic progenitors and eventually pancreatic β cells in vitro.

6.2.2 Differentiation into Pancreatic Progenitors

Pancreatic lineage differentiation is stimulated by two contrary effects of BMP signaling pathway [86]. The first effect is an inhibitory one where those signals are suppressed in the dorsal endoderm to direct the differentiation of the cells into the pancreatic lineage; however, the other effect is reflected by the activation of BMP signaling after pancreatic cells formation. Activation of BMP signaling has been found to be required for the regular expression of the pancreatic and duodenal homeobox 1 gene (PDX1) [86], a transcription factor that plays a vital role in early pancreatic development [87]. The expression of PDX1 has been detected in all pancreatic precursor cells and was found to be associated with different stages during the development of the pancreas. At the initial phases of endocrine specification, cells would not express PDX1, while at later stages when cells are committed to pancreatic lineage specification, PDX1 expression increases. This increase has been found to be essential in pancreatic development, enhance β cell function, and is engaged with the secretion of insulin [87]. The essential role of PDX1 during pancreatic development has been demonstrated by the failure of Pdx1 knockout mice to grow a pancreas during embryonic development [88], whereas its ectopic expression leads to the formation of pancreatic progenitors from the epithelium [89]. This role has been also confirmed by other studies that reported the generation of insulin-secreting cells from mESCs overexpressing PDX1 [90, 91]. Therefore PDX1 expression is known to be a hallmark of switching from the endocrine stage to pancreatic progenitors formation.

It has been previously shown that several factors regulate the differentiation of PDX1-expressing cells in vitro. These factors induce such differentiation process by either activation or inhibition of different signaling pathways. One of these signaling pathways that has shown a notable involvement in DE differentiation into pancreatic cells is HEDGEHOG signaling pathways [92]. During DE induction HEDGEHOG signals were upregulated whereas PDX1 expression was suppressed [93, 94], indicating that using compounds and/or factors that repress HEDGEHOG signaling would induce the expression of PDX1. Indeed, the natural occurring compound, Cyclopamine or KAAD cyclopamine, has been found to induce the generation of PDX1-expressing cells through the inhibition of HEDGEHOG-signaling in both human and mouse ESCs [33, 36, 38, 40, 42, 95]. Also, the basic growth factor, FGF2, has been used extensively in pancreatic progenitors expansion protocols as it inhibits sonic hedgehog (Shh) expression, which in turn stimulates PDX1 expression [32, 37, 39, 91, 96]. Interestingly, this regulatory mechanism was found to be concentration dependent, where high concentrations of FGF2 induce Shh expression that block the expression of PDX1 while treating cells with low concentrations of FGF2 leads to adverse effects [97]. Although collectively this data indicate that PDX1 activation is associated with Shh inhibition, one controversial study reported the significant activation of both PDX1 and Shh expression by Activin B in differentiating hESCs as EBs [98].

Other pathways that were found to play a role in pancreatic progenitors development is NOTCH, epidermal growth factor (EGF), TGFβ, and protein kinase C (PKC) signaling pathways. NOTCH signals are activated by Fibroblast growth factor 10 (FGF10) that subsequently lead to the proliferation of PDX1-expressing pancreatic progenitors [99]. Similarly the induction of EGF pathway enhances the expansion of these cells [21]. Although the involvement of TGFβ signaling in pancreatic precursors generation has been previously reported, the exact possible role(s) of this pathway need to be elucidated. It has been found that TGFβ2 significantly induces the expression of PDX1 in mESCs, whereas same family members such as TGFα and TGFβ1 did not induce the formation of PDX1-positive cells [100]. Despite the inability of TGFβ1 to generate PDX1-positive cells, an old report had demonstrated its role in improving the generation of endocrine cells from the pancreatic cells of fetal mouse [101]. On the other hand, the PDX1-positive cells generated by TGFβ2 were incapable to secrete either glucagon or insulin despite their ability to express known endodermal markers [100]. This might reflect a distinct role of TGFβ1 and TGFβ2 in pancreatic development where the first may help in endocrine cells development whereas the later is involved in the early stages of pancreatic lineage specification. Like the previously mentioned pathways, the activation of PKC pathway leads to the generation of PDX1 pancreatic progenitors in hESCs [33]. This activation was induced by a small molecule, Indolactam V, and enhanced by treating the cells with retinoic acid (RA) and dorsomorphin (a BMP type 1 receptor inhibitor) [41]. Moreover, the inducible effect of PKC on PDX1 pancreatic progenitors generation was further confirmed by Rezania and colleagues who found that another two PKC activators (TBP and PBDu) enhances PDX1 expression during the late stages of pancreatic differentiation in hESCs [102]. As pancreatic progenitors have incessant needs for PDX1 expression, the interaction between signaling pathways that regulate its expression is vital for successful pancreatic differentiation.

6.2.3 Differentiation into Endocrine Cells

Neurogenin 3 (NGN3) is another well-known marker that is detected during late pancreatic development and has shown to play an important role in the growth of endocrine precursors of the pancreas. Such critical role has been confirmed by the mice knockout studies that were done on the gene expressing this transcription factor and showed the inability of *Ngn3* deficient mice to initiate the growth of the known pancreatic endocrine cells that secrete insulin, glucagon, pancreatic polypeptide, or somatostatin [103]. Indeed, during endocrine differentiation, NGN3-positive cells were generated after the formation of PDX1 pancreatic progenitors and were shown to give rise to those islets of pancreatic endocrine cells [104], thus NGN3-positive cells are considered islet progenitors. Similar to PDX1, the expression of NGN3 is regulated by different signaling pathways, however, the mechanisms in their regulation is different than PDX1. Among these pathways NOTCH signaling stands out as the one most well-known critical pathway in regulating the switch from pancreatic progenitors to endocrine cells development. As mentioned above, PDX1 expression is stimulated by the activation of NOTCH signaling, which will also inhibit NGN3 expression to sustain the expansion of pancreatic progenitors. Once NOTCH signaling is blocked, NGN3 expression is enhanced and the endocrine lineage is initiated as indicated by the formation of NGN3-positive cells [105, 106]. This role of NOTCH signaling during pancreatic development has been reflected by an enhanced differentiation of endocrine cells in NGN3-overexpression mouse embryos or the inhibition of this differentiation by the continuous activation of NOTCH signaling [107, 108]. Interestingly, NOTCH signaling effector genes, Hes1 [103, 104, 109], and NGN3 gene activator, Sox9 [110], have been found to control the regulatory function of NOTCH during pancreatic differentiation. High levels of NOTCH induce Hes1 gene expression where Hes1 bind to *Ngn3* and block its expression to interfere with endocrine differentiation, whereas in conditions where NOTCH levels are low SOX9 over rides the binding effect of HES1 to *Ngn3* and stimulates its expression, which in turn stimulate endocrine cell differentiation. This indicates that NOTCH regulates pancreatic differentiation fate in dose-dependent manner rather than a switch on/off mode. The effect of NOTCH signaling on endocrine progenitors generation had been also demonstrated in in vitro pancreatic differentiation protocols [33, 36, 40], where cells were treated with a gamma secretase inhibitor (DAPT) after pancreatic progenitors formation. This treatment enhances the expression of NGN3 by the direct inhibition of NOTCH and thus directs the cells towards endocrine fate. However, formation of NGN3-positive cells was not consistent as it depends on the cell line used.

It is worth to note that several studies had linked the differentiation of PDX1-positive cells into NGN3-positive cells to different types of specific treatments. Treatment of hESC-derived PDX1-positive pancreatic cells with an inhibitor of TGFβ type 1 receptor inhibitor known as SB431542 stimulates the differentiation of those cells into NGN3-positive cells [41, 111]. Reserpine and tetrabenazine (TBZ), two vesicular monoamine transporter 2 (VMAT2) inhibitors, display the formation of NGN3-positive endocrine precursors from PDX1-positive cells [112]. In line with this, treating iPSCs with high concentrations of NOGGIN induces the differentiation of PDX1-positive pancreatic progenitors into NGN3-positive pancreatic endocrine progenitor cells [46]. It is worth to note that initial culture cell density affects drastically the differentiation ability of PSCs into pancreatic endocrine cells. For example, it has been previously shown that hESCs seeded in high densities showed a significant increase in cell differentiation rate into PDX1- and NGN3-positive cells as compared to those cultures with low number of cells

[113]. The link between PDX1 and NGN3 has been also shown on the studies done on mESCs that demonstrated a significant increase in insulin secretion in cells co-expressing PDX1 and NGN3. This effect was only seen in endoderm populations derived from EB indicating the specificity of PDX1 and NGN3 to pancreatic endocrine [114].

6.2.4 Differentiation into Pancreatic β Cells

The terminal phase of pancreatic differentiation includes the transfer of endocrine cells from the immature to the mature phase that is characterized by the formation of functional β cells. Mature and functional β cells are known to be cells that secret a single hormone (insulin) in response to glucose. Mature pancreatic β cells generation from hESCs as well as hiPSCs has been previously reported and is indicated by the expression of different markers such as PDX1, MAFA, NKX6.1, NEUROD, ISL-1, and GLUT2, C-peptide, and INS (insulin) [21]. The homebox transcription factor NKX6 homebox 1 (NKX6.1) is the most well known among these factors to potentially induce the generation of mature β cells and maintain their function. The in vivo ablation of NKX6.1 was sufficient to interfere with the development of pancreatic cells in the knockout mice, where as the development of these cells were restored when NKX6.1 was re-expressed in pancreatic progenitor cells [115]. In accordance with this, diabetic mice transplanted with NKX6.1 expressing cells showed a dramatic decrease in glucose levels after transplantation; however, in those that harbor cells expressing low levels of NKX6.1, no noticeable changes in hyperglycemia were observed [116]. Such significant role of NKX6.1 has been further confirmed by parallel studies done by Taylor and colleagues who showed that inactivation of NKX6.1 gene from the β cells of adult mice leads to the development of diabetes, which is associated with an insufficient production of insulin. Such gene inactivation leads also to a significant effect on the genes responsible for regulating insulin synthesis and secretion in β cells [117]. In addition, NKX6.1-positive cells generated from hESCs treated with EGF, NOG-GIN, nicotinamide, and BMP and HEDGEHOG inhibitors then transplanted into SCID mice were able to generate insulin-secreting cells as well as other types of endocrine cells in vivo [118]. Moreover, a recent study showed that the expression of two members from the nuclear receptor subfamily 4 (Nr4a1 and Nr4a3) is regulated by NKX6.1 and their expression is correlated to β cell proliferation [119]. Collectively these results reflect the vital role of NKX6.1 as a master regulator in β cell maturation and insulin secretion. Interestingly, this has been in line with the low expression levels of NKX6.1 in pancreatic β cells of patients with type 2 diabetes [120].

In addition to NKX6.1, the role of other transcription factors in enhancing the differentiation of pancreatic β cells has been previously reported [90, 121, 122]. Those factors are known to play a role in pancreatic development and promoting cell proliferation in embryos. One of these factors, paired box4

(PAX4), one of the *Pax* gene family that is known to play an important role in pancreatic endocrine cell development [123], is expressed mainly in pancreatic islets specifically β and δ endocrine cells indicating its significant role in those cells [124, 125]. In mice lacking *Pax4* gene, neither β cells nor δ cells are formed, where as α cells formation increases as indicated by the high expression levels of ARX, a specific marker for α cells generation [125, 126]. It has been previously reported that during embryonic development PAX4 represses ARX expression to enable the development of pancreatic β cells [127, 128]. Consistent with this, PAX4 overexpression in pancreatic progenitors generated from hESCs, interfere with ARX and glucagon expression and efficiently formed β cells that are able to secrete insulin only [129]. The enhancement of pancreatic β cell differentiation is specific after PAX4 overexpression [130], because the overexpression of PDX1 in hESCs failed to generate β cells and only stimulates the formation of pancreatic endocrine cell during differentiation within EB [131].

Importantly, genetic studies had correlated well different mutations in *Pax4* gene with T1D, T2D, and MODY in different populations [132–137]. The common feature between T1D and T2D is pancreatic β cell destruction; therefore it is logical to point out the vital role of PAX4 in β cell maintenance and survival. This was confirmed by the in vivo experiments that showed that mice overexpressing PAX4 within their β cells did not develop hyperglycemia when they were treated with streptozotocin (STZ), a toxic compound that destructs insulin-secreting cells, whereas hyperglycemic animals expressing *Pax4* mutation (R129W), that is linked to T2D, develop high glucose levels and showed noticeable degree of β cell death [138]. Moreover, a recent study showed the presence of genuine population of PAX4 expressing cells within mice pancreatic islets and its existence was linked with the active functional status of β cells [139]. It is noteworthy that the effect of PAX4 on β cell differentiation is reversed after long periods of the protein overexpression in vivo, where β cells loses its defined structure as well as its ability to secrete insulin [138]. Overall this data define PAX4 as a prominent factor that plays a critical role in maintaining the functionality and maturity of pancreatic β cells.

For several years, tremendous efforts have been directed towards the production of functional and mature pancreatic β cells, which has been defined as the main challenge during in vitro differentiation. This has been done by treating cells with different compounds and/or factors such as forskolin (an adenylate cyclase activator) and dexamethasone (a synthetic adrenocortical steroid) [41], hepatocyte growth factor (HGF), insulin growth factor 1 (IGF-1), and glucagon-like peptide 1 (GLP-1) [140]. Although both hESCs and hiPSCs have been shown as a reproducible generation of pancreatic β cells that secrete insulin in vitro [20, 21, 32, 36–38, 42, 47, 61, 80, 141, 142], these cells are not recognized as mature or functional β cells as they did not respond to the glucose challenge test and did not express the main markers that reflect β cell maturity such as NKX6.1 and MAFA [20]. In addition, the differentiated cells derived from these studies are multi-hormonal secretory cells, where they have shown the ability to simultaneously secrete insulin, glucagon, and C-peptide. Therefore, they lack a hallmark feature of functional pancreatic β cells, which is the mono-hormonal secretion of insulin. Despite the fact that these cells were not functional in vitro, pancreatic progenitors expressing PDX1 were able to generate mature endocrine cells in vivo, as reflected by their ability to secrete insulin and show an expression profile similar to that at the comparable stage during pancreatic development [102]. This data leads to a controversial opinion on the capability of PSCs to generate mature and functional β cells that are able to respond to glucose and secret insulin [143].

Recently several research groups were able to produce β cells from PSCs both in vitro and in vivo. A combined treatment of a cell-permeable cAMP analog (dibutyryl adenosine 3′,5′-cyclic AMP) and two VMAT2 inhibitors (reserpine and tetrabenazine) efficiently promotes the differentiation endocrine precursors derived ESCs into pancreatic β cells that respond to glucose in vitro and combat hyperglycemia in vivo [112]. In addition, a stepwise protocol for β cell differentiated from hESCs successfully produced cells that secrete insulin in response to glucose in vitro and were able to reverse diabetes in vivo [144]. However, those cells were not yet fully mature as compared to normal pancreatic β cells in human. Remarkably, successful generation of massive numbers of functional pancreatic β cells that fully resemble those of the human pancreas has been recently achieved in vitro. These differentiated pancreatic β cells were capable to significantly decrease high glucose levels when transplanted into diabetic mice [24]. Moreover, Russ and colleagues recently developed a simple and fast protocol that omit BMP inhibitors, commonly used during pancreatic differentiation, use retinoic acid to produce PDX1-positive cells, and subsequently add EGF and KGF to generate PDX1/NKX6.1-positive progenitors with high efficiency (~90 %). PDX1/NKX6.1-positive progenitors are induced to differentiate into NEUROG3-positive endocrine cells. These treatments avoid polyhormonal endocrine cell production and lead to an efficient and large scale in vitro differentiation into pancreatic beta cells that secrete insulin only and sustain its mature and functional status after transplantation into diabetic mice [145]. The recent data on the successful generation of functional pancreatic β cells in vitro renew the hope in developing an efficient cell therapy for diabetes.

6.3 Maturation of Pancreatic β Cells

The mechanisms initiating the conversion of immature pancreatic β cells into maturity during development are not known. Functionality and maturity of pancreatic β cell-derived PSCs are crucial to for cell replacement therapy as well as to understand the pathophysiology of the disease in vitro. As mentioned above, several reports showed the differentiation of PSCs into pancreatic β cells that are glucose-responsive in vivo, but they have very limited response to glucose in vitro and are polyhormonal [19–21, 32, 33, 146] indicating that the in vivo microenvironment may contain specific factors enhancing the maturation process. The difficulties to obtain fully functional pancreatic β cells in vitro, which are highly responsive to glucose, may be because the differentiated cells are closely similar to those of human fetal β cells (not adult β cells) as previously reported [146]. It has been reported that fetal pancreatic β cells secrete insulin regardless of alterations in glucose levels [147, 148].

Transplantation of pancreatic progenitors (PDX1-positive cells) or immature pancreatic β cells into healthy [38, 47] or diabetes mice [102] leads to their differentiation in vivo into mature and functional β cells (Fig. 6.2). Also, pancreatic progenitors can differentiate into functional β cells inside the macrocapsules after transplantation, where they can secrete insulin, glucagon, and somatostatin [149]. Furthermore, transplantation of pancreatic β cells derived from iPSCs into mouse models, recapitulating T1D and T2D, leads to their differentiation into glucose-responsive β cells in vivo and reduces hyperglycemia in those mice [111, 150, 151]. The mechanism of maturation is still not clear. However, several factors have been found to be involved in the maturity of pancreatic β cells. Previous reports demonstrated that the process of changing from immature to mature of β cells is associated with chromatin remodeling [141, 152–154]. It has been found that MAFB is expressed in pancreatic β cells only during the early development. However, MAFA is increased with the maturity of β cells [155–157]. MAFA and NeuroD have been found to be involved in the maturation of β cells [155, 156, 158]. Also, TGF-β and thyroid hormone are also involved in the maturation process of β cells [159, 160]. Furthermore, loss of the important transcription factors such as PDX1, NKX6.1, and MAFA leads to immaturity of β cells because these factors are involved in insulin production and its response to glucose [36, 38, 161]. In addition, a corticotropin-releasing factor known as urocortin 3 (Ucn3) is secreted by insulin-secreting β cells and is linked to insulin secretion in response to glucose stimulation [162]. A previous study showed inability of pancreatic β cells to secrete Ucn3 in vitro; however, it is expressed during in vivo maturation [147].

Three recent studies reported the ability of PSCs to differentiate into fully functional pancreatic β cells, which are similar to human adult pancreatic β cells. The generated β cells secrete only one hormone (insulin) and respond to glucose stimulation [24, 144, 145]. Interestingly, it has been indicated that the polyhormonal cells are produced from the pancreatic progenitors (PDX1-positive cells), which are not expressing NKX6.1. Removing BMP inhibitors during specification stage of the pancreas can prevent this. Thus, generation of PDX1-positive progenitor cells, which are also positive for NKX6.1, before NEUROG3 induction (endocrine progenitors) leads to the generation of functional pancreatic β cells in vitro (glucose-responsive cells) [145].

6.4 Patient-Specific Pluripotent Stem Cells for In Vitro Modeling of Diabetes

In the past few years, several studies reported the generation of patient-specific PSCs from the somatic cells of diabetic patients. The generated PSCs can be differentiated into insulin-secreting β cells that are genetically identical to the patient profile. This is a great advantage that protects these cells from being rejected by the immune system and in turn becomes an attractive tool for future cell therapy. Furthermore, it is now possible to model diabetes by culturing insulin-secreting β cells generated from a specific patient with a known form of diabetes and studying the disease pathogenesis in vitro. Disease modeling using patient-specific iPSCs has the potential to give more understanding into the cellular and molecular defects of diabetes and to enable new cell-based drug discovery [163, 164]. The generation of iPSCs from diabetic patients has been well documented. Importantly, it did not cover only one type of diabetes, but its production spread out to include a broad range of patients who suffers from different types of diabetes including T1D and T2D [19, 22, 23, 140, 165–167] (Fig. 6.3).

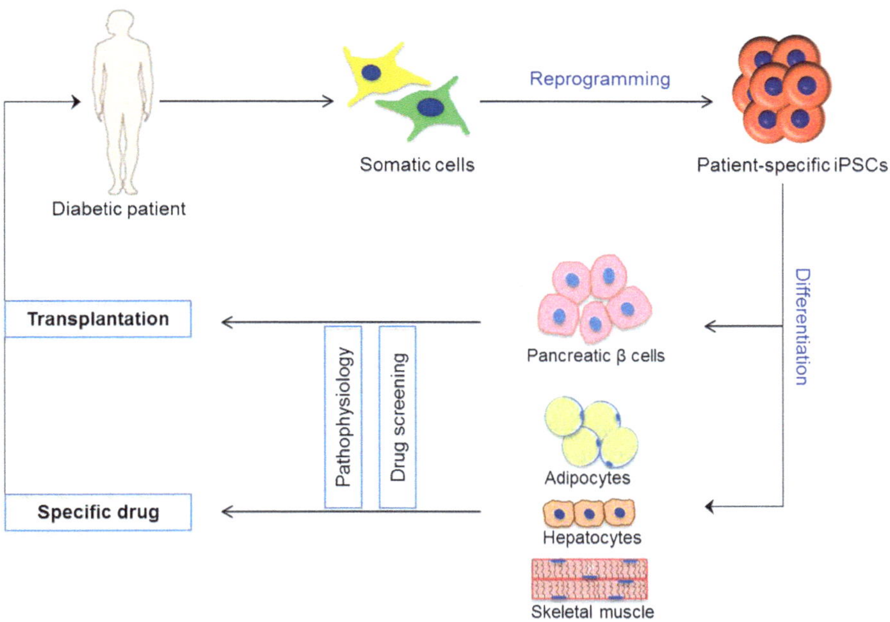

Fig. 6.3 Generation of patient-specific iPSCs from diabetic patients. Patient-specific iPSCs can be differentiated into functional pancreatic beta cells, which can be used for transplantation therapy. Also, they can be differentiated into insulin target cells, such as adipocytes, hepatocytes, and skeletal myocytes. Those cells can be used to study the pathophysiology of the disease as well as for the drug screening

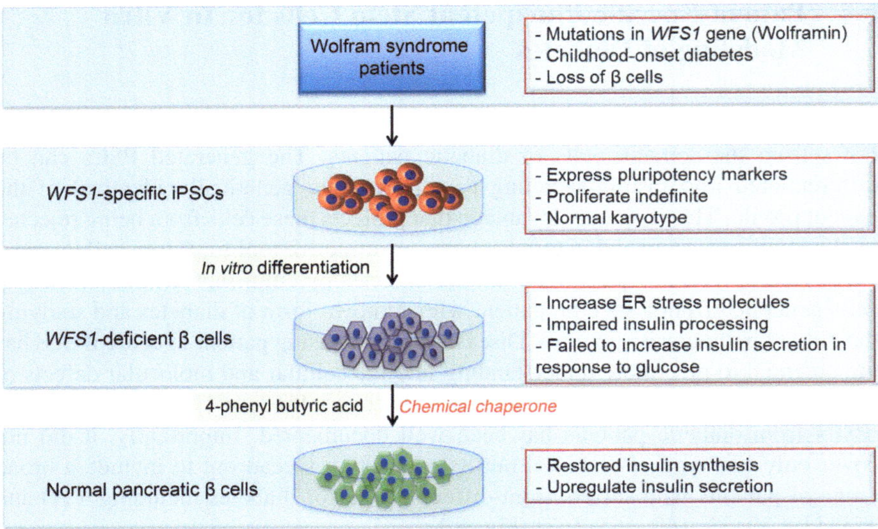

Fig. 6.4 hiPSC-based model of Wolfram syndrome. hiPSCs have been generated from patients suffering from mutations in *WFS1* gene (Wolframin). Pancreatic β cells derived from *WFS1*-specific hiPSCs showed an increase in ER stress and inability to respond to glucose. However, treating the cells with a *chemical chaperone* (4-phenyl butyric acid) leads to generation of functional pancreatic β cells, responding to glucose stimulation

Maehr et al. have generated the first patient-specific hiPSC from T1D patients using three TFs [19]. Interestingly, Bhatt et al. reported very low reprogramming efficiency of fibroblasts isolated from long-standing T1D patients (with T1D for more than 50 years) with severe (Medalist + C) complications. iPSCs generated from those patients showed impairment in their proliferation and differentiation ability due to an increased levels of miR200 in the parental cells and the generated iPSCs [168]. In a recent study, patient-specific ESCs have been successfully generated from somatic cells of T1D patients [163]. Also, hiPSC lines have been generated from T2D elderly patients (56–78 years old) and are able to differentiate into pancreatic β cells [140]. Interestingly, hiPSCs generated from patients with severe insulin resistance due to mutations in the insulin receptor (INSR) showed defects in self-renewal ability and gene expression of undifferentiated hiPSCs, indicating that genetic defects in the insulin signaling can change iPSC characteristics [169]. Furthermore, hiPSC lines have been generated from patients suffering from Wolfram syndrome, which is characterized by insulin-dependent diabetes due to mutations in WFS1 [170]. Pancreatic β cells differentiated from WFS1-iPSCs exhibited elevated levels of endoplasmic reticulum (ER) stress mediators and reduced insulin signals. Also, in vitro exposure of WFS1 iPSC-derived β cells into ER stress leads to impairment in insulin signaling and inability to respond to glucose. Interestingly, treatment of β cells with 4PBA, a chemical chaperone, is able to rescue pancreatic β cells from the adverse effect of ER stress [170] (Fig. 6.4).

The establishment of patient-specific iPSCs from monogenic diabetes, MODY, is essential to understand functions of MODY genes in the development of pancreatic beta cells as well as their roles in the pathogenesis of diabetes. Recent studies reported the generation of several hiPSC lines from different types of MODY patients, including MODY1 (*HNF4A*), MODY2 (*GCK*), MODY3 (*HNF1A*), MODY5 (*HNF1B*), and MODY8 (*CEL*) patients [23, 165]. hiPSCs generated from MODY2 patients with two inactive GCK alleles are not able to differentiate into pancreatic beta cells; however, *GCK* gene correction rescues the ability of MODY2-specific iPSCs to differentiate into pancreatic β cells that respond to glucose [23]. Recently, hiPSC lines have been generated from Japanese MODY5 patients with R177X mutation [167]. During the differentiation of Japanese MODY5-IPSCs into pancreatic β cells, it has been found that R177X mutant mRNAs are disrupted by nonsense-mediated mRNA decay [167].

The reprogramming efficiency is very crucial because producing iPSCs with different qualities might affect the obtained results. For example, the ability of patient-specific iPSCs to differentiate into insulin-secreting β cells showed intrapatient variations in several studies [20, 22, 42]. There are several factors involved in the reprogramming process, which may be the cause for these variations. One of these factors is the genetic background of the somatic cells. ESCs and iPSCs generated from nonobese diabetic (NOD) mice, which develop diabetes similar to human T1D, have defects in their pluripotent abilities [171]. This indicates that the genetic background of the patients can affect the reprogramming process as well as the pluripotent state. Furthermore, the reprogramming method may affect the efficiency. Using viral vectors, integrating into the genome, can induce mutations and subsequently affect pluripotency and differentiation of iPSCs [2, 4, 172]. However, recently several studies showed the generation of iPSCs using non-integrating vectors, such as using Adeno viral vectors [173, 174] and Sendai viral vectors [166]. Transgene-free patient-specific iPSCs have been produced from T1D and T2D patients with Sendai viral vectors [166]. Some reports showed that Cre/LoxP recombination [175, 176] and seamless excision of piggyback transposons could be used to produce transgene-free iPSCs [177]. Also, iPSCs are generated directly using recombinant proteins [178, 179].

6.5 Therapeutic Application of Pluripotent Stem Cells in Diabetes

There is a progress toward the treatment of T1D using PSCs. In case of T1D, the transplanted cells must be protected from the immune system to avoid their damage, even if they are originated from the same patient, as a result of autoimmune defects.

Recently, Viacyte Company developed encapsulation device, which can protect the transplanted cells from the immunological attack. The company obtained FDA approval in 2014 and started phase 1/2 of the clinical trials. Encapsulated hESC-derived pancreatic progenitors (PDX1-positive cells) are transplanted under the skin of T1D patients. These progenitor cells can differentiate in vivo into different pancreatic cells expressing insulin, glucagon, and somatostatin. On the other hand, after the success of Melton and his colleagues to obtain fully functional insulin-secreting β cells from PSCs [24], they are currently developing new encapsulation device to be able to use them for the treatment of T1D. Taken together, these steps indicate that we are very close to see approved treatment for T1D.

A previous study showed that transplantation of hESC-derived pancreatic epithelium (hESC-PE) in encapsulation device leads to their differentiation into functional pancreatic β cells [180]. Therefore, encapsulation technology is an important way to protect the transplanted cells. However, future studies should focus on how to treat the deviations in the immune system to be able to transplant insulin-secreting cells without protection devices.

6.6 Conclusion and Future Directions

There is no doubt that the field of stem cell research related to diabetes and pancreatic β cell development has substantially developed. However, several studies are needed to address the challenging facing the field. Maturation of iPSC-derived pancreatic β cells is essential to study the pathophysiology of the disease as well as to be used for cellular therapies. The maturation of pancreatic β cells is identified with their ability to secrete insulin in response to glucose stimulation. Several studies reported the ability of PSCs to be differentiated into pancreatic β cells, which are glucose-responsive in vivo, but they have very limited response to glucose in vitro [19–21, 23, 32, 33, 116, 141, 146, 152–154]. Recently, three studies reported the ability of PSCs to differentiate into fully functional pancreatic β cells, which are similar to human adult pancreatic β cells. The generated β cells secrete only one hormone (insulin) and respond to glucose stimulation [24, 144, 145]. However, further studies are needed to simplify the method of generating fully functional pancreatic β cells in vitro through understanding pathways involved in the maturation process. In addition, the tumorigenicity of iPSCs should be considered carefully, because some genes used to reprogram somatic cells into pluripotency are oncogenic (c-MYC and KLF4) [181, 182]. Recent studies have reported that iPSCs can be generated without MYC, which is an oncogenic gene [19, 183, 184].

To use pancreatic β cells for cell replacement therapy, it is essential to differentiate them into a pure population of differentiated cells to avoid development of teratoma formation after transplantation into patients because the contamination with undifferentiated pluripotent cells induces teratoma. However, in case of using encapsulation technology, the growth of unwanted pluripotent cells is controlled within the capsule [180, 185].

Using of hESCs in regenerative medicine faces a lot of concerns in several countries in the world, because of the ethical and religious issues. Also, using hESCs for cell therapy faces the problem of immune rejection as the differentiated cells are not genetically identical to the patients. However, recent studies have solved the immune rejection issue through generation of patient-specific hESCs using somatic cell nuclear transfer (SCNT) method [163, 186], but this technology remains ethically more complicated. Therefore, using iPSC technology is more appropriate since it avoids ethical and religious concerns and can provide cells immunologically identical to those of the patients.

Future studies are needed to improve our understanding of the pathophysiology of different forms of diabetes as well as providing new therapies. Detailed transcriptional analysis using the genomic approaches should be done during the differentiation process to identify signaling pathways, which are involved in maturation and functionality of pancreatic β cells. Also, identifying defects responsible for the development of different forms of diabetes will help in discovery of new drugs and tools to treat diabetes. It has been found that animal models do not completely reflect the diabetes phenotype in humans, for example, in several types of MODY (mice with heterozygous mutations have no diabetes) [187] and Wolfram Syndrome [188]. Thus, generation of hiPSCs from patients suffering from those forms of the disease and their differentiation into beta cells can serve as appropriate substitute human in vitro models to study diabetes. Genome editing technology has been used to model MODY2, where the pancreatic beta cells generated from hiPSCs with GCK mutation are not responsive to glucose [165]. Furthermore, insulin resistance can be studied using patient-specific iPSCs. Generation of hiPSCs from patients with genetic defects in insulin signaling components such as INSR, AKT, and TBC1D4 and their differentiation into target cells such as skeletal muscle cells, adipocytes, and hepatocytes would be helpful to study defects during development. Also, it will give insights on the mechanisms underlying hyperglycemia and hyperinsulinemia. In case of T1D, the defects in autoimmunity lead to an immune-mediated damage of pancreatic beta cells. Therefore, generation of hiPSCs from T1D patients and their differentiation into T lymphocytes and pancreatic beta cells enable us to examine the interaction between lymphocytes and beta cells in vitro.

References

1. Thomson JA, Itskovitz-Eldor J, Shapiro SS, Waknitz MA, Swiergiel JJ, Marshall VS, et al. Embryonic stem cell lines derived from human blastocysts. Science. 1998;282 (5391):1145–7.
2. Takahashi K, Tanabe K, Ohnuki M, Narita M, Ichisaka T, Tomoda K, et al. Induction of pluripotent stem cells from adult human fibroblasts by defined factors. Cell. 2007;131 (5):861–72.
3. Hanna J, Markoulaki S, Schorderet P, Carey BW, Beard C, Wernig M, et al. Direct reprogramming of terminally differentiated mature B lymphocytes to pluripotency. Cell. 2008;133(2):250–64.

4. Yu J, Vodyanik MA, Smuga-Otto K, Antosiewicz-Bourget J, Frane JL, Tian S, et al. Induced pluripotent stem cell lines derived from human somatic cells. Science. 2007;318(5858):1917–20.
5. Abdelalim EM. Molecular mechanisms controlling the cell cycle in embryonic stem cells. Stem Cell Rev. 2013;9(6):764–73.
6. Ruiz S, Panopoulos AD, Herrerias A, Bissig KD, Lutz M, Berggren WT, et al. A high proliferation rate is required for cell reprogramming and maintenance of human embryonic stem cell identity. Curr Biol. 2011;21(1):45–52.
7. Gillespie KM. Type 1 diabetes: pathogenesis and prevention. Can Med Assoc J. 2006;175(2):165–70.
8. Joost HG. Pathogenesis, risk assessment and prevention of type 2 diabetes mellitus. Obes Facts. 2008;1(3):128–37.
9. Yang L, Calay ES, Fan J, Arduini A, Kunz RC, Gygi SP, et al. Metabolism. S-Nitrosylation links obesity-associated inflammation to endoplasmic reticulum dysfunction. Science. 2015;349(6247):500–6.
10. Doria A, Patti ME, Kahn CR. The emerging genetic architecture of type 2 diabetes. Cell Metab. 2008;8(3):186–200.
11. Mathis D, Vence L, Benoist C. Beta-cell death during progression to diabetes. Nature. 2001;414(6865):792–8.
12. Donath MY, Halban PA. Decreased beta-cell mass in diabetes: significance, mechanisms and therapeutic implications. Diabetologia. 2004;47(3):581–9.
13. Vaxillaire M, Froguel P. Monogenic diabetes in the young, pharmacogenetics and relevance to multifactorial forms of type 2 diabetes. Endocr Rev. 2008;29(3):254–64.
14. Bonnefond A, Froguel P, Vaxillaire M. The emerging genetics of type 2 diabetes. Trends Mol Med. 2010;16(9):407–16.
15. Martello G, Smith A. The nature of embryonic stem cells. Annu Rev Cell Dev Biol. 2014;30:647–75.
16. Abdelalim EM, Emara MM. Advances and challenges in the differentiation of pluripotent stem cells into pancreatic β cells. World J Stem Cells. 2015; 7(1):174-81.
17. Takahashi K, Yamanaka S. Induction of pluripotent stem cells from mouse embryonic and adult fibroblast cultures by defined factors. Cell. 2006;126(4):663–76.
18. Evans M. Discovering pluripotency: 30 years of mouse embryonic stem cells. Nat Rev Mol Cell Biol. 2011;12(10):680–6.
19. Maehr R, Chen S, Snitow M, Ludwig T, Yagasaki L, Goland R, et al. Generation of pluripotent stem cells from patients with type 1 diabetes. Proc Natl Acad Sci U S A. 2009;106(37):15768–73.
20. Tateishi K, He J, Taranova O, Liang G, D'Alessio AC, Zhang Y. Generation of insulin-secreting islet-like clusters from human skin fibroblasts. J Biol Chem. 2008;283(46):31601–7.
21. Zhang D, Jiang W, Liu M, Sui X, Yin X, Chen S, et al. Highly efficient differentiation of human ES cells and iPS cells into mature pancreatic insulin-producing cells. Cell Res. 2009;19(4):429–38.
22. Thatava T, Kudva YC, Edukulla R, Squillace K, De Lamo JG, Khan YK, et al. Intrapatient variations in type 1 diabetes-specific iPS cell differentiation into insulin-producing cells. Mol Ther. 2013;21(1):228–39.
23. Hua H, Shang L, Martinez H, Freeby M, Gallagher MP, Ludwig T, et al. iPSC-derived beta cells model diabetes due to glucokinase deficiency. J Clin Invest. 2013;123(7):3146–53.
24. Pagliuca FW, Millman JR, Gurtler M, Segel M, Van Dervort A, Ryu JH, et al. Generation of functional human pancreatic beta cells in vitro. Cell. 2014;159(2):428–39.
25. Haegel H, Larue L, Ohsugi M, Fedorov L, Herrenknecht K, Kemler R. Lack of beta-catenin affects mouse development at gastrulation. Development. 1995;121(11):3529–37.
26. Liu P, Wakamiya M, Shea MJ, Albrecht U, Behringer RR, Bradley A. Requirement for Wnt3 in vertebrate axis formation. Nat Genet. 1999;22(4):361–5.

27. Kelly OG, Pinson KI, Skarnes WC. The Wnt co-receptors Lrp5 and Lrp6 are essential for gastrulation in mice. Development. 2004;131(12):2803–15.
28. Conlon FL, Lyons KM, Takaesu N, Barth KS, Kispert A, Herrmann B, et al. A primary requirement for nodal in the formation and maintenance of the primitive streak in the mouse. Development. 1994;120(7):1919–28.
29. Osada SI, Wright CV. Xenopus nodal-related signaling is essential for mesendodermal patterning during early embryogenesis. Development. 1999;126(14):3229–40.
30. Vincent SD, Dunn NR, Hayashi S, Norris DP, Robertson EJ. Cell fate decisions within the mouse organizer are governed by graded Nodal signals. Genes Dev. 2003;17(13):1646–62.
31. D'Amour KA, Agulnick AD, Eliazer S, Kelly OG, Kroon E, Baetge EE. Efficient differentiation of human embryonic stem cells to definitive endoderm. Nat Biotechnol. 2005;23 (12):1534–41.
32. Jiang J, Au M, Lu K, Eshpeter A, Korbutt G, Fisk G, et al. Generation of insulin-producing islet-like clusters from human embryonic stem cells. Stem Cells. 2007;25(8):1940–53.
33. Chen S, Borowiak M, Fox JL, Maehr R, Osafune K, Davidow L, et al. A small molecule that directs differentiation of human ESCs into the pancreatic lineage. Nat Chem Biol. 2009;5 (4):258–65.
34. Osafune K, Caron L, Borowiak M, Martinez RJ, Fitz-Gerald CS, Sato Y, et al. Marked differences in differentiation propensity among human embryonic stem cell lines. Nat Biotechnol. 2008;26(3):313–5.
35. Chin MH, Mason MJ, Xie W, Volinia S, Singer M, Peterson C, et al. Induced pluripotent stem cells and embryonic stem cells are distinguished by gene expression signatures. Cell Stem Cell. 2009;5(1):111–23.
36. D'Amour KA, Bang AG, Eliazer S, Kelly OG, Agulnick AD, Smart NG, et al. Production of pancreatic hormone-expressing endocrine cells from human embryonic stem cells. Nat Biotechnol. 2006;24(11):1392–401.
37. Jiang W, Shi Y, Zhao D, Chen S, Yong J, Zhang J, et al. In vitro derivation of functional insulin-producing cells from human embryonic stem cells. Cell Res. 2007;17(4):333–44.
38. Kroon E, Martinson LA, Kadoya K, Bang AG, Kelly OG, Eliazer S, et al. Pancreatic endoderm derived from human embryonic stem cells generates glucose-responsive insulin-secreting cells in vivo. Nat Biotechnol. 2008;26(4):443–52.
39. Lumelsky N, Blondel O, Laeng P, Velasco I, Ravin R, McKay R. Differentiation of embryonic stem cells to insulin-secreting structures similar to pancreatic islets. Science. 2001;292 (5520):1389–94.
40. Thatava T, Nelson TJ, Edukulla R, Sakuma T, Ohmine S, Tonne JM, et al. Indolactam V/GLP-1-mediated differentiation of human iPS cells into glucose-responsive insulin-secreting progeny. Gene Ther. 2011;18(3):283–93.
41. Kunisada Y, Tsubooka-Yamazoe N, Shoji M, Hosoya M. Small molecules induce efficient differentiation into insulin-producing cells from human induced pluripotent stem cells. Stem Cell Res. 2012;8(2):274–84.
42. Nostro MC, Sarangi F, Ogawa S, Holtzinger A, Corneo B, Li X, et al. Stage-specific signaling through TGFbeta family members and WNT regulates patterning and pancreatic specification of human pluripotent stem cells. Development. 2011;138(5):861–71.
43. Micallef SJ, Janes ME, Knezevic K, Davis RP, Elefanty AG, Stanley EG. Retinoic acid induces Pdx1-positive endoderm in differentiating mouse embryonic stem cells. Diabetes. 2005;54(2):301–5.
44. Schulz TC, Young HY, Agulnick AD, Babin MJ, Baetge EE, Bang AG, et al. A scalable system for production of functional pancreatic progenitors from human embryonic stem cells. PLoS One. 2012;7(5):e37004.
45. Micallef SJ, Li X, Schiesser JV, Hirst CE, Yu QC, Lim SM, et al. INS(GFP/w) human embryonic stem cells facilitate isolation of in vitro derived insulin-producing cells. Diabetologia. 2012;55(3):694–706.

46. Shahjalal HM, Shiraki N, Sakano D, Kikawa K, Ogaki S, Baba H, et al. Generation of insulin-producing beta-like cells from human iPS cells in a defined and completely xeno-free culture system. J Mol Cell Biol. 2014;6(5):394–408.
47. Shim JH, Kim SE, Woo DH, Kim SK, Oh CH, McKay R, et al. Directed differentiation of human embryonic stem cells towards a pancreatic cell fate. Diabetologia. 2007;50 (6):1228–38.
48. Hammar EB, Irminger JC, Rickenbach K, Parnaud G, Ribaux P, Bosco D, et al. Activation of NF-kappaB by extracellular matrix is involved in spreading and glucose-stimulated insulin secretion of pancreatic beta cells. J Biol Chem. 2005;280(34):30630–7.
49. Weber LM, Hayda KN, Anseth KS. Cell–matrix interactions improve beta-cell survival and insulin secretion in three-dimensional culture. Tissue Eng Part A. 2008;14(12):1959–68.
50. Parnaud G, Hammar E, Ribaux P, Donath MY, Berney T, Halban PA. Signaling pathways implicated in the stimulation of beta-cell proliferation by extracellular matrix. Mol Endocrinol. 2009;23(8):1264–71.
51. Speier S, Gjinovci A, Charollais A, Meda P, Rupnik M. Cx36-mediated coupling reduces beta-cell heterogeneity, confines the stimulating glucose concentration range, and affects insulin release kinetics. Diabetes. 2007;56(4):1078–86.
52. Lu CC, Brennan J, Robertson EJ. From fertilization to gastrulation: axis formation in the mouse embryo. Curr Opin Genet Dev. 2001;11(4):384–92.
53. Lawson KA, Meneses JJ, Pedersen RA. Clonal analysis of epiblast fate during germ layer formation in the mouse embryo. Development. 1991;113(3):891–911.
54. Rodaway A, Patient R. Mesendoderm. An ancient germ layer? Cell. 2001;105(2):169–72.
55. Rodaway A, Takeda H, Koshida S, Broadbent J, Price B, Smith JC, et al. Induction of the mesendoderm in the zebrafish germ ring by yolk cell-derived TGF-beta family signals and discrimination of mesoderm and endoderm by FGF. Development. 1999;126(14):3067–78.
56. Tada S, Era T, Furusawa C, Sakurai H, Nishikawa S, Kinoshita M, et al. Characterization of mesendoderm: a diverging point of the definitive endoderm and mesoderm in embryonic stem cell differentiation culture. Development. 2005;132(19):4363–74.
57. Kubo A, Shinozaki K, Shannon JM, Kouskoff V, Kennedy M, Woo S, et al. Development of definitive endoderm from embryonic stem cells in culture. Development. 2004;131 (7):1651–62.
58. Bakre MM, Hoi A, Mong JC, Koh YY, Wong KY, Stanton LW. Generation of multipotential mesendodermal progenitors from mouse embryonic stem cells via sustained Wnt pathway activation. J Biol Chem. 2007;282(43):31703–12.
59. Shiraki N, Harada S, Ogaki S, Kume K, Kume S. Identification of DAF1/CD55, a novel definitive endoderm marker. Cell Struct Funct. 2010;35(2):73–80.
60. Wang P, McKnight KD, Wong DJ, Rodriguez RT, Sugiyama T, Gu X, et al. A molecular signature for purified definitive endoderm guides differentiation and isolation of endoderm from mouse and human embryonic stem cells. Stem Cells Dev. 2012;21(12):2273–87.
61. Mfopou JK, Chen B, Mateizel I, Sermon K, Bouwens L. Noggin, retinoids, and fibroblast growth factor regulate hepatic or pancreatic fate of human embryonic stem cells. Gastroenterology. 2010;138(7):2233–45. 45 e1-14.
62. Johannesson M, Stahlberg A, Ameri J, Sand FW, Norrman K, Semb H. FGF4 and retinoic acid direct differentiation of hESCs into PDX1-expressing foregut endoderm in a time- and concentration-dependent manner. PLoS One. 2009;4(3):e4794.
63. Niakan KK, Ji H, Maehr R, Vokes SA, Rodolfa KT, Sherwood RI, et al. Sox17 promotes differentiation in mouse embryonic stem cells by directly regulating extraembryonic gene expression and indirectly antagonizing self-renewal. Genes Dev. 2010;24(3):312–26.
64. Koutsourakis M, Langeveld A, Patient R, Beddington R, Grosveld F. The transcription factor GATA6 is essential for early extraembryonic development. Development. 1999;126 (4):723–32.

65. Cai KQ, Capo-Chichi CD, Rula ME, Yang DH, Xu XX. Dynamic GATA6 expression in primitive endoderm formation and maturation in early mouse embryogenesis. Dev Dyn. 2008;237(10):2820–9.
66. Champeris TS, Jones PM. Generating pancreatic beta-cells from embryonic stem cells by manipulating signaling pathways. J Endocrinol. 2010;206(1):13–26.
67. Tian T, Meng AM. Nodal signals pattern vertebrate embryos. Cell Mol Life Sci. 2006;63 (6):672–85.
68. Zhou X, Sasaki H, Lowe L, Hogan BL, Kuehn MR. Nodal is a novel TGF-beta-like gene expressed in the mouse node during gastrulation. Nature. 1993;361(6412):543–7.
69. Pfendler KC, Catuar CS, Meneses JJ, Pedersen RA. Overexpression of Nodal promotes differentiation of mouse embryonic stem cells into mesoderm and endoderm at the expense of neuroectoderm formation. Stem Cells Dev. 2005;14(2):162–72.
70. Barrow JR, Howell WD, Rule M, Hayashi S, Thomas KR, Capecchi MR, et al. Wnt3 signaling in the epiblast is required for proper orientation of the anteroposterior axis. Dev Biol. 2007;312(1):312–20.
71. McLean AB, D'Amour KA, Jones KL, Krishnamoorthy M, Kulik MJ, Reynolds DM, et al. Activin a efficiently specifies definitive endoderm from human embryonic stem cells only when phosphatidylinositol 3-kinase signaling is suppressed. Stem Cells. 2007;25 (1):29–38.
72. Sui L, Mfopou JK, Geens M, Sermon K, Bouwens L. FGF signaling via MAPK is required early and improves Activin A-induced definitive endoderm formation from human embryonic stem cells. Biochem Biophys Res Commun. 2012;426(3):380–5.
73. Vallier L, Touboul T, Chng Z, Brimpari M, Hannan N, Millan E, et al. Early cell fate decisions of human embryonic stem cells and mouse epiblast stem cells are controlled by the same signalling pathways. PLoS One. 2009;4(6):e6082.
74. Hansson M, Olesen DR, Peterslund JM, Engberg N, Kahn M, Winzi M, et al. A late requirement for Wnt and FGF signaling during activin-induced formation of foregut endoderm from mouse embryonic stem cells. Dev Biol. 2009;330(2):286–304.
75. Yasunaga M, Tada S, Torikai-Nishikawa S, Nakano Y, Okada M, Jakt LM, et al. Induction and monitoring of definitive and visceral endoderm differentiation of mouse ES cells. Nat Biotechnol. 2005;23(12):1542–50.
76. Gadue P, Huber TL, Paddison PJ, Keller GM. Wnt and TGF-beta signaling are required for the induction of an in vitro model of primitive streak formation using embryonic stem cells. Proc Natl Acad Sci U S A. 2006;103(45):16806–11.
77. Tam PP, Kanai-Azuma M, Kanai Y. Early endoderm development in vertebrates: lineage differentiation and morphogenetic function. Curr Opin Genet Dev. 2003;13(4):393–400.
78. Schier AF. Nodal signaling in vertebrate development. Annu Rev Cell Dev Biol. 2003;19:589–621.
79. Hay DC, Fletcher J, Payne C, Terrace JD, Gallagher RC, Snoeys J, et al. Highly efficient differentiation of hESCs to functional hepatic endoderm requires ActivinA and Wnt3a signaling. Proc Natl Acad Sci U S A. 2008;105(34):12301–6.
80. Xu X, Browning VL, Odorico JS. Activin, BMP and FGF pathways cooperate to promote endoderm and pancreatic lineage cell differentiation from human embryonic stem cells. Mech Dev. 2011;128(7–10):412–27.
81. Teo AK, Ali Y, Wong KY, Chipperfield H, Sadasivam A, Poobalan Y, et al. Activin and BMP4 synergistically promote formation of definitive endoderm in human embryonic stem cells. Stem Cells. 2012;30(4):631–42.
82. Bruin JE, Erener S, Vela J, Hu X, Johnson JD, Kurata HT, et al. Characterization of polyhormonal insulin-producing cells derived in vitro from human embryonic stem cells. Stem Cell Res. 2014;12(1):194–208.
83. Bone HK, Nelson AS, Goldring CE, Tosh D, Welham MJ. A novel chemically directed route for the generation of definitive endoderm from human embryonic stem cells based on inhibition of GSK-3. J Cell Sci. 2011;124(Pt 12):1992–2000.

84. Takeuchi H, Nakatsuji N, Suemori H. Endodermal differentiation of human pluripotent stem cells to insulin-producing cells in 3D culture. Sci Rep. 2014;4:4488.
85. Borowiak M, Maehr R, Chen S, Chen AE, Tang W, Fox JL, et al. Small molecules efficiently direct endodermal differentiation of mouse and human embryonic stem cells. Cell Stem Cell. 2009;4(4):348–58.
86. Wandzioch E, Zaret KS. Dynamic signaling network for the specification of embryonic pancreas and liver progenitors. Science. 2009;324(5935):1707–10.
87. Bernardo AS, Cho CH, Mason S, Docherty HM, Pedersen RA, Vallier L, et al. Biphasic induction of Pdx1 in mouse and human embryonic stem cells can mimic development of pancreatic beta-cells. Stem Cells. 2009;27(2):341–51.
88. Jonsson J, Carlsson L, Edlund T, Edlund H. Insulin-promoter-factor 1 is required for pancreas development in mice. Nature. 1994;371(6498):606–9.
89. Grapin-Botton A, Majithia AR, Melton DA. Key events of pancreas formation are triggered in gut endoderm by ectopic expression of pancreatic regulatory genes. Genes Dev. 2001;15 (4):444–54.
90. Blyszczuk P, Czyz J, Kania G, Wagner M, Roll U, St-Onge L, et al. Expression of Pax4 in embryonic stem cells promotes differentiation of nestin-positive progenitor and insulin-producing cells. Proc Natl Acad Sci U S A. 2003;100(3):998–1003.
91. Miyazaki S, Yamato E, Miyazaki J. Regulated expression of pdx-1 promotes in vitro differentiation of insulin-producing cells from embryonic stem cells. Diabetes. 2004;53(4):1030–7.
92. Mfopou JK, Bouwens L. Hedgehog signals in pancreatic differentiation from embryonic stem cells: revisiting the neglected. Differentiation. 2008;76(2):107–17.
93. Mfopou JK, Willems E, Leyns L, Bouwens L. Expression of regulatory genes for pancreas development during murine embryonic stem cell differentiation. Int J Dev Biol. 2005;49 (8):915–22.
94. Mfopou JK, De Groote V, Xu X, Heimberg H, Bouwens L. Sonic hedgehog and other soluble factors from differentiating embryoid bodies inhibit pancreas development. Stem Cells. 2007;25(5):1156–65.
95. Skoudy A, Rovira M, Savatier P, Martin F, Leon-Quinto T, Soria B, et al. Transforming growth factor (TGF)beta, fibroblast growth factor (FGF) and retinoid signalling pathways promote pancreatic exocrine gene expression in mouse embryonic stem cells. Biochem J. 2004;379(Pt 3):749–56.
96. Segev H, Fishman B, Ziskind A, Shulman M, Itskovitz-Eldor J. Differentiation of human embryonic stem cells into insulin-producing clusters. Stem Cells. 2004;22(3):265–74.
97. Hebrok M, Kim SK, Melton DA. Notochord repression of endodermal Sonic hedgehog permits pancreas development. Genes Dev. 1998;12(11):1705–13.
98. Frandsen U, Porneki AD, Floridon C, Abdallah BM, Kassem M. Activin B mediated induction of Pdx1 in human embryonic stem cell derived embryoid bodies. Biochem Biophys Res Commun. 2007;362(3):568–74.
99. Hart A, Papadopoulou S, Edlund H. Fgf10 maintains notch activation, stimulates proliferation, and blocks differentiation of pancreatic epithelial cells. Dev Dyn. 2003;228(2):185–93.
100. Shiraki N, Lai CJ, Hishikari Y, Kume S. TGF-beta signaling potentiates differentiation of embryonic stem cells to Pdx-1 expressing endodermal cells. Genes Cells. 2005;10(6):503–16.
101. Sanvito F, Herrera PL, Huarte J, Nichols A, Montesano R, Orci L, et al. TGF-beta 1 influences the relative development of the exocrine and endocrine pancreas in vitro. Development. 1994;120(12):3451–62.
102. Rezania A, Bruin JE, Riedel MJ, Mojibian M, Asadi A, Xu J, et al. Maturation of human embryonic stem cell-derived pancreatic progenitors into functional islets capable of treating pre-existing diabetes in mice. Diabetes. 2012;61(8):2016–29.
103. Gradwohl G, Dierich A, LeMeur M, Guillemot F. Neurogenin3 is required for the development of the four endocrine cell lineages of the pancreas. Proc Natl Acad Sci U S A. 2000;97 (4):1607–11.

104. Gu G, Dubauskaite J, Melton DA. Direct evidence for the pancreatic lineage: NGN3+ cells are islet progenitors and are distinct from duct progenitors. Development. 2002;129 (10):2447–57.
105. Apelqvist A, Li H, Sommer L, Beatus P, Anderson DJ, Honjo T, et al. Notch signalling controls pancreatic cell differentiation. Nature. 1999;400(6747):877–81.
106. Jensen J, Pedersen EE, Galante P, Hald J, Heller RS, Ishibashi M, et al. Control of endodermal endocrine development by Hes-1. Nat Genet. 2000;24(1):36–44.
107. Hald J, Hjorth JP, German MS, Madsen OD, Serup P, Jensen J. Activated notch1 prevents differentiation of pancreatic acinar cells and attenuate endocrine development. Dev Biol. 2003;260(2):426–37.
108. Murtaugh LC, Stanger BZ, Kwan KM, Melton DA. Notch signaling controls multiple steps of pancreatic differentiation. Proc Natl Acad Sci U S A. 2003;100(25):14920–5.
109. Lee JC, Smith SB, Watada H, Lin J, Scheel D, Wang J, et al. Regulation of the pancreatic pro-endocrine gene neurogenin3. Diabetes. 2001;50(5):928–36.
110. Shih HP, Kopp JL, Sandhu M, Dubois CL, Seymour PA, Grapin-Botton A, et al. A notch-dependent molecular circuitry initiates pancreatic endocrine and ductal cell differentiation. Development. 2012;139(14):2488–99.
111. Zhu FF, Zhang PB, Zhang DH, Sui X, Yin M, Xiang TT, et al. Generation of pancreatic insulin-producing cells from rhesus monkey induced pluripotent stem cells. Diabetologia. 2011;54(9):2325–36.
112. Sakano D, Shiraki N, Kikawa K, Yamazoe T, Kataoka M, Umeda K, et al. VMAT2 identified as a regulator of late-stage beta-cell differentiation. Nat Chem Biol. 2013;10(2):141–8.
113. Gage BK, Webber TD, Kieffer TJ. Initial cell seeding density influences pancreatic endocrine development during in vitro differentiation of human embryonic stem cells. PLoS One. 2013;8(12):e82076.
114. Kubo A, Stull R, Takeuchi M, Bonham K, Gouon-Evans V, Sho M, et al. Pdx1 and Ngn3 overexpression enhances pancreatic differentiation of mouse ES cell-derived endoderm population. PLoS One. 2011;6(9):e24058.
115. Nelson SB, Schaffer AE, Sander M. The transcription factors Nkx6.1 and Nkx6.2 possess equivalent activities in promoting beta-cell fate specification in Pdx1+ pancreatic progenitor cells. Development. 2007;134(13):2491–500.
116. Rezania A, Bruin JE, Xu J, Narayan K, Fox JK, O'Neil JJ, et al. Enrichment of human embryonic stem cell-derived NKX6.1-expressing pancreatic progenitor cells accelerates the maturation of insulin-secreting cells in vivo. Stem Cells. 2013;31(11):2432–42.
117. Taylor BL, Liu FF, Sander M. Nkx6.1 is essential for maintaining the functional state of pancreatic beta cells. Cell Rep. 2013;4(6):1262–75.
118. Nostro MC, Sarangi F, Yang C, Holland A, Elefanty AG, Stanley EG, et al. Efficient generation of NKX6-1+ pancreatic progenitors from multiple human pluripotent stem cell lines. Stem Cell Reports. 2015;4(4):591–604.
119. Tessem JS, Moss LG, Chao LC, Arlotto M, Lu D, Jensen MV, et al. Nkx6.1 regulates islet beta-cell proliferation via Nr4a1 and Nr4a3 nuclear receptors. Proc Natl Acad Sci U S A. 2014;111(14):5242–7.
120. Guo S, Dai C, Guo M, Taylor B, Harmon JS, Sander M, et al. Inactivation of specific beta cell transcription factors in type 2 diabetes. J Clin Invest. 2013;123(8):3305–16.
121. Kwon YD, Oh SK, Kim HS, Ku SY, Kim SH, Choi YM, et al. Cellular manipulation of human embryonic stem cells by TAT-PDX1 protein transduction. Mol Ther. 2005;12 (1):28–32.
122. Soria B, Roche E, Berna G, Leon-Quinto T, Reig JA, Martin F. Insulin-secreting cells derived from embryonic stem cells normalize glycemia in streptozotocin-induced diabetic mice. Diabetes. 2000;49(2):157–62.
123. St-Onge L, Sosa-Pineda B, Chowdhury K, Mansouri A, Gruss P. Pax6 is required for differentiation of glucagon-producing alpha-cells in mouse pancreas. Nature. 1997;387 (6631):406–9.

124. Greenwood AL, Li S, Jones K, Melton DA. Notch signaling reveals developmental plasticity of Pax4(+) pancreatic endocrine progenitors and shunts them to a duct fate. Mech Dev. 2007;124(2):97–107.
125. Sosa-Pineda B, Chowdhury K, Torres M, Oliver G, Gruss P. The Pax4 gene is essential for differentiation of insulin-producing beta cells in the mammalian pancreas. Nature. 1997;386 (6623):399–402.
126. Wang J, Elghazi L, Parker SE, Kizilocak H, Asano M, Sussel L, et al. The concerted activities of Pax4 and Nkx2.2 are essential to initiate pancreatic beta-cell differentiation. Dev Biol. 2004;266(1):178–89.
127. Collombat P, Hecksher-Sorensen J, Broccoli V, Krull J, Ponte I, Mundiger T, et al. The simultaneous loss of Arx and Pax4 genes promotes a somatostatin-producing cell fate specification at the expense of the alpha- and beta-cell lineages in the mouse endocrine pancreas. Development. 2005;132(13):2969–80.
128. Collombat P, Mansouri A, Hecksher-Sorensen J, Serup P, Krull J, Gradwohl G, et al. Opposing actions of Arx and Pax4 in endocrine pancreas development. Genes Dev. 2003;17(20):2591–603.
129. Gage BK, Baker RK, Kieffer TJ. Overexpression of PAX4 reduces glucagon expression in differentiating hESCs. Islets. 2014;6(2):e29236.
130. Liew CG, Shah NN, Briston SJ, Shepherd RM, Khoo CP, Dunne MJ, et al. PAX4 enhances beta-cell differentiation of human embryonic stem cells. PLoS One. 2008;3(3):e1783.
131. Lavon N, Yanuka O, Benvenisty N. The effect of overexpression of Pdx1 and Foxa2 on the differentiation of human embryonic stem cells into pancreatic cells. Stem Cells. 2006;24 (8):1923–30.
132. Gong ZC, Huang Q, Dai XP, Lei GH, Lu HB, Yin JY, et al. NeuroD1 A45T and PAX4 R121W polymorphisms are associated with plasma glucose level of repaglinide monotherapy in Chinese patients with type 2 diabetes. Br J Clin Pharmacol. 2012;74(3):501–9.
133. Jo W, Endo M, Ishizu K, Nakamura A, Tajima T. A novel PAX4 mutation in a Japanese patient with maturity-onset diabetes of the young. Tohoku J Exp Med. 2011;223(2):113–8.
134. Plengvidhya N, Kooptiwut S, Songtawee N, Doi A, Furuta H, Nishi M, et al. PAX4 mutations in Thais with maturity onset diabetes of the young. J Clin Endocrinol Metab. 2007;92 (7):2821–6.
135. Tokuyama Y, Matsui K, Ishizuka T, Egashira T, Kanatsuka A. The Arg121Trp variant in PAX4 gene is associated with beta-cell dysfunction in Japanese subjects with type 2 diabetes mellitus. Metabolism. 2006;55(2):213–6.
136. Zhang Y, Xiao XH, Wang H, Wang T, Sun Q, Yang GH, et al. Association between A1168C polymorphism in PAX4 gene and type 1 diabetes in Han Chinese. Zhongguo Yi Xue Ke Xue Yuan Xue Bao. 2007;29(3):370–3.
137. Brun T, Gauthier BR. A focus on the role of Pax4 in mature pancreatic islet beta-cell expansion and survival in health and disease. J Mol Endocrinol. 2008;40(2):37–45.
138. Hu He KH, Lorenzo PI, Brun T, Jimenez Moreno CM, Aeberhard D, Vallejo Ortega J, et al. In vivo conditional Pax4 overexpression in mature islet beta-cells prevents stress-induced hyperglycemia in mice. Diabetes. 2011;60(6):1705–15.
139. Lorenzo PI, Fuente-Martin E, Brun T, Cobo-Vuilleumier N, Jimenez-Moreno CM, G Herrera Gomez I, et al. PAX4 defines an expandable beta-cell subpopulation in the adult pancreatic islet. Sci Rep. 2015;5:15672.
140. Ohmine S, Squillace KA, Hartjes KA, Deeds MC, Armstrong AS, Thatava T, et al. Reprogrammed keratinocytes from elderly type 2 diabetes patients suppress senescence genes to acquire induced pluripotency. Aging. 2012;4(1):60–73.
141. Kelly OG, Chan MY, Martinson LA, Kadoya K, Ostertag TM, Ross KG, et al. Cell-surface markers for the isolation of pancreatic cell types derived from human embryonic stem cells. Nat Biotechnol. 2011;29(8):750–6.

142. Cai J, Yu C, Liu Y, Chen S, Guo Y, Yong J, et al. Generation of homogeneous PDX1(+) pancreatic progenitors from human ES cell-derived endoderm cells. J Mol Cell Biol. 2010;2 (1):50–60.
143. Teo AK, Wagers AJ, Kulkarni RN. New opportunities: harnessing induced pluripotency for discovery in diabetes and metabolism. Cell Metab. 2013;18(6):775–91.
144. Rezania A, Bruin JE, Arora P, Rubin A, Batushansky I, Asadi A, et al. Reversal of diabetes with insulin-producing cells derived in vitro from human pluripotent stem cells. Nat Biotechnol. 2014;32(11):1121–33.
145. Russ HA, Parent AV, Ringler JJ, Hennings TG, Nair GG, Shveygert M, et al. Controlled induction of human pancreatic progenitors produces functional beta-like cells in vitro. EMBO J. 2015;34(13):1759–72.
146. Hrvatin S, O'Donnell CW, Deng F, Millman JR, Pagliuca FW, DiIorio P, et al. Differentiated human stem cells resemble fetal, not adult, beta cells. Proc Natl Acad Sci U S A. 2014;111 (8):3038–43.
147. Blum B, Hrvatin SS, Schuetz C, Bonal C, Rezania A, Melton DA. Functional beta-cell maturation is marked by an increased glucose threshold and by expression of urocortin 3. Nat Biotechnol. 2012;30(3):261–4.
148. Jermendy A, Toschi E, Aye T, Koh A, Aguayo-Mazzucato C, Sharma A, et al. Rat neonatal beta cells lack the specialised metabolic phenotype of mature beta cells. Diabetologia. 2011;54(3):594–604.
149. Bruin JE, Rezania A, Xu J, Narayan K, Fox JK, O'Neil JJ, et al. Maturation and function of human embryonic stem cell-derived pancreatic progenitors in macroencapsulation devices following transplant into mice. Diabetologia. 2013;56(9):1987–98.
150. Alipio Z, Liao W, Roemer EJ, Waner M, Fink LM, Ward DC, et al. Reversal of hyperglycemia in diabetic mouse models using induced-pluripotent stem (iPS)-derived pancreatic beta-like cells. Proc Natl Acad Sci U S A. 2010;107(30):13426–31.
151. Jeon K, Lim H, Kim JH, Thuan NV, Park SH, Lim YM, et al. Differentiation and transplantation of functional pancreatic beta cells generated from induced pluripotent stem cells derived from a type 1 diabetes mouse model. Stem Cells Dev. 2012;21(14):2642–55.
152. Rezania A, Riedel MJ, Wideman RD, Karanu F, Ao Z, Warnock GL, et al. Production of functional glucagon-secreting alpha-cells from human embryonic stem cells. Diabetes. 2011;60(1):239–47.
153. Basford CL, Prentice KJ, Hardy AB, Sarangi F, Micallef SJ, Li X, et al. The functional and molecular characterisation of human embryonic stem cell-derived insulin-positive cells compared with adult pancreatic beta cells. Diabetologia. 2012;55(2):358–71.
154. Xie R, Everett LJ, Lim HW, Patel NA, Schug J, Kroon E, et al. Dynamic chromatin remodeling mediated by polycomb proteins orchestrates pancreatic differentiation of human embryonic stem cells. Cell Stem Cell. 2013;12(2):224–37.
155. Artner I, Blanchi B, Raum JC, Guo M, Kaneko T, Cordes S, et al. MafB is required for islet beta cell maturation. Proc Natl Acad Sci U S A. 2007;104(10):3853–8.
156. Nishimura W, Kondo T, Salameh T, El Khattabi I, Dodge R, Bonner-Weir S, et al. A switch from MafB to MafA expression accompanies differentiation to pancreatic beta-cells. Dev Biol. 2006;293(2):526–39.
157. Artner I, Hang Y, Mazur M, Yamamoto T, Guo M, Lindner J, et al. MafA and MafB regulate genes critical to beta-cells in a unique temporal manner. Diabetes. 2010;59(10):2530–9.
158. Gu C, Stein GH, Pan N, Goebbels S, Hornberg H, Nave KA, et al. Pancreatic beta cells require NeuroD to achieve and maintain functional maturity. Cell Metab. 2010;11 (4):298–310.
159. Aguayo-Mazzucato C, Zavacki AM, Marinelarena A, Hollister-Lock J, El Khattabi I, Marsili A, et al. Thyroid hormone promotes postnatal rat pancreatic beta-cell development and glucose-responsive insulin secretion through MAFA. Diabetes. 2013;62(5):1569–80.

160. Blum B, Roose AN, Barrandon O, Maehr R, Arvanites AC, Davidow LS, et al. Reversal of beta cell de-differentiation by a small molecule inhibitor of the TGFbeta pathway. Elife. 2014;3:e02809.
161. Schaffer AE, Taylor BL, Benthuysen JR, Liu J, Thorel F, Yuan W, et al. Nkx6.1 controls a gene regulatory network required for establishing and maintaining pancreatic beta cell identity. PLoS Genet. 2013;9(1):e1003274.
162. Li C, Chen P, Vaughan J, Lee KF, Vale W. Urocortin 3 regulates glucose-stimulated insulin secretion and energy homeostasis. Proc Natl Acad Sci U S A. 2007;104(10):4206–11.
163. Yamada M, Johannesson B, Sagi I, Burnett LC, Kort DH, Prosser RW, et al. Human oocytes reprogram adult somatic nuclei of a type 1 diabetic to diploid pluripotent stem cells. Nature. 2014;510(7506):533–6.
164. Abdelalim EM, Bonnefond A, Bennaceur-Griscelli A, Froguel P. Pluripotent stem cells as a potential tool for disease modelling and cell therapy in diabetes. Stem Cell Rev. 2014;10 (3):327–37.
165. Teo AK, Windmueller R, Johansson BB, Dirice E, Njolstad PR, Tjora E, et al. Derivation of human induced pluripotent stem cells from patients with maturity onset diabetes of the young. J Biol Chem. 2013;288(8):5353–6.
166. Kudva YC, Ohmine S, Greder LV, Dutton JR, Armstrong A, De Lamo JG, et al. Transgene-free disease-specific induced pluripotent stem cells from patients with type 1 and type 2 diabetes. Stem Cells Transl Med. 2012;1(6):451–61.
167. Yabe SG, Iwasaki N, Yasuda K, Hamazaki TS, Konno M, Fukuda S, et al. Establishment of maturity-onset diabetes of the young-induced pluripotent stem cells from a Japanese patient. J Diabetes Investig. 2015;6(5):543–7.
168. Bhatt S, Gupta MK, Khamaisi M, Martinez R, Gritsenko MA, Wagner BK, et al. Preserved DNA damage checkpoint pathway protects against complications in long-standing type 1 diabetes. Cell Metab. 2015;22(2):239–52.
169. Iovino S, Burkart AM, Kriauciunas K, Warren L, Hughes KJ, Molla M, et al. Genetic insulin resistance is a potent regulator of gene expression and proliferation in human iPS cells. Diabetes. 2014;63(12):4130–42.
170. Shang L, Hua H, Foo K, Martinez H, Watanabe K, Zimmer M, et al. Beta-cell dysfunction due to increased ER stress in a stem cell model of Wolfram syndrome. Diabetes. 2014;63 (3):923–33.
171. Hanna J, Markoulaki S, Mitalipova M, Cheng AW, Cassady JP, Staerk J, et al. Metastable pluripotent states in NOD-mouse-derived ESCs. Cell Stem Cell. 2009;4(6):513–24.
172. Okita K, Ichisaka T, Yamanaka S. Generation of germline-competent induced pluripotent stem cells. Nature. 2007;448(7151):313–7.
173. Stadtfeld M, Nagaya M, Utikal J, Weir G, Hochedlinger K. Induced pluripotent stem cells generated without viral integration. Science. 2008;322(5903):945–9.
174. Okita K, Nakagawa M, Hyenjong H, Ichisaka T, Yamanaka S. Generation of mouse induced pluripotent stem cells without viral vectors. Science. 2008;322(5903):949–53.
175. Soldner F, Hockemeyer D, Beard C, Gao Q, Bell GW, Cook EG, et al. Parkinson's disease patient-derived induced pluripotent stem cells free of viral reprogramming factors. Cell. 2009;136(5):964–77.
176. Kaji K, Norrby K, Paca A, Mileikovsky M, Mohseni P, Woltjen K. Virus-free induction of pluripotency and subsequent excision of reprogramming factors. Nature. 2009;458 (7239):771–5.
177. Woltjen K, Michael IP, Mohseni P, Desai R, Mileikovsky M, Hamalainen R, et al. piggyBac transposition reprograms fibroblasts to induced pluripotent stem cells. Nature. 2009;458 (7239):766–70.
178. Zhou H, Wu S, Joo JY, Zhu S, Han DW, Lin T, et al. Generation of induced pluripotent stem cells using recombinant proteins. Cell Stem Cell. 2009;4(5):381–4.

179. Kim D, Kim CH, Moon JI, Chung YG, Chang MY, Han BS, et al. Generation of human induced pluripotent stem cells by direct delivery of reprogramming proteins. Cell Stem Cell. 2009;4(6):472–6.
180. Kirk K, Hao E, Lahmy R, Itkin-Ansari P. Human embryonic stem cell derived islet progenitors mature inside an encapsulation device without evidence of increased biomass or cell escape. Stem Cell Res. 2014;12(3):807–14.
181. Yamanaka S. Strategies and new developments in the generation of patient-specific pluripotent stem cells. Cell Stem Cell. 2007;1(1):39–49.
182. Knoepfler PS. Why myc? An unexpected ingredient in the stem cell cocktail. Cell Stem Cell. 2008;2(1):18–21.
183. Nakagawa M, Koyanagi M, Tanabe K, Takahashi K, Ichisaka T, Aoi T, et al. Generation of induced pluripotent stem cells without Myc from mouse and human fibroblasts. Nat Biotechnol. 2008;26(1):101–6.
184. Wernig M, Meissner A, Cassady JP, Jaenisch R. c-Myc is dispensable for direct reprogramming of mouse fibroblasts. Cell Stem Cell. 2008;2(1):10–2.
185. Yakhnenko I, Wong WK, Katkov II, Itkin-Ansari P. Cryopreservation of human insulin expressing cells macro-encapsulated in a durable therapeutic immunoisolating device theracyte. Cryo Letters. 2012;33(6):518–31.
186. Tachibana M, Amato P, Sparman M, Gutierrez NM, Tippner-Hedges R, Ma H, et al. Human embryonic stem cells derived by somatic cell nuclear transfer. Cell. 2013;153(6):1228–38.
187. Servitja JM, Ferrer J. Transcriptional networks controlling pancreatic development and beta cell function. Diabetologia. 2004;47(4):597–613.
188. Riggs AC, Bernal-Mizrachi E, Ohsugi M, Wasson J, Fatrai S, Welling C, et al. Mice conditionally lacking the Wolfram gene in pancreatic islet beta cells exhibit diabetes as a result of enhanced endoplasmic reticulum stress and apoptosis. Diabetologia. 2005;48 (11):2313–21.

Chapter 7
Clinical Applications of Induced Pluripotent Stem Cells in Cancer

Teresa de Souza Fernandez, André Luiz Mencalha, and Cecília de Souza Fernandez

7.1 Introduction

Cancer pathogenesis has been studied through different approaches, as animal models and cell cultures, using mainly cell lines. Much of our understanding of cancer cell biology, including the aspects of gene regulation and signaling pathways, has come from studies of cancer cells in culture. But, theoretically, the best model to study cancer is the primary patient samples, although the amount of obtained cells may be inadequate for various analyses [1–3]. Despite some studies initiated a research in genomic analyses in a single-cell of cancer trying to define the clonal architecture of tumors [4, 5], the discovery of the human induced pluripotent stem cells, hiPSCs, opens a new perspective to study the biology of different diseases, including cancer [2, 3, 6].

It is very important to study the pathogenesis of cancer because this disease is a major cause of mortality through the world. Cancer evolves by a process of clonal expansion, genetic diversification, and clonal selection. The dynamics are complex and with highly variable patterns of genetic diversity and resultant clonal architecture [7]. Cancer cells have diverse biological capabilities that are conferred by

T. de Souza Fernandez, Ph.D. (✉)
Laboratory Division, National Cancer Institute (INCA), Bone Marrow Transplantation Center (CEMO), Praça Cruz Vermelha 23, 6° andar, 20230-130 Rio de Janeiro, RJ, Brazil
e-mail: teresafernandez@inca.gov.br

A.L. Mencalha, Ph.D.
Laboratory of Cancer Biology (LABICAN), State University of Rio de Janeiro (UERJ), Roberto Alcantara Gomes Biology Institute (IBRAG), 20551-030 Rio de Janeiro, RJ, Brazil
e-mail: andre.mencalha@uerj.br

C. de Souza Fernandez, Ph.D.
Institute of Mathematics and Statistics, Federal Fluminense University (UFF), 24020-140 Niterói, RJ, Brazil
e-mail: gancsfz@vm.uff.br

E.M. Abdelalim (ed.), *Recent Advances in Stem Cells*, Stem Cell Biology and Regenerative Medicine, DOI 10.1007/978-3-319-33270-3_7

numerous genetic and epigenetic modifications [1]. Classical cancer therapies, as surgery, radiotherapy and chemotherapy, are the first therapeutic choice against cancer for many patients [8]. However, many challenges have been emerged to cancer treatment. For the development of new molecular target therapies, several studies have been done with the aim of identifying biomarkers involved in cancer. High-throughput platforms have been used for the genomic, transcriptomic, proteomic and epigenomic analyses to search for new biomarkers involved in cancer and to bring new insights into the several aspects of cancer pathophysiology including angiogenesis, immune evasion, metastasis, altered cell growth, death and metabolism [1, 9–14]. However many studies are still necessary to better understand the development and evolution of cancer, such as the molecular characterization of resistant cancer cells. The resistant cancer cells emerged in different kinds of tumors and research groups are studying these molecular mechanisms, especially in cancer stem cells (CSC) because of their dual role, as a tumor-initiating cell and as a source of treatment resistance cells [15–17].

The hiPSCs open new opportunities in biomedical sciences, since these cells may be useful for understanding the mechanisms of diseases. The hiPSCs are being used to make disease models, to develop new drugs and test toxicity and in regenerative medicine. Reprogramming technology offers the potential to treat many diseases, including neurodegenerative diseases, cardiovascular diseases and diabetes. In theory, easily accessible cell types (such as skin fibroblasts) could be obtained from a patient and reprogrammed, effectively recapitulating the patients' disease in a culture system. Therefore, such cells could serve as the basis for autologous cell replacement. Human iPSCs have the potential to become a platform for personalized medicine by allowing a patient's own cells to become a source of therapeutic tissue. However, depending on the methods used, reprogramming adult cells to obtain hiPSCs may pose significant risks that could limit their use in clinical practice. For example, if viruses are used to genomically alter the cells, the expression of cancer-causing genes, "oncogenes," may potentially be triggered [18]. Many different groups have successfully generated iPSCs, but due to different techniques, their methods of calculating efficiency of conversion are varied [19–21]. In this chapter, we show the recent advances in hiPSCs basic research and some potential clinical applications in cancer. We also present the importance in using statistical methods to evaluate the validation of the hiPSCs for future therapeutic use.

7.2 Discovery of Human Induced Pluripotent Stem Cells

In 2006, induced pluripotent stem cells (iPSCs) were first developed by the research group from Yamanaka's laboratory at Kyoto University, Japan. Initially, researchers have performed iPSCs derived from somatic mice cells, from where DNA vectors containing cloned embryonic expressed genes were transfected, by retroviral methodology [22]. These genes encoded transcription factors (TFs) expressed in undifferentiated embryonic inner cell mass (ICM). Since these genes are expressed in undifferentiated cells, being able to differentiate into any adult tissue, their forced expression could promote cellular pluripotency capacity. The TF-reprogramming genes, *Oct-4*, *Sox2*, *Klf4*, and *c-Myc*, were used for iPSC establishment and induced pluripotency phenotype of adult somatic cell to undifferentiated cell [22]. The transcriptional factor Oct-4, encoded by *POUF5F1* gene, is temporal-spatially expressed in ICM and is promptly downregulated in gastrulation stage. Oct-4 is essential for preserving the pluripotent state of embryonic cells [23]. Sox-2 is a transcriptional factor, which belongs to the high mobility group (HMG) superfamily, responsible for regulating genes involved with maintenance of undifferentiated phenotype of ICM. Sox-2 interacts with Oct-4. Both of them work on DNA binding sites and regulate the expression of a dozen of genes involved in embryonic cells differentiation [24]. KLF4 (*Kruppel-Like Factor 4*) acts as transcription factor controlling expression of genes during embryonic development that play an important role in maintaining pluripotent-state of embryonic stem cells [25]. *c-Myc* gene was discovered in aggressive chicken tumors and was identified as one of the first gene described as oncogene function [26, 27]. In embryonic development, c-Myc works as transcriptional factor involved in maintenance of undifferentiated phenotype. In 2007, human iPSCs were first generated by the same group (group from Yamanaka's laboratory) by transducing adult human dermal fibroblasts with viral vectors carrying the key pluripotency genes, *Oct3/4*, *Sox2*, *Klf4*, and *c-Myc* (Yamanaka factors), using a retroviral system [28].

In 2007, Thomson's group at the University of Wisconsin-Madison, EUA, also generated human iPSCs. They used the factors *Oct4*, *Sox2*, *Nanog*, and *LIN28* and a lentiviral system to reprogram human somatic cells to pluripotent stem cells that exhibit the essential characteristics of embryonic stem cells (ESCs) [29]. The ESCs are pluripotent cells derived from the inner cell mass of the preimplantation blastocyst. These cells are potential renewable sources of all human tissues for regenerative medicine and, for this reason, it is very valuable to understand the early events of human development, for gene therapy and for new drug discovery. However, the usage of ESCs is a highly controversial issue on moral, social and ethical grounds. This is because the process involves the destruction of a blastocyst, which is considered a human embryo with the potential of developing into a person. The research using the ESCs is prohibited in some countries, while in other countries the research using the ESCs is allowed under legislation, but remains tightly restricted [20]. So, the research using hiPSCs, which are derived from human somatic cells, does not present the ethical dilemmas as the research using the ESCs.

The hiPSCs technology represents an important platform with the potential to advance in medical therapy by personalizing regenerative medicine and by creating new human disease models for research and therapeutic tests. The discovery that adult somatic stem cells can be reprogrammed into pluripotent cells is so important that, in 2012, Dr. Yamanaka was awarded with the Nobel Prize in Physiology or Medicine [22, 28, 30].

7.2.1 Methods Used to Generate hiPSCs

In the experiment of Dr. Yamanaka, it was cloned and promoted the ectopic expression of "embryonic factors" in the differentiated human cells. Initially, 24 genes were analyzed and selected. Among these genes, there were genes involved in the maintenance of pluripotency like *Oct3/4*, *Nanog*, and *Sox2*; there were genes overexpressed in the tumors related with fast proliferation and maintenance of undifferentiated stage like *STAT-3*, *Ras*, *c-Myc*, *Klf4*, and *Beta-catenin* and genes expressed in the early stages of development such as *FGF4*, *Zfp296*, *Utf1*, and others. For the expression of these genes, they were selectively amplified from cDNA template by PCR, cloned into plasmid and in vitro introduced in fibroblast cells through retroviral transduction. After infections and confirmation of expression of the introduced genes, the fibroblast cells were analyzed to observe cell phenotype. Dr. Yamanaka performed a series of evaluations in a single or combined gene to verify which ones were essential or able to induce alterations in the differentiated fibroblast cell morphology, growth, and gene expression profile similar to ESCs. Among the initial genes studied, only the *Oct3/4*, *Sox2*, *c-Myc*, and *Klf4* appeared to be important, generating the iPSCs. This study established a new concept in the science scenario: the in vitro induced pluripotent stem cells [28].

Basically, the methodology used to generate hiPSCs implies in the specific gene amplification by PCR, insertion of this product in a DNA vector and introduction of this cloned gene in the host cell. The foreign DNA vector can be inserted in the receptor by several different ways, like the viral transduction. The method using viral transduction has efficiency to introduce the DNA vector inside cell and successful to integrate the cloned in the host cell's genome and this is the main advantage of viral method. The DNA vector viral integrates in host genome cell particularly due to long terminal repeats (LTR) present in the both extremities of virus genome. These LTRs are compound by hundreds of nucleotides repetitions that, by recombination, attach the DNA inner contained in genomes [31].

Many approaches have used viral particles carrying DNA constructions that can be integrated in the genome's cell randomly. In fact, it is the main counterpart of iPSCs utilization. Therefore, reprogramming by cloning with the usage of viral strategies and long-term culture can also induce abnormalities in these pluripotent cells. In some in vitro cultures, iPSCs have demonstrated genomic instability. Unlike other stem cell cultures, the genomic instability is more common in early passages [32]. It is believed that this phenomenon is due to genetic reprogramming [32, 33]. This enhanced genomic instability in iPSCs can involve p53 protein inactivation, which is important to proliferation and DNA repair machinery activation in response to DNA damage [34].

Additionally, the viral DNA that carries cloned gene of interest can integrate in any *loci* in genome host cells. This implies many consequences, such as: (1) integration into DNA sequence that encodes essential gene, disrupting its function which can cause loss of cell viability; (2) disrupt regions that coordinate expression of important genes, like promoter or enhancers regions, mainly if these genes contain "tumor suppression functions"; and (3) the viral DNA may integrate in DNA regions that are responsible for negative regulation of "oncogenes," allowing their constitutive expressions [35, 36]. Chromosomal instability, mutational possibilities and use of known oncogenes to produce iPSCs have implicated in high incidence of cancer development in preclinical tests [37]. These observations have increased the discussion about the possibility of the usage of iPSCs in cellular therapies.

Another point is that stimulation of loss of differentiation state to generate iPSCs also involves epigenetics reprogramming process and differential expression of noncoding functional RNA (ncRNA). Expressed ncRNA represents approximately 1 % of mRNA in human [38]. A recent study discovered that there are more miRNA upregulated in the iPSCs than in the ESCs. These miRNAs have been frequently found related in the cancer development [39]. Noncoding RNA (ncRNA) is a group of untranslated RNA related to posttranscriptional gene expression control. ncRNAs are represented mostly by the microRNAs (miRNA) and long noncoding RNA (lncRNA). Long noncoding RNA (lncRNA) is a class of functional ncRNA longer than 200 nucleotides that harbor many possibilities to act. LncRNA can regulate gene expression by interacting with transcriptional machinery, with transcriptional factors, controlling spliceosomes, and interfering in translational process [40]. As lncRNA is a recent discovery, data about lncRNA and iPSC remain restricted to *Xist*, an lncRNA involved with X chromosome inactivation. A recent study has suggested that X chromosome is reactivated in reprogramming cells. This process involves *Txist*, also lncRNA acts as *Xist* anti-sense and for transcriptional activation of factor PRDM14. *Txist* and PRDM14 are directly involved in X chromosome reactivation in iPSC, repressing *Xist* and recruiting chromatin regulator proteins, such as Polycomb Complex, respectively [41]. A study performed in mouse showed that iPSC exhibited different epigenetic and ncRNA profiles when compared to ESC. These data reinforce a deeper iPSC molecular analysis to better understanding these cells phenotype before clinical application [42].

Most strategies currently under use to generate iPSCs are based on gene delivery via retroviral or lentiviral vectors. Adenovirus and transposable DNA elements had alternatively been used in place of retrovirus and lentivirus. However, most experiments involved integration in the host cell genome with an identified risk for insertional mutagenesis and oncogenic transformation. To avoid such risks, which are incompatible with therapeutic prospects, significant progress has been made with transgene-free reprogramming methods based, for example, on Sendai virus (SeV) direct mRNA or protein delivery to achieve conversion of adult cells into hiPSCs [43].

Alternatively, specific class of transposons, minicircle DNA vectors, or episomal systems have been established for iPSC development. PiggyBac (PB) and Slepping Beauty (SP) are methodological strategies based on transposable DNA elements [44]. Natural transposable elements are functional DNA segments evolutionarily conserved along various organisms, including human [45]. Tol2, a zebrafish transposable element, has also emerged to transducing gene in human cells [46]. Although it is an integrating-DNA method, the transposon/transposase system is transient. They carry desired DNA allowing insertion and excision from genomic DNA. This system requires an inverted DNA terminal repeats flanking a TF-reprogramming genes. PB and SB had been applied as cell therapy and DNA vaccine in many diseases, including cancer [45]. For while, few studies had focused in using transposable DNA elements to generate human iPSC. A recent study using transposable DNA elements to carrier *c-Myc*, *Klf4*, *Oct4*, and *Sox2* genes showed that the individual gene PB insertions can be detached from DNA's established iPSCs [47]. This find allows including transposable DNA elements as a valuable tool for iPSC development, where these elements can replace the use of virus. However, there are few data about transposons in iPSC and these DNA elements still been included in a class of potential insertional mutagenesis inducers.

The expression of transposable elements can be controlled, for instance expression of transposable elements can be dependent of doxycycline in cell medium [48], or could have many possibilities for controlling its expression and its picturing by chimeric gene-reporter fusion in transfected genes [49]. Thus, PB and SB can have their transcriptional activity time and dose-dependent fine controlled. In a study realized by Cadiñanos and Bradley, it was demonstrated effective TF-reprogramming genes expression in mouse and human embryonic fibroblasts using doxycycline-inducible delivered by PB transposition [48].

The use of minicircle and episomal DNA has been assayed as a strategy to replace host genome integrating methods to generate iPSC. Minicircles and episomal DNA, known as plasmids, are circular DNA and they are obtained from prokaryotes. Initially, minicircles and episomal DNA were considered distinct molecular structure, the first one had a non-self-replicative ability and second was replicative DNA circular. However, molecular strategies provided self-replication capacity to minicircle DNA [50]. These DNA molecules work as vectors where, by DNA recombinant technology, a gene of interest can be cloned. These DNA constructions are easily transfected inside target cell by lipofectamine or electroporation methods. Once inside, these DNA constructions express the cloned gene, for hiPSC episomal TF-reprogramming genes trigger expression profile gene that induce the undifferentiated cell phenotype [51].

Together with TF-reprogramming factors, some additional gene transfection had shown improvement in the iPSC establishment. For instance, combinatory transfection of TF-reprogramming genes and human telomerase gene, *hTERT*, had improved iPSC efficiency and maintenance [52].

So, several improvements in the gene transduction method for making safe iPSCs have been done. Because of an intense discussion about the use of hiPSCs in cellular therapies, many works, trying to establish *in vitro* stem cells derived from a variety of sources, have emerged. For example, bone marrow-derived hematopoietic stem cells and multipotent mesenchymal stromal cells derived from bone marrow, umbilical cord blood, and adipose tissue. The ideal source of the cell to be isolated from the patients and used for reprogramming must have easy accessibility. This means it is not necessary to have surgery to get the cells. It is possible to obtain them from a skin biopsy, for example, with minimal risk procedures, availability in large quantities, relatively high reprogramming efficiency, and fast iPSCs derivation speed [43]. Thus, beyond new sources to obtain stem cell had emerged, new strategies to induce cell reprogramming without the use of viral particles have been used aiming safety and efficiency to generate hiPSCs with the purpose of their use in clinical practice [53–58].

Now, basic research should be focused to characterize the hiPSCs at cytogenetic and molecular levels to observe if these cells retain the genetic stability. It is necessary to understand how the cellular reprogramming works at molecular level, generating new knowledge in cell signaling pathways, comparing the different cell sources and the different methods used to generate the hiPSCs with the basic requirements of high quality and safety for their use in patients [18].

7.3 Potential Clinical Applications of hiPSCs in Cancer

Cancer is a complex disease, characterized by genetic and epigenetic alterations. Additionally, cancer complexity also includes distinct cellular proliferation and survival signaling pathways, which are triggered by different stimulus from intra or extracellular microenvironment. It is well characterized that over a period of time many tumors become more aggressive and acquire malignant potential. There is an orderly evolution from preneoplastic lesions to benign tumors and, ultimately, invasive cancer. This phenomenon is referred to as tumor progression. It occurs in a multistep process (Fig. 7.1). At molecular level, tumor progression and associated heterogeneity result from multiple mutations that accumulate independently in different cells, thus generating subclones with different characteristics. Mutations can be divided into two broad classes: those whose products "drive" tumorigenesis in a dominant fashion and "passengers" with no obvious role in the tumor causation [59, 60].

Many researchers are trying to identify biomarkers involved in tumor initiation as well as the steps involved during the evolution of disease. The main purpose in using biomarkers is the development of new drugs for cancer therapy. Biological markers (biomarkers) have been defined as "cellular, biochemical, or molecular alterations that are measurable in biological media such as human tissues, cells, or fluids" [61]. Furthermore, the identification of biomarkers can be used for early diagnosis and for therapeutic stratification groups aiding the medical staff to choose the appropriate treatment for the patient [1, 62].

Theoretically, the best model to study cancer pathogenesis is the primary patient samples, but the amount of obtained cells may be inadequate for various analyses. Recently, it has been reported that iPSCs can be generated not only from normal tissue cells but also from malignant cells [3, 63–65]. So, the hiPSCs are important to study the multiple stages of oncogenesis, from the initial cellular transformation to the hierarchical organization of established malignancies providing a human cell model to study the stages of disease [66, 67].

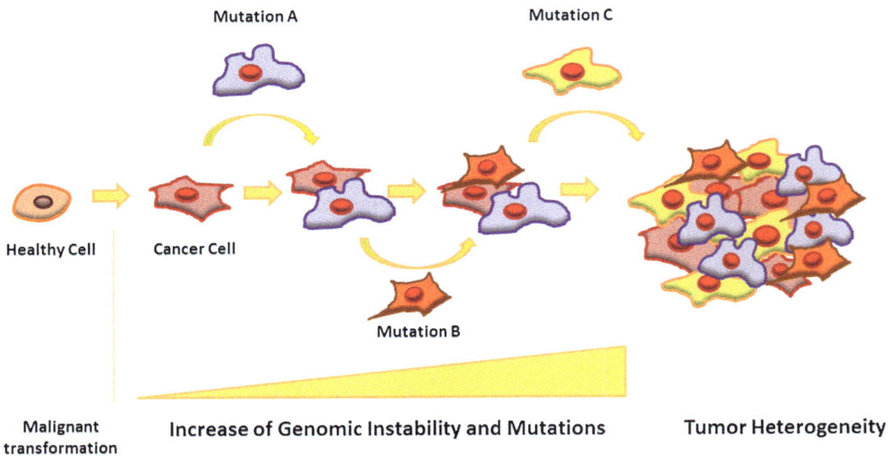

Fig. 7.1 Clonal evolution of cancer and its heterogeneity

7.3.1 Use of iPSCs for Cancer Modeling

The generation of iPSCs from human somatic cells heralds a new era in disease modeling, allowing the development of patient-specific models. As previously mentioned, despite improvements in cancer treatment, the disease is still a major cause of morbidity and mortality. The lack of a relevant model to study the development of cancer and its progression has limited research, which is suitable for translation to the clinical setting. Generation of iPSCs from human cancer cells represents an opportunity to develop in vitro models of carcinogenesis for specific cancer types [68].

Using patient-derived iPSCs to recapitulate the conditions of cancer differentiation could help identify significant molecular events responsible for disease initiation and progression directly in a susceptible cell type. Also, understanding the niche in which cancer develop will be crucial for recreating the cancer-initiating context and building a more physiologically relevant disease model. Therefore, iPSC cancer models have numerous potential clinical applications, including the identification of early biomarkers to stage disease progression and better risk groups stratification of patients [69].

In this sense, there are some examples. Kim et al. [66] used the hiPSCs as a model to study the pancreatic ductal adenocarcinoma (PDAC). This cancer carries a dismal prognosis and lacks a human cell model of early disease progression. In this study, the authors made the following hypothesis: if human PADC cells were converted to pluripotency and then allowed to differentiate back into pancreatic tissue, they might undergo early stages of cancer [66]. So, the iPSCs technology provides a live human cell model of early pancreatic cancer and disease progression [18].

Another example for the potential clinical applications of hiPSCs in disease modeling for studying cancer is in hematological malignancies [18]. Primary samples of hematologic malignancy are usually difficult to be expanded in cultures. However, after they are reprogrammed to iPSCs, they can expand unlimitedly. The iPSCs technology has been used to study myeloproliferative diseases as chronic myeloid leukemia (CML) [3] and juvenile myelomonocytic leukemia (JMML) [70]. Many studies are being performed to elucidate the mechanisms of tyrosine kinase inhibitor (TKI) resistance in CML stem cells and to overcome the resistance in these patients. Kumano et al. [3] established the CML-iPSCs by Sendai virus system and confirmed the resistance of these cells to imatinib [3]. So, they developed a model to study the CML disease and the TKI resistance. Another example for the use of iPSCs is the JMML. JMML is an aggressive myeloproliferative neoplasm of young children initiated by mutations that deregulated cytokine receptor signaling. Children with this disease have a poor prognosis. Gandre-Babbe et al. [70] generated iPSCs from two JMML patients. In this study, the authors suggested the relevance of this method to explore the pathophysiology and treatment of JMML [70].

Chromosomal deletions associated with human diseases, such as cancer, are common, but it is complicate modeling these deletions in mice. Myelodysplastic syndrome (MDS) comprises a heterogeneous group of clonal bone marrow disorders characterized by varying degrees of cytopenias, morphological and functional abnormalities of hematopoietic cells and an increased risk of transformation into acute myeloid leukemia (AML). Loss of one copy of the long arm of chromosome 7 [del(7q)] or the entire chromosome 7 (−7) is a cytogenetic abnormality, frequently observed in pediatric MDS, well recognized as a biomarker of unfavorable prognosis [71, 72]. Kotini et al. [73] used the cellular reprogramming and genome engineering to functionally dissect the loss of chromosome 7q [del(7q)], a somatic cytogenetic abnormality present in MDS. They derived del(7q) and isogenic karyotypically normal induced pluripotent stem cells (iPSCs) from hematopoietic cells of MDS patients and showed that the del(7q) iPSCs recapitulate disease-associated phenotypes, including impaired hematopoietic differentiation. In this study, the authors highlight the utility of human iPSCs for functional mapping of disease-associated large-scale chromosomal deletions and for discovery of haploinsufficient genes [73].

Another example for the use of iPSCs in modeling cancer is in familial cancer. Li-Fraumeni Syndrome patient-derived iPSCs have been used revealing a role of mutant p53 in regulating the imprinted gene network whose dysregulation results in osteoblast differentiation defects and tumorigenesis. In this study, Lee et al. [74] demonstrated that the model system using iPSCs not only serves as an alternative tool to study p53 mutation-associated disorders, but also provides substantial benefits for studying the role of p53 in the early stages of tumor development [74].

Emerging developments of iPSCs, research can be used as a tool in modeling hematopoietic disorders and could lead to new clinical applications in gene and cell therapies. The advantage of using disease modeling with iPSCs technology is that it allows the generation of pluripotent cells from any individual in the context of his/her own particular genetic identity including individuals with simple forms of disease and those with complex multifactorial diseases of unknown genetic identity [18, 43].

7.3.2 Generation of iPSCs from Cancer Cells

The cancer-derived hiPSCs represent important systems for modeling cancer pathogenesis, aiding in the discovery of new diagnostic and prognostic biomarkers, and for the development of new therapies for cancer. However, reprogramming cancer cells has been demonstrated to be harder than generating normal iPSCs, because of genetic and epigenetic status of these cells. So, some researchers are testing other possibilities to generate cancer-derived hiPSCs as the application of other factors in addition to the Yamanaka factors, such as exogenous expression of miRNA302; chemical compounds, as azacitidine (DNA methyltransferase inhibitor); and knockdown of p53, p21, and Ink4/Arf [3, 75]. Another point here, for normal and cancer cells, is the gene delivery systems for the iPSCs generation. The integration site of retrovirus in the iPSCs may affect the gene expression and change the disease phenotype after redifferentiating them into the original lineages. So, efficient induction of transgene-free iPSCs such as using Sendai virus and episomal systems has been reported [3, 55, 63]. But, we must have in mind, as mentioned by Ramos-Mejia et al. [76], that the difficulties in reprogramming cancer cells are not exclusively due to technical barriers or the need for improved reprogramming technologies. It seems that biological barriers such as cancer-specific genetic mutations, epigenetic remodeling, and accumulation of DNA damage may influence the reprogramming of human cancer cells [76].

The cancer stem cells (CSCs) play a critical role in the origin and propagation of cancer. These CSCs, which have the tumor initiating characteristics, have been identified in several types of cancer (hematologic neoplasms and solid tumors). They are responsible for tumor relapses and metastasis. However, the molecular mechanisms of CSCs origin are difficult to study, mainly in solid tumors, because these cells represent a rare population of undifferentiated tumor cells that retain the ability of self-renewal, proliferation and develop into more differentiated tumor cells. One hypothesis about the origin of the CSCs in solid tumors is that these cells may arise through a genetic/epigenetic reprogramming-like mechanism. The ability of certain cancer cells to be reprogrammed to pluripotency might allow the in vitro generation of pluripotent cancer stem cell lines from human tumors, which would provide an important research in studying the molecular process of CSCs [77].

There are key factors essential for ES cell maintenance, possibly able to reprogram cancer cell into a more ES-like state, for example, mir-302s. The mir-302 microRNA family is expressed, most abundantly, as slow-growing human embryonic stem (ES) cells and decreases after cell differentiation and proliferation [78]. To test the function of mir-302s, Lin et al. [78] developed a retroviral Pol

II-based intronic mi-RNA expressing system namely, pLNCX2-rT-spRNAi, and used it to generate transgenic mi-RNA-expressing cell lines named mir-PS-Colo and mir PS-PC3 derived from human melanoma colo and prostate cancer PC3 cells, respectively. Using this strategy, it was observed that mir-302 does not function to reprogram cancer into an ES-like pluripotent state, but it also maintains this state under a feeder-free condition, which may offer an opportunity for therapeutic intervention [78].

Several experiments have been done in order to generate iPSCs more effectively identifying somatic cells that are easily accessible and possibly require fewer factors for conversion into iPSCs. Utikal et al. [79] demonstrated that in contrast to skin fibroblasts (the initial cell type report of reprogramming into iPSCs), the melanocytes and melanoma cells offer advantages. These cells did not require ectopic Sox2 expression for conversion into iPSCs and might be an appropriate source of cells for attempt to replace viral gene delivery systems with transient expression approaches such as plasmids or adenoviruses. Lastly, melanocytes can be easily obtained by skin punch biopsies, which make them an accessible cell type for clinical applications [79].

Many solid tumors contain poorly vascularized regions that are severely hypoxic and contribute to cancer progression by activating transcription factors that promote cell survival, tumor angiogenesis, and metastasis. Tumor hypoxia is also associated with more aggressive disease course and poor clinical outcomes. It has been suggested that hypoxia could contribute to the formation of cancer stem cell niche within the tumor [80]. Mathieu et al. [80] showed that hypoxia inducible factor (HIF) can induce hESC like transcriptional program, including the induced pluripotent stem cell (iPSCs) inducers OCT4, NANOG, SOX2, KLF4, c-MYC, and microRNA 302 in cancer cell lines, as example in lung cancer. This study suggested that HIF targets are critical for stemness in malignant cells [80].

The study of molecular characterization of CSCs is necessary to facilitate the potential discovery of new targets that are specifically involved in tumor initiation. Accumulated evidence suggests that changes in the cellular bioenergetics may be a novel prerequisite for acquired stemness [77]. Another example for in vitro generation of pluripotent cancer stem cell lines from human tumors was the study done by Corominas-Faja and colleagues [77], who studied whether the nuclear reprogramming of breast cancer cells (MCF-7 human breast cancer cell line) to Sox-2 overexpressing CSC-like states involves the remodeling of bioenergetics and biosynthetic metabolism. It was studied the AMPK/mTOR pathway, which plays a critical role in the regulation of energy metabolism. In this study it was showed the first characterization of the mTOR signaling-related transcriptome during the conversion of differentiated MCF-7 tumor cells to CSC-like MCF-7 cells. It was observed that the acquisition of the stem cell-like states appears to utilize molecular mechanisms involved in the transcriptional suppression of mTOR repressors and activation of mTOR enhancers. The remodeling of the AMPK/mTOR regulated the bioenergetics and biosynthetic metabolism and may be an active contributor that defines cancer cell fate and it is responsible for the acquisition of CSC-like status in breast cancer. The dysfunction of negative metabolic regulators, including defects in the AMPK-mTOR pathway, could result in permissive metabolic reprogramming that allows a differentiated cancer cell to be reprogrammed to regain stem cell characteristics in a process of tumorigenic reprogramming to pluripotency. This study may provide a new path for obtaining molecular information about preventing the appearance of CSCs through the modulation of AMPK/ mTOR pathway [77].

Studying the nuclear reprogramming, it is possible to demonstrate that pluripotent cells can be derived from various types of somatic cells by nuclear reprogramming using defined transcription factors. But, it is unclear whether human cancer cells can be similarly reprogrammed and subsequently terminally differentiated with abrogation of tumorigenicity [81]. Using sarcomas as models to study this unclear question, Zhang et al. [81] showed that human-derived complex karyotypes solid tumors can be reprogrammed into a pluripotent-like state and they can be terminally differentiated into mature connective and red blood cells and terminal differentiation is accompanied with loss of proliferation and tumorigenicity. In this study, the reprogramming decreased the aggressiveness of cancer (as measured by growth/size/cellularity). Interestingly, no tumors formed upon subcutaneous inoculation of the entire cell culture obtained from differentiated reprogrammed-sarcomas into mice and followed for up to 16 weeks. The results of this study suggest that nuclear reprogramming may be a broadly applicable therapeutic strategy for the treatment of cancer, but further studies are necessary to investigate the genetic and epigenetic basis of direct cancer reprogramming [81].

Some studies have shown that cancer cell reprogramming may be possible with the introduction of fewer reprogramming factors since some cancer cell lines often express some of the reprogramming factors at baseline levels equivalent to ESC or IPSCs [79, 81]. Therefore, reprogramming cancer cells may be simpler than reprogramming somatic cells [81].

Another example of reprogramming cancer cells is in Ewing sarcoma. The Ewing sarcoma (EWS) is the second most common type of primary bone malignancy in children and adolescents. It is a highly invasive, undifferentiated tumor of unknown histogenic origin. In approximately 85 % of tumors it is observed the expression of EWS-FLI1 fusion product generated from the chromosomal translocation t(11;22)(q24;q12). Although EWS typically responds to initial combination chemotherapy treatment, approximately one-third of patients will have recurrent disease and metastatic disease despite aggressive multimodal therapeutic approaches. The discovery of novel molecularly target therapies to improve patient outcomes will require a greater understanding of the molecular mechanism driving EWS oncogenesis, metastasis, and drug resistance. So the EWS-iPSCs may provide an expandable disease model that could be used to investigate processes modulating oncogenesis, metastasis, and chemotherapeutic resistance in EWS [82]. In Table 7.1 we present some examples of cancer-derived hiPSCs mentioned in Sect. 7.3.1 and in this section.

Table 7.1 Summary of cancer-derived hiPSCs

Type of cancer (hematologic malignancies and solid tumors)	Aim of study	Method of generation of the cancer-hiPSCs	References
Myeloproliferative disorder (MPD) with JAK2-V617F somatic mutation	Generate iPS cells to provide a renewable cell source and a prospective hematopoiesis model for investigating MPD pathogenesis	Frozen peripheral blood $CD34^+$ cells from two patients with MPD/retroviral transduction	Ye et al. [65]
Chronic myeloid leukemia (CML)	To address whether human cancer cells can be reprogrammed into iPSCs	Cell line, KBM7, derived from blast crisis stage of CML/retroviral transduction	Carette et al. [83]
Chronic myeloid leukemia (CML)	To eliminate the genomic integration and background transgene expression, toward advancing iPSCs technology for the modeling of blood diseases	Bone marrow mononuclear cells from a patient with CML (chronic phase)/episomal vectors	Hu et al. [63]
Chronic myeloid leukemia (CML)	Investigate CML pathogenesis on the basis of patient-derived samples	Two patients samples of CML (chronic phase) bone marrow cells, retrovirus and Sendai virus system	Kumano et al. [3]
Juvenile myelomonocytic leukemia (JMML)	Explore the pathophysiology and treatment of JMML	Two pediatric patient's samples from bone marrow or peripheral blood/ lentivirus	Gandre-Babbe et al. [70]
Myelodysplastic syndrome (MDS)	Functionally dissect the loss of chromosome 7q for discovery of haploinsufficient genes	Two patients with MDS with del(7q)/lentiviral	Kotini et al. [73]
Gastrointestinal cancer	Study new cancer therapies via reprogramming approaches in cancer cells	Gastrointestinal cell lines of cancers from esophageal, stomach, colorectal, pancreas, liver and bile ducts/lentiviral and retroviral	Miyoshi et al. [64]
Gastrointestinal cancer	Generate a human cell model of early pancreatic cancer and disease progression for biomarkers detection for useful diagnosis	Tissue from the center of pancreatic ductal adenocarcinoma (PDAC) sample of patient/lentivirus system	Kim et al. [66]
Melanoma and prostate cancer	Generate two mir-302-expressing mirPS cell lines, namely, mirPS-Colo and mirPS-PC3	Melanoma and prostate cancer cell lines/retroviral Pol-II-based intronic miR-302 expression system, namely, *pLNCX2-rT-SpRNAi*	Lin et al. [78]

(continued)

Table 7.1 (continued)

Type of cancer (hematologic malignancies and solid tumors)	Aim of study	Method of generation of the cancer-hiPSCs	References
Melanoma	Generate and characterize of human iPSCs derived from malignant melanoma cell line	Malignant melanoma cell line/lentiviruses containing a reverse tetracycline transactivator (rtTA) and the four reprogramming factors (Oct4, Sox2, c-Myc, and Klf4) and doxycycline	Utikal et al. [79]
Lung cancer	Study the role of HIF as a inducer of hESC markers including the critical iPSC factors in cancer cells and the tumor aggressiveness	Lung adenocarcinoma cell line/retroviruses with or without nondegradable forms of HIF/lentiviruses expressing Oct4/Sox2 and Nanog/Lin28	Mathieu et al. [80]
Breast cancer	Create stable cancer stem cells lines to study the transcriptional control of mTOR	MCF-7 cells were transduced with retroviruses containing Oct-4, Sox2, Klf4, and c-Myc	Corominas-Faja et al. [77]
Osteosarcoma	To show that direct reprogramming of sarcomas is feasible and allows for recapitulation of terminal differentiation into varied connective tissues with cessation of tumorigenicity	Human osteosarcoma cells lines and lentivectors expressing cDNAs of human Oct4, Nanog, Sox2, Lin28, Klf4, c-Myc	Zhang et al. [81]
Ewing sarcoma (EWS)	Generate iPSCs from EWS cell lines for improving the understanding of the molecular mechanisms driving oncogenesis and metastasis and to investigate chemotherapeutic resistance	CHLA-10 or HEK293T cell lines were induced to pluripotency, episomal vector containing OCT4, SOX2, NANOG, and KLF4 together with a reporter plasmid	Moore et al. [82]

Adapted from Fernandez et al. [18]

7.3.3 The Use of iPSCs for Drug Screening and Predictive Cytotoxicity

During all of the steps of drug development, models play a decisive role. The first to be used are models of pathology that enable pathogenesis mechanisms to be investigated and a relevant target(s) to be identified to screen chemical compound libraries in the search for drug candidates. These so-called "hits" are then evaluated again in models for their pharmacokinetic and safety properties [84]. Animals or in vitro animal-derived cells are used as testing systems, but are limited by their inability to replicate the "exact" human physiological conditions and related phenotypic attributions. For carcinogenic agents, different agents pose different levels of carcinogenicity in different animals. For these reasons, being able to use the systems closer to human is very important [85].

In drug screening, hiPSCs would be used to verify the response to a specific target gene, to research the single nucleotide polymorphism-related of each individual that influences the ability of an individual to effectively metabolize and clear drugs and toxins. In particular, hepatotoxicity and cardiotoxicity are two principal causes of drug failure during preclinical testing. The variability in individual responses to potential therapeutic agents is also a major problem in effective drug development. The advantage of iPSCs technology is that it allows the generation of various cell lines that may represent the genetic and potentially epigenetic variation of a broad spectrum of the population. This approach used the in vitro model of disease to identify new drugs to treat disease [18, 43].

Cellular assays can be developed for large-throughput drug screening by converting cancer-cell-specific iPSCs into the cell types of interest. If directed differentiation can recapitulate tumor formation in vitro, drugs that can selectively eliminate the cancerous cells may be identified and also tested in a range of other cell types [69].

Human iPSCs can be obtained at large scale and exhibit remarkable application prospects in drug selection, mechanism research, and organ regeneration. Nevertheless, few studies have reported the use of human iPSCs as tumor therapeutic reagents. Human iPSCs cells are considered suitable for in vivo therapy. First, human iPSCs are effective gene delivery agents because they can deliver siRNA or drugs into tumor sites and inhibit the growth of tumor cells in vivo. Second, human iPSCs can differentiate into immunological cells in tumor sites and thus kill tumor cells. Finally, human iPSCs can destroy the niche of tumor cell proliferation and repress tumor growth. Therefore, the development of human iPSCs for in vivo tumor therapy provides considerable potential for clinical translation [86].

The human iPSCs have been used labeled with fluorescent magnetic nanoparticles (FMNPs) for targeted imaging and synergistic therapy of gastric cancer cells in vivo [86]. The mechanism of FMNP-labeled iPSCs targeting gastric cancer cells in vivo includes the secretion of cytokines, chemokines, and/or growth factors into the blood or lymph circulation, which serve as candidate migration stimulatory signals. Some receptors on the iPSC surface or iPSCs may secrete cytokines and chemokines, which combine with factors secreted by tumor cells; this phenomenon induces iPSCs to move to the tumor sites. As iPSCs can actively target and recognize gastric cancer cells *in vivo* and may localize around the tumor site, FMNPs inside iPSCs can also localize around the tumor cells. FMNPs can produce heat energy when subjected under external magnetic field; in tumor sites, a high temperature of 62 °C can kill and inhibit the growth of tumor cells. However, in important organs, such as liver or kidney or lung, a temperature of 30 °C was generated, which cannot damage important organs. In this study, Li et al. [86] concluded that the prepared FMNPs-labeled iPSCs could achieve the cancer therapy effect, which presents good clinical application prospects. The therapeutic effects of FMNP-labeled iPSCs coupled with the hyperthermal effects of FMNPs demonstrate a significant potential for clinical treatment of cancer [86].

The cancer-derived hiPSCs represents important systems for modeling cancer pathogenesis, aiding in the discovery of new diagnostic and prognostic biomarkers, and for the development of new therapies for cancer. Yang et al. [87] demonstrated a tumor tropism of intravenously injected human iPSC-derived neural stem cells and their gene therapy application in a metastatic breast cancer mouse model. In this study, the authors used a lentiviral transduction method to derive hiPSCs from primary human fibroblasts and then generate neural stem cells (NSCs) from the iPSCs. The NSCs are able to home in on not just brain tumors, but also solid tumors of a non-neural origin. This intrinsic tropism occurs because of the presence of cytokines, chemokines, and growth factors released from the tumor cells. Yang and collaborators investigated whether the iPSCs-derived NCS can be used as a cellular delivery vehicle for cancer gene therapy. For this propose, the cells were transduced with a baculoviral vector containing the herpes simplex virus thymidine kinase suicide gene and injected through tail vein into tumor-bearing mice. The transduced NCSs were effective in inhibiting the growth of the breast tumor and the metastatic spread of the cancer cells in the presence of ganciclovir, leading to prolonged survival of the tumor bearing mice. This study demonstrated the use of iPSC-derived NSCs for cancer gene therapy [87].

7.3.4 iPSCs and Cancer Immunotherapy

A potential clinical application of hiPSCs in cancer is in the field of immunotherapy ([18, 88–91]. Traditional treatment modalities are all based on destroying cancer cell by irradiation, chemotherapy or surgery. Although they can effectively kill or remove cancer cells, the use of these treatments is often limited because a number of health cells also tend to be destroyed and, in some cases, may occur the recidive of cancer. In the case of cancer, the immune system alone often fails to effectively fight the tumor for the following reasons: (1) the normal immune system is "blind" to tumor cells because the tumor cells are derived from the body's own cells. The body "thinks" about the tumor as "self," a phenomenon known as tumor tolerance; (2) the immune system may recognize certain cancer cells, but the response may not be strong enough to destroy cancer; (3) the tumor has the ability to defend itself secreting some substances that allow its survival and expansion. In the case of cancer, the immune system needs a boost to strengthen its response to become more effective. So, immunotherapy strategies include antitumor monoclonal antibodies, cancer vaccines, adoptive transfer of ex vivo activated T or natural killer cells, and administration of antibodies that either stimulate immune cells or block immune inhibitory pathways. The impact of immunotherapy was initially demonstrated in patients with advanced cancer, and then translated to the adjuvant setting of patients with operable disease at high risk for postoperative recurrence [18, 92].

The immunotherapy based on the adoptive transfer or gene-engineered T cells can mediate tumor regression in patients with metastatic cancer [93]. Adoptive T cell immune therapy is based on the isolation of tumor-specific T cells from a cancer patient, in vitro activation, expansion of these T cells, and reinfusion of the T cells to the patient [94]. The adoptive immunotherapy with T cells is an effective therapeutic strategy for combating many types of cancer. However, the limitations associated with the number of antigen-specific T cells represent a major challenge to this approach [89]. The recent iPSCs technology and the development of an in vitro system for gene delivery are able to generate iPSCs from patients. The iPSCs have a great potential to be used in adoptive cell transfer of antigen-specific CD8(+) cytotoxic T lymphocytes [95, 96]. Some research groups are studying methods to generate T-lymphocytes from iPSCs in vitro and in vivo programming antigen-specific T cells from iPSCs for promoting cancer immune surveillance [95]. Given the low frequency of tumor-specific T cells in the periphery of individuals and difficulties surrounding their identification, it has been demonstrated the use of iPS cells for genetic modification to introduce a bicistronic lentiviral vector encoding 19–28z, a CAR specific for CD19, expressed by the majority of leukemias and lymphomas [97, 98]. Themeli et al. [98] were able to optimize differentiation conditions to allow for serum and feeder-free generation of hematopoietic progenitor cells which, when co-cultured with OP9-DL1 stromal cells in the presence of SCF, Flt3L, and interleukin-7 (IL-7), differentiated into T cells expressing the CD19-specific CAR. T cells produced in this way were activated by CD19C APCs and, upon infusion into mice, potently inhibited tumor progression [97, 98].

Therapies based on the use of autologous immune cells are among the best candidates for cancer immunotherapy. The dendritic cell vaccines have demonstrated very encouraging responses for some solid tumors, while in melanoma T-cell therapies have exceeded 70 % objective response rates in selected Phase I trial [99]. However, it is difficult to obtain a sufficient number of functional dendritic cells (DCs) in DC-based immunotherapy. In this sense, some studies are being performed using the iPSCs. Iwamoto et al. [88] used the iPS cell-derived DCs (iPSDCs) and compared the therapeutic efficacy of iPSDCs and the equivalent to that of bone marrow-derived DCs (BMDCs). In this study, the authors examined the capacity for maturation of iPSDCs compared with that of BMDCs in addition to the capacity for migration of iPSDCs to regional lymph nodes. The therapeutic efficacy of the vaccination was examined in a subcutaneous tumor model. The vaccination with genetically modified iPSDCs achieved a level of therapeutic efficacy as high as vaccination with BMDCs. This study showed experimentally that genetically modified iPSDCs have an equal capacity of BMDCs in terms of tumor-associated antigen-specific therapeutic antitumor immunity. Therefore, vaccination strategy may be useful for future clinical application as a cancer vaccine [18, 88].

Natural killer (NK) cells play critical role in host immunity against cancer. In response, cancer develops mechanisms to escape NK cell attack or induce defective

NK cells. Current NK cell-based cancer immunotherapy aims to overcome NK cell paralysis using several approaches. One approach is the genetic modification of fresh NK cells or NK cell lines to highly express cytokines, Fc receptors, and/or chimeric tumor-antigen receptors. Therapeutic NK cells can be derived from various sources, including peripheral or cord blood cells, stem cells or even induced pluripotent stem cells (iPSCs) and a variety of stimulators can be used for large-scale production in laboratories or good manufacturing practice [18, 100].

Adult stem cell therapies have provided success for more than 50 years, through reconstitution of the hematopoietic system using bone marrow, umbilical cord blood, and mobilized peripheral blood transplantation. Mesenchymal stem cell (MSC) mediated therapy is a fast-growing field that has showed safe and effective in the treatment of various degenerative diseases and tissues injuries. The expansion and manipulation of human MSCs are important approaches to immune regulatory and regenerative cell therapies. MSCs are fibroblast-like cells of the BM microenvironment called "marrow stromal cells," which was able to support hematopoiesis. These cells have adult stem cell properties as they could differentiate into cartilage, bone, adipocytes, and muscle cells. MSCs are a promising tool for cell therapies because they are easily accessible from various tissue sources as bone marrow (BM-MSC), fat, and umbilical cord [101]. These cells have been widely tested and showed efficacious in preclinical and clinical studies for cardiovascular and neurodegenerative diseases, orthopedic injuries, graft-versus-host disease (GvHD) following bone marrow transplantation, autoimmune diseases, and liver diseases [101, 102].

Because BM-MSC can be easily harvested from adult sources and cultured in vitro, many preclinical and clinical studies have used BM-MSC. Although these cells show great potential for clinical use, there are some problems. The need for extensive cell number for use poses a risk of accumulating genetic and epigenetic abnormalities that could lead malignant cell transformation. Binato et al. [103] studied the stability of human MSCs during in vitro culture in several passages using cytogenetic, cellular, and molecular methods and it was observed that these cells demonstrated chromosomal instability and molecular changes during passage 5 [103]. Although easy access to BM-MSC is recognized as a great advantage, extended in vitro cultures reduce the differentiation potential of MSC, which limits their therapeutic efficacy [101]. So, to overcome this problem, MSCs derived from iPSC may be considered for human cell and gene therapy applications as iPSCs have the potential to be expanded indefinitely without senescence. It is observed a greater regenerative potential of MSCs derived from iPSCs, which may be attributed to superior survival and engraftment after transplantation, because of higher telomerase activity and less senescence as compared to BM-MSC. Genetically manipulated MSCs may also serve as cellular therapeutics since MSCs can be used as target drug delivery vehicles [18, 101].

7.4 Considering Probability Models to Evaluate the Possible Use of the hiPSCs for Therapeutic Procedures

7.4.1 Probability: An Important Mathematical Concept in Clinical Research

An important mathematical concept used in clinical research is the concept of probability. In fact, clinical outcomes such as the occurrence of disease, death or symptoms can be counted and expressed as numbers. In most clinical situations, diagnosis, prognosis and treatment results are uncertain for an individual patient. A person will experiment a clinical outcome or not: the prediction is rarely accurate. Therefore, *the prediction needs to be expressed as a probability.*

Probability is used when the research selects a probability model. This is the case when it is necessary to make predictions about the frequency with which certain results can be expected to occur when the experiment is repeated a number of times. For example, the mathematical model that should be used to predict the percentage of a false negative outcome for tests used to diagnose a certain disease should be a probability model.

Probability models lead to *hypothesis tests*. Hypothesis tests are used to draw inferences and reach conclusions about data, when only a part of a population, a sample, has been studied. A hypothesis test can be parametric or nonparametric. If we decide to approximate clinical measurements by a normal curve, we are deciding to use a *parametric test*. A hypothesis test asks if an effect (difference) exists or not. It works with two hypothesis: the null hypothesis (designated H_0) and the alternative hypothesis (designated H_A).

The hypothesis that there is no difference is the null hypothesis. The hypothesis that contradicts H_0 is H_A. When we retain H_A (equivalently reject H_0), we say the results are significant and when we retain H_0 (equivalently reject H_A), we say the results are not significant. Because we are dealing with probabilities, this implies in making two possible errors from four possible relations between the conclusions obtained using a hypothesis test and real situations, as shown in Table 7.2.

The two errors mentioned in the previous paragraph are known as Type I error and Type II error. A Type I error leads to a false positive conclusion. The probability of such an error occurs is noted by α. Mathematically, α is a conditional probability: it is the probability of reject H_0 when there is no real difference. A Type II error leads to a false negative conclusion. The probability of such an error occurs is noted by β. Mathematically, β is a conditional probability: it is the probabilities of retain H_0 when there is a real difference.

Hypothesis tests are used to estimate the probability of a Type I error. In the literature, we usually use $\alpha < 0.05$. This means we are assuming a probability less than 0.05 of rejecting H_0 when there is no real difference between treatments, drugs,

Table 7.2 Relations between statistical conclusions and real situations

	Real difference	
Conclusion of the hypothesis test	Presence	Absence
Results are significant	True	Type I error
Results are not significant	Type II error	True

or procedures. In other words, if the study were repeated 100 times, we probably would find five outcomes showing H_0 should be accepted. For those who would like to study this subject, we recommend the book [104].

7.4.2 *Probability: Its Use to Evaluate hiPSCs for Therapeutic Procedures*

The iPSCs are undifferentiated cells that have the capacity to proliferate in undifferentiated cells both in vitro and in vivo (self-renewal) and to differentiate into mature specialized cells. Because this is a new discovery, there are open questions regarding, mainly, the safe application of stem cell therapy using the iPSCs. As we have presented in this chapter, many different groups have successfully generated iPSCs, but due to different techniques, until now, there is no standard information about the safety and effectiveness of the use of iPSCs in the clinical practice.

Investigators aim to answer a question that arises by observations or the results of previous studies. Structuring a study helps that this question can be answered in a systematic way (Fig. 7.2). A well-formulated question is of great importance to the success of a study.

In order to have a better understanding of how we can minimize the problems, which occur with the use of iPSCs, we think it is important to consider some questions as if there is an association between cell sources (fibroblasts from skin, stem cells from bone marrow, umbilical cord blood, adipose tissue) and self-renewal capacity and how the cellular reprogramming works at molecular level. Investigations about which kind of tissues can make easier the introduction of the hiPSCs are also very important.

There are several hypothesis tests commonly used in the medical literature; they are resumed in Table 7.3. When we use such tests, we compute a *p-value*, which is the probability of obtaining a result as extreme as or more extreme than the sample value, assuming the null hypothesis is true. The sample value is calculated. Depending on the test we use, there is a specific formula to calculate the sample value. Appropriate computer software can do such a calculation.

Further basic research on each aspect of reprogramming is required in order to understand how reprogramming leads to pluripotency. Even with improvements in the virus-free and transgene-free reprogramming technology, the "safe" iPSCs still

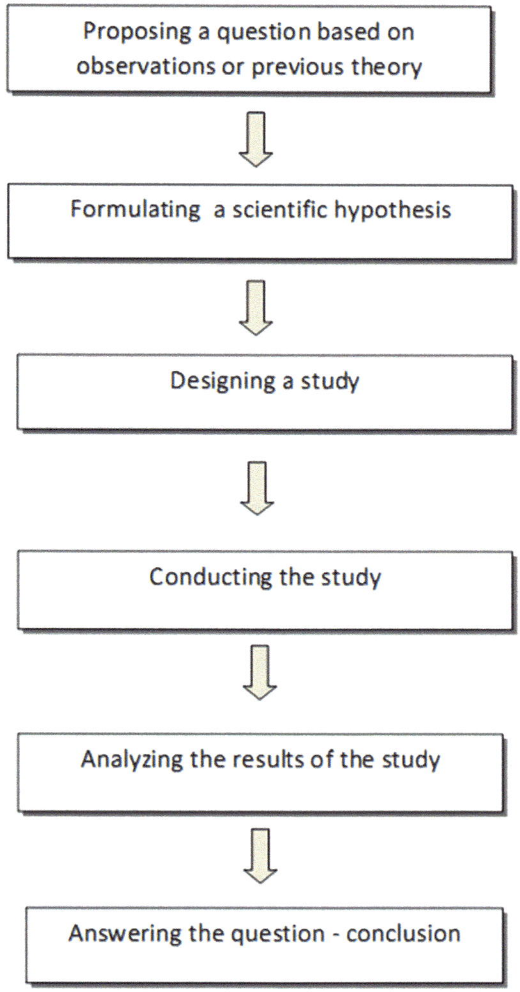

Fig. 7.2 Steps of a clinical study

needs to be evaluated in animals models, for example, before these products be used clinically for cancer therapy.

We finish saying that probability models are important tools that *can help* making decisions and must be used if the numerical outcomes are clinically meaningful. Of course, medical professionals should put away the complexity of the mathematical concepts behind on probability techniques, although only Mathematics could explain rigorously why these techniques really work.

Table 7.3 Hypothesis tests usually used in the medical literature

To test the statistical significance of the difference between		
Two proportions	Fisher's exact test	Nonparametric
Two or more proportions	Chi-square	Nonparametric
Two medians	Mann–Whitney	Nonparametric
Two means	t-Student	Parametric
More than two means	Kruskal–Wallis	Nonparametric
	ANOVA	Parametric
More than two variances	Bartlett	Parametric
To test the correlation between two variables	Spearman's rank correlation test	Nonparametric
	Pearson's correlation test	Parametric

7.5 Conclusion and Future Perspective

Several approaches have been used to understand cancer pathogenesis. The discovery of the hiPSCs opens a new perspective to study different diseases, including cancer. Cancer cells have many biological characteristics that are conferred by numerous genetic and epigenetic modifications. Cancer evolves by a process of clonal expansion, genetic diversification and clonal selection. Despite improvements in cancer treatment, the disease is still a major cause of morbidity and mortality. The lack of a relevant model to study the development and the progression of cancer has limited the research, which is indispensable for translation to the clinical setting. Generation of iPSCs from human cancer cells represents a new paradigm in cancer modeling (hematologic malignancies and solid tumors) in order to study the multiple stages of cancer, for the discovery of new drugs designed for specific biomarkers and for testing drugs' toxicity. Cancer-derived iPSCs have been used to study CML disease and tyrosine kinase resistance;to study JMML pathology and treatment. In MDS, cellular reprogramming and genome engineering have been used to functionally dissect the loss of chromosome 7, a somatic cytogenetic abnormality, considered a biomarker of unfavorable prognosis, recapitulating phenotypes associated with the disease. In solid tumors, for example, it has been demonstrated in sarcomas that cancer cells can be reprogrammed and subsequently terminally differentiated with loss of proliferation and tumorigenicity, so reprogramming may decrease the aggressiveness of cancer. Another example of reprogramming cancer cells is in Ewing sarcoma, the second most common type of primary bone malignancy in children and adolescents. In this solid tumor, despite aggresive multimodal therapeutic approaches, one-third of patients will have recurrent disease and metastatic disease. The EWS-iPSCs may provide an expandable disease model that could be used to investigate processes modulating oncogenesis, metastasis and chemotherapeutic resistance. Another potential clinical application of hiPSCs in cancer is in the field of immunotherapy. Since the first description of iPSCs generation, there has been a great improvement in the methods to generate these cells. The main problem in using these cells is the possibility of developing tumors. It is also very important to obtain a characterization of these cells at cytogenetic and molecular levels, in order to understand how reprogramming works in signaling pathways. To generate iPSCs, different sources of cells have been used and compared. Hypothesis tests and estimates may be used to validate the safe and efficacy of hiPSCs for therapeutic use. As future perspective, we must have in mind that the discovery of novel molecularly target therapies to improve patient outcomes will require a greater understanding of the molecular mechanism of cancer. Technical and basic knowledge are necessary before using iPSCs in clinical practice. But, the possibility to induce pluripotency in somatic cells or, even further, to induce transdifferentiation through the forced expression of reprogramming factors has offered a new field for cancer research and new insights in cancer origin and progression. This may be translated in clinical practice allowing the development of a better drug screening platforms, less toxic therapies and different future applications in the clinical practice. So, the use of hiPSCs may contribute to the development of future personalized cell therapies and opens new possibilities for the treatment of cancer patients.

Acknowledgments The authors thank Dr. Essam M. Abdelalim for the invitation to participate in this book.

Conflict of Interests The authors declare no conflict of interests.

References

1. Chin L, Gray JW. Translating insights from the cancer genome into clinical practice. Nature. 2008;452:553–63.
2. Grob B, Pittermann E, Reinhardt D, Cantz T, Klusmann JH. Prospects and challenges of reprogrammed cells in hematology and oncology. Pediatr Hematol Oncol. 2012;29:507–28.
3. Kumano K, Arai S, Hosoi M, Taoka K, Takayama N, Otsu M, Nagae G, Ueda K, Nakazaki K, Kamikubo Y, Eto K, Aburatani H, Nakauchi H, Kurokawa M. Generation of induced pluripotent stem cells from primary chronic myelogenous leukemia patient samples. Blood. 2012;119:6234–42.
4. Suzuki A, Matsushima K, Makinoshima H, Sugano S, Kohno T, Tsuchihara K, Suzuki Y. Single-cell analysis of lung adenocarcinoma cell lines reveals diverse expression patterns of individual cells invoked by a molecular target drug treatment. Genome Biol. 2015;16:66.
5. Wills QF, Mead AJ. Application of single-cell genomics in cancer: promise and challenges. Hum Mol Genet. 2015;24:R74–84.
6. Takahashi K, Yamanaka S. Induced pluripotent stem cells in medicine and biology. Development. 2013;140:2457–61.
7. Greaves M, Maley CC. Clonal evolution in cancer. Nature. 2012;481:306–13.
8. Urruticoechea A, Alemany R, Balart J, Villanueva A, Viñals F, Capellá G. Recent advances in cancer therapy: an overview. Curr Pharm Des. 2010;16:3–10.
9. Chung L, Baxter RC. Breast cancer biomarkers: proteomic discovery and translation to clinically relevant assays. Expert Rev Proteomics. 2012;9:599–614.
10. Fang WJ, Zheng Y, Wu LM, Ke QH, Shen H, Yuan Y, Zheng SS. Genome-wide analysis of aberrant DNA methylation for identification of potential biomarkers in colorectal cancer patients. Asian Pac J Cancer Prev. 2012;13:1917–21.

11. Fenderico N, Casamichele A, Profumo V, Zaffaroni N, Gandellini P. MicroRNA-mediated control of prostate cancer metastasis: implications for the identification of novel biomarkers and therapeutic targets. Curr Med Chem. 2013;20:1566–84.
12. Kalari S, Pfeifer GP. Identification of driver and passenger DNA methylation in cancer by epigenomic analysis. Adv Genet. 2010;70:277–308.
13. Pixberg CF, Schulz WA, Stoecklein NH, Neves RPL. Characterization of DNA methylation in circulating tumor cells. Genes. 2015;6:1053–75.
14. Rodrigues EF, Santos-Rebouças CB, Gonçalves Pimentel MM, Mencalha AL, Dobbin J, Da Costa ES, Fernandez CS, Bouzas LF, Abdelhay E, Fernandez TS. Epigenetic alterations of p15(INK4B) and p16(INK4A) genes in pediatric primary myelodysplastic syndrome. Leuk Lymphoma. 2010;10:1887–94.
15. Frame FM, Maitland NJ. Cancer stem cells, models of study and implications of therapy resistance mechanisms. Adv Exp Med Biol. 2011;720:105–18.
16. Ito T. Stem cell maintenance and disease progression in chronic myeloid leukemia. Int J Hematol. 2013;98:641–7.
17. Zhou BB, Zhang H, Damelin M, Geles KG, Grindley JC, Dirks PB. Tumour-initiating cells: challenges and opportunities for anticancer drug discovery. Nat Rev Drug Discov. 2009;8:806–23.
18. Fernandez TS, de Souza FC, Mencalha AL. Human induced pluripotent stem cells from basic research to potential clinical applications in cancer. Biomed Res Int. 2013;13:430290.
19. Hussein SM, Nagy AA. Progress made in the reprogramming field: new factors, new strategies and a new outlook. Curr Opin Genet Dev. 2012;22:435–43.
20. Teoh HK, Cheong SK. Induced pluripotent stem cells in research and therapy. Malays J Pathol. 2012;34:1–13.
21. Walia B, Satija N, Tripathi RP, Gangenahalli GU. Induced pluripotent stem cells: fundamentals and applications of the reprogramming process and its ramifications on regenerative medicine. Stem Cell Rev. 2012;8:100–15.
22. Takahashi K, Yamanaka S. Induction of pluripotent stem cells from mouse embryonic and adult fibroblast cultures by defined factors. Cell. 2006;126:663–76.
23. Niwa H, Miyazaki J, Smith AG. Quantitative expression of Oct-3/4 defines differentiation, dedifferentiation or self-renewal of ES cells. Nat Genet. 2000;24:372–6.
24. Rodda DJ, Chew JL, Lim LH, Loh YH, Wang B, Ng HH, Robson P. Transcriptional regulation of nanog by OCT4 and SOX2. J Biol Chem. 2005;280:24731–7.
25. Jiang J, Chan YS, Loh YH, Cai J, Tong GQ, Lim CA, Robson P, Zhong S, Ng HH. A core Klf circuitry regulates self-renewal of embryonic stem cells. Nat Cell Biol. 2008;10:353–60.
26. Coll J, Saule S, Martin P, Raes MB, Lagrou C, Graf T, Beug H, Simon IE, Stehelin D. The cellular oncogenes c-myc, c-myb and c-erb are transcribed in defined types of avian hematopoietic cells. Exp Cell Res. 1983;149:151–62.
27. Hayward WS, Neel BG, Astrin SM. Activation of a cellular oncogene by promoter insertion in ALV-induced lymphoid leukosis. Nature. 1981;290:475–80.
28. Takahashi K, Tanabe K, Ohnuki M, Narita M, Ichisaka T, Tomoda K, Yamanaka S. Induction of pluripotent stem cells from adult human fibroblasts by defined factors. Cell. 2007;131:861–72.
29. Yu J, Vodyanik MA, Smuga-Otto K, Antosiewicz-Bourget J, Frane JL, Tian S, Nie J, Jonsdottir GA, Ruotti V, Stewart R, Slukvin II, Thomson JA. Induced pluripotent stem cell lines derived from human somatic cells. Science. 2007;318:1917–20.
30. Nobel Media AB Web. The 2012 Nobel Prize in Physiology or Medicine—Press Release, Nobelprize.org. http://www.nobelprize.org/nobel_prizes/medicine/laureates/2012/press.html (2013). Accessed 2 Aug 2013
31. Shoemaker C, Goff S, Gilboa E, Paskind M, Mitra SW, Baltimore D. Structure of a cloned circular Moloney murine leukemia virus DNA molecule containing an inverted segment: implications for retrovirus integration. Proc Natl Acad Sci U S A. 1980;77:3932–6.

32. Laurent LC, Ulitsky I, Slavin I, Tran H, Schork A, Morey R, Lynch C, Harness JV, Lee S, Barrero MJ, Ku S, Martynova M, Semechkin R, Galat V, Gottesfeld J, Izpisua Belmonte JC, Murry C, Keirstead HS, Park HS, Schmidt U, Laslett AL, Muller FJ, Nievergelt CM, Shamir R, Loring JF. Dynamic changes in the copy number of pluripotency and cell proliferation genes in human ESCs and iPSCs during reprogramming and time in culture. Cell Stem Cell. 2011;8:106–18.
33. Pasi CE, Dereli-Öz A, Negrini S, Friedli M, Fragola G, Lombardo A, Van Houwe G, Naldini L, Casola S, Testa G, Trono D, Pelicci PG, Halazonetis TD. Genomic instability in induced stem cells. Cell Death Differ. 2011;18:745–53.
34. Marión RM, Strati K, Li H, Murga M, Blanco R, Ortega S, Fernandez-Capetillo O, Serrano M, Blasco MA. A p53-mediated DNA damage response limits reprogramming to ensure iPS cell genomic integrity. Nature. 2009;460:1149–53.
35. Harui A, Suzuki S, Kochanek S, Mitani K. Frequency and stability of chromosomal integration of adenovirus vectors. J Virol. 1999;73:6141–6.
36. Okita K, Ichisaka T, Yamanaka S. Generation of germline-competent induced pluripotent stem cells. Nature. 2007;448:313–7.
37. Halazonetis TD, Gorgoulis VG, Bartek J. An oncogene-induced DNA damage model for cancer development. Science. 2008;319:1352–5.
38. Lim LP, Glasner ME, Yekta S, Burge CB, Bartel DP. Vertebrate microRNA genes. Science. 2003;299:1540.
39. Malchenko S, Galat V, Seftor EA, Vanin EF, Costa FF, Seftor REB, Soares MB, Hendrix MJC. Cancer hallmarks in induced pluripotent cells: new insights. J Cell Physiol. 2010;225:390–3.
40. Mercer TR, Dinger ME, Mattick JS. Long non-coding RNAs: insights into functions. Nat Rev Genet. 2009;10:155–9.
41. Payer B, Rosenberg M, Yamaji M, Yabuta Y, Koyanagi-Aoi M, Hayashi K, Yamanaka S, Saitou M, Lee JT. Tsix RNA and the germline factor, PRDM14, link X reactivation and stem cell reprogramming. Mol Cell. 2013;52:805–18.
42. Fort A, Yamada D, Hashimoto K, Koseki H, Carninci P. Nuclear transcriptome profiling of induced pluripotent stem cells and embryonic stem cells identify non-coding loci resistant to reprogramming. Cell Cycle. 2015;14:1148–55.
43. Chun YS, Byun K, Lee B. Induced pluripotent stem cells and personalized medicine: current progress and future perspectives. Anat Cell Biol. 2011;44:245–55.
44. Talluri TR, Kumar D, Glage S, Garrels W, Ivics Z, Debowski K, Behr R, Kues WA. Non-viral reprogramming of fibroblasts into induced pluripotent stem cells by Sleeping Beauty and PiggyBac transposons. Biochem Biophys Res Commun. 2014;450:581–7.
45. Vand Rajabpour F, Raoofian R, Habibi L, Akrami SM, Tabrizi M. Novel trends in genetics: transposable elements and their application in medicine. Arch Iran Med. 2014;17:702–12.
46. Ishibashi M, Mechaly AS, Becker TS, Rinkwitz S. Using zebrafish transgenesis to test human genomic sequences for specific enhancer activity. Methods. 2013;62:216–25.
47. Woltjen K, Michael IP, Mohseni P, Desai R, Mileikovsky M, Hämäläinen R, Cowling R, Wang W, Liu P, Gertsenstein M, Kaji K, Sung HK, Nagy A. Piggyback transposition reprograms fibroblasts to induced pluripotent stem cells. Nature. 2009;458:766–70.
48. Cadiñanos J, Bradley A. Generation of an inducible and optimized piggyback transposon system. Nucleic Acids Res. 2007;35:e87.
49. Kowarz E, Löscher D, Marschalek R. Optimized sleeping beauty transposons rapidly generate stable transgenic cell lines. Biotechnol J. 2015;10:647–53.
50. Kay MA, He CY, Chen ZY. A robust system for production of minicircle DNA vectors. Nat Biotechnol. 2010;28:1287–9.
51. Cheng L, Hansen NF, Zhao L, Du Y, Zou C, Donovan FX, Chou BK, Zhou G, Li S, Dowey SN, Ye Z, NISC Comparative Sequencing Program, Chandrasekharappa SC, Yang H, Mullikin JC, Liu PP. Low incidence of DNA sequence variation in human induced

pluripotent stem cells generated by nonintegrating plasmid expression. Cell Stem Cell. 2012;10:337–44.
52. Ruiz S, Lopez-Contreras AJ, Gabut M, Marion RM, Gutierrez-Martinez P, Bua S, Ramirez O, Olalde I, Rodrigo-Perez S, Li H, Marques-Bonet T, Serrano M, Blasco MA, Batada NN, Fernandez-Capetillo O. Limiting replication stress during somatic cell reprogramming reduces genomic instability in induced pluripotent stem cells. Nat Commun. 2015;6:8036.
53. Ban H, Nishishita N, Fusaki N, Tabata T, Saeki K, Shikamura M, Takada N, Inoue M, Hasegawa M, Kawamata S, Nishikawa S. Efficient generation of transgene-free human induced pluripotent stem cells (iPSCs) by temperature-sensitive Sendai virus vectors. Proc Natl Acad Sci U S A. 2011;108:14234–9.
54. Churko JM, Burridge PW, Wu JC. Generation of human iPSCs from human peripheral blood mononuclear cells using non-integrative Sendai virus in chemically defined conditions. Methods Mol Biol. 2013;1036:81–8.
55. Hu K, Slukvin I. Generation of transgene-free iPSC lines from human normal and neoplastic blood cells using episomal vectors. Methods Mol Biol. 2013;997:163–76.
56. Kudva YC, Ohmine S, Greder LV, Dutton JR, Armstrong A, De Lamo JG, Khan YK, Thatava T, Hasegawa M, Fusaki N, Slack JM, Ikeda Y. Transgene-free disease-specific induced pluripotent stem cells from patients with type 1 and type 2 diabetes. Stem Cells Transl Med. 2012;1:451–61.
57. Narsinh KH, Jia F, Robbins RC, Kay MA, Longaker MT, Wu JC. Generation of adult human induced pluripotent stem cells using nonviral minicircle DNA vectors. Nat Protoc. 2011;6:78–88.
58. Zhou H, Ding S. Evolution of induced pluripotent stem cell technology. Curr Opin Hematol. 2010;17:276–80.
59. Salk JJ, Fox EJ, Loeb LA. Mutational heterogeneity in human cancers: origin and consequences. Annu Rev Pathol. 2010;5:51–75.
60. Vogelstein B, Papadopoulos N, Velculescu VE, Zhou S, Diaz Jr LA, Kenneth W, Kinzler KW. Cancer genome landscapes. Science. 2013;339:1546–58.
61. Karley D, Gupta D, Tiwari A. Biomarker for cancer: a great promise for future. World J Oncol. 2011;2:151–7.
62. Gonzalez-Angulo AM, Hennessy BT, Mills GB. Future of personalized medicine in oncology: a systems biology approach. J Clin Oncol. 2010;28:2777–83.
63. Hu K, Yu J, Suknuntha K, Tian S, Montgomery K, Choi KD, Stewart R, Thomson JA, Slukvin II. Efficient generation of transgene-free induced pluripotent stem cells from normal and neoplastic bone marrow and cord blood mononuclear cells. Blood. 2011;117:e109–19.
64. Miyoshi N, Ishii H, Nagai K, Hoshino H, Mimori K, Tanaka F, Nagano H, Sekimoto M, Doki Y, Mori M. Defined factors induce reprogramming of gastrointestinal cancer cells. Proc Natl Acad Sci U S A. 2010;107:40–5.
65. Ye Z, Zhan H, Mali P, Dowey S, Williams DM, Jang YY, Dang CV, Spivak JL, Moliterno AR, Cheng L. Human-induced pluripotent stem cells from blood cells of healthy donors and patients with acquired blood disorders. Blood. 2009;114:5473–80.
66. Kim J, Hoffman JP, Alpaugh RK, Rhim AD, Reichert M, Stanger BZ, Furth EE, Sepulveda AR, Yuan CX, Won KJ, Donahue G, Sands J, Gumbs AA, Zaret KS. An iPSC line from human pancreatic ductal adenocarcinoma undergoes early to invasive stages of pancreatic cancer progression. Cell Rep. 2013;3:2088–99.
67. Suvà ML, Riggi N, Bernstein BE. Epigenetic reprogramming in cancer. Science. 2013;339:1567–70.
68. Curry EL, Moad M, Robson CN, Heer R. Using induced pluripotent stem cells as a tool for modeling carcinogenesis. World J Stem Cells. 2015;26:461–9.
69. Kim JJ. Applications of iPSCs in cancer research. Biomark Insights. 2015;10(S1):125.
70. Gandre-Babbe S, Paluru P, Aribeana C, Chou ST, Bresolin S, Lu L, Sullivan SK, Tasian SK, Weng J, Favre H, Choi JK, French DL, Loh ML, Weiss MJ. Patient-derived induced

pluripotent stem cells recapitulate hematopoietic abnormalities of juvenile myelomonocytic leukemia. Blood. 2013;121:4925–9.
71. Fernandez TS, Ornellas MH, Otero de Carvalho L, Tabak D, Abdelhay E. Chromosomal alterations associated with evolution from myelodysplastic syndrome to acute myeloid leukemia. Leuk Res. 2000;24:839–48.
72. Fernandez TS, Mencalha AL, Fernandez CS. Epigenetics in cancer: the myelodysplastic syndrome as a model to study epigenetic alterations as diagnostic and prognostic biomarkers. In: Khan TK, editor. Biomarker. 1st ed. Rijeka, Croatia: InTech; 2012.
73. Kotini AG, Chang CJ, Boussaad I, Delrow JJ, Dolezal EK, Nagulapally AB, Perna F, Fishbein GA, Klimek VM, Hawkins RD, Huangfu D, Murry CE, Graubert T, Nimer SD, Papapetrou EP. Functional analysis of a chromosomal deletion associated with myelodysplastic syndromes using isogenic human induced pluripotent stem cells. Nat Biotechnol. 2015;33:646–55.
74. Lee DF, Su J, Schaniel D, Lemischka IR. Modeling familial cancer with induced pluripotent stem cells. Cell. 2015;161:240–54.
75. Miyazaki S, Yamamoto H, Miyoshi N, Takahashi H, Suzuki Y, Haraguchi N, Ishii H, Doki Y, Mori M. Emerging methods for preparing iPS cells. Jpn J Clin Oncol. 2012;42:773–9.
76. Ramos-Mejia V, Fraga MF, Menendez P. iPSCs from cancer cells: challenges and opportunities. Trends Mol Med. 2012;18:245–7.
77. Corominas-Faja B, Cufí S, Oliveras-Ferraros C, Cuyàs E, López-Bonet E, Lupu R, Alarcón T, Vellon L, Iglesias JM, Leis O, Martín AG, Vazquez-Martin A, Menendez JA. Nuclear reprogramming of luminal-like breast cancer cells generates Sox2-overexpressing cancer stem-like cellular states harboring transcriptional activation of the mTOR pathway. Cell Cycle. 2013;12:3109–24.
78. Lin SL, Chang DC, Chang-Lin S, Lin CH, Wu DT, Chen DT, Ying SY. Mir-302 reprograms human skin cancer cells into a pluripotent ES-cell-like state. RNA. 2008;14:2115–24.
79. Utikal J, Maherali N, Kulalert W, Hochedlinger K. Sox2 is dispensable for the reprogramming of melanocytes and melanoma cells into induced pluripotent stem cells. J Cell Sci. 2009;122:3502–10.
80. Mathieu J, Zhang Z, Zhou W, Wang AJ, Heddleston JM, Pinna CM, Hubaud A, Stadler B, Choi M, Bar M, Tewari M, Liu A, Vessella R, Rostomily R, Born D, Horwitz M, Ware C, Blau CA, Cleary MA, Rich JN, Ruohola-Baker H. HIF induces human embryonic stem cell markers in cancer cells. Cancer Res. 2011;71:4640–52.
81. Zhang X, Dela Cruz F, Terry M, Remotti F, Matushansky I. Terminal differentiation and loss of tumorigenicity of human cancers via pluripotency based reprogramming. Oncogene. 2013;32:2249–60.
82. Moore JB, Loeb DM, Hong KU, Sorensen PH, Triche TJ, Lee DW, Barbato MI, Arceci RJ. Epigenetic reprogramming and re-differentiation of a Ewing sarcoma cell line. Front Cell Dev Biol. 2015;3:15.
83. Carrette JE, Pruszak J, Varadarajan M, Blomen VA, Gokhale S, Camargo FD, Wernig M, Jaenisch R, Brummelkamp TR. Generation of iPSCs from cultured human malignant cells. Blood. 2010;115:4039–42.
84. Laustriat D, Gide J, Peschanski M. Human pluripotent stem cells in drug discovery and predictive toxicology. Biochem Soc Trans. 2010;38:1051–7.
85. Singh VK, Kalsan M, Kumar N, Saini A, Chandra R. Induced pluripotent stem cells: applications in regenerative medicine, disease modeling, and drug discovery. Front Cell Dev Biol. 2015;3:1–18.
86. Li C, Ruan J, Yang M, Pan F, Gao G, Qu S, Shen YL, Dang YJ, Wang K, Jin W, Cui W. Human induced pluripotent stem cells labeled with fluorescent magnetic nanoparticles for targeted imaging and hyperthermia therapy for gastric cancer. Cancer Biol Med. 2015;12:163–74.
87. Yang J, Lam DH, Goh SS, Lee EX, Zhao Y, Tay FC, Chen C, Du S, Balasundaram G, Hahbazi M, Tham CK, Ng WH, Toh HC, Wang S. Tumor tropism of intravenously injected

human-induced pluripotent stem cell-derived neural stem cells and their gene therapy application in a metastatic breast cancer model. Stem Cells. 2012;30:1021–9.
88. Iwamoto H, Ojima T, Hayata K, Katsuda M, Miyazawa M, Iida T, Nakamura M, Nakamori M, Iwahashi M, Yamaue H. Antitumor immune response of dendritic cells (DCs) expressing tumor-associated antigens derived from induced pluripotent stem cells: in comparison to bone marrow-derived DCs. Int J Cancer. 2014;134:332–41.
89. Nishimura T, Kaneko S, Kawana-Tachikawa A, Tajima Y, Goto H, Zhu D, Nakayama-Hosoya K, Iriguchi S, Uemura Y, Shimizu T, Takayama N, Yamada D, Nishimura K, Ohtaka M, Watanabe N, Takahashi S, Iwamoto A, Koseki H, Nakanishi M, Eto K, Nakauchi H. Generation of rejuvenated antigen-specific T cells by reprogramming to pluripotency and redifferentiation. Cell Stem Cell. 2013;12:114–26.
90. Stroncek DF, Berger C, Cheever MA, Childs RW, Dudley ME, Flynn P, Gattinoni L, Heath JR, Kalos M, Marincola FM, Miller JS, Mostoslavsky G, Powell Jr DJ, Rao M, Restifo NP, Rosenberg SA, O'Shea J, Melief CJ. New directions in cellular therapy of cancer: a summary of the summit on cellular therapy for cancer. J Transl Med. 2012;15:10–48.
91. Watarai H, Yamada D, Fujii S, Taniguchi M, Koseki H. Induced pluripotency as a potential path towards iNKT cell-mediated cancer immunotherapy. Int J Hematol. 2012;95:624–31.
92. Kirkwood JM, Butterfield LH, Tarhini AA, Zarour H, Kalinski P, Ferrone S. Immunotherapy of cancer in 2012. CA Cancer J Clin. 2012;62:309–35.
93. Restifo NP, Dudley ME, Rosenberg SA. Adoptive immunotherapy for cancer: harnessing the T cell response. Nat Rev Immunol. 2012;12:269–81.
94. McKee MD, Fichera A, Nishimura MI. T cell immunotherapy. Front Biosci. 2007;12:919–32.
95. Lei F, Haque G, Xiong X, Song JJ. Directed differentiation of induced pluripotent stem cells towards T lymphocytes. J Vis Exp. 2012;63:e3986.
96. Vizcardo R, Masuda K, Yamada D, Ikawa D, Shimizu K, Fujii S, Koseki H, Kawamoto H. Regeneration of human tumor antigen-specific T cells from iPSCs derived from mature CD8(+) T cells. Cell Stem Cell. 2013;12:31–6.
97. Sachamitr P, Hackett S, Fairchild PJ. Induced pluripotent stem cells: challenges and opportunities for cancer immunotherapy. Front Immunol. 2014;5:176.
98. Themeli M, Kloss CC, Ciriello G, Fedorov VD, Perna F, Gonen M, et al. Generation of tumor targeted human T lymphocytes from induced pluripotent stem cells for cancer therapy. Nat Biotechnol. 2013;31:928–33.
99. Copier J, Bodman-Smith M, Dalgleish A. Current status and future applications of cellular therapies for cancer. Immunotherapy. 2011;3:507–16.
100. Cheng M, Chen Y, Xiao W, Sun R, Tian Z. NK cell-based immunotherapy for malignant diseases. Cell Mol Immunol. 2013;10:230–52.
101. Jung Y, Bauer G, Nolta JA. Concise review: induced pluripotent stem cell-derived mesenchymal stem cells: progress toward safe clinical products. Stem Cells. 2012;30:42–7.
102. Kim N, Cho SG. Clinical applications of mesenchymal stem cells. Korean J Intern Med. 2013;28:387–402.
103. Binato R, de Souza FT, Lazzarotto-Silva C, Du Rocher B, Mencalha A, Pizzatti L, Bouzas LF, Abdelhay A. Stability of human mesenchymal stem cells during in vitro culture: considerations for cell therapy. Cell Prolif. 2013;46:10–22.
104. Zar JH. Biostatistical analysis. 5th ed. Upper Saddle River, NJ: Prentice Hall; 2010.

Chapter 8
Banking of Human Umbilical Cord Blood Stem Cells and Their Clinical Applications

Dunia Jawdat

8.1 Introduction

Umbilical cord blood (UCB) is the remaining blood in the umbilical cord and placenta after the birth of a baby. It used to be discarded as medical waste until it was shown to possess a highly enriched stem cell source. UCB is now recognized as an alternative source of hematopoietic progenitor/stem cell (HPSC) to treat many malignant and nonmalignant diseases such as acute [1] and chronic leukemia [2], myelodysplastic syndromes [3], β thalassemia [4], aplastic anemia, Fanconi anemia [5], bone marrow failures, immune deficiencies [6], and metabolic diseases [7].

UCB contains both hematopoietic and non-hematopoietic progenitor cells. CD34, an integral membrane glycoprotein, is defined as the hallmark of HPSC with a frequency of 1 % within UCB's total nucleated cells (TNC) [8, 9]. The non-hematopoietic cell population includes endothelial progenitor cells and mesenchymal stem cells (MSCs) that under certain conditions have the capability to differentiate into osteoblasts, adipocytes, and chondroblasts. Today MSCs are used widely as a source for regenerative cell therapy and immune modulation in many diseases as reviewed by Zarrabi et al. [10].

The first evidence of human UCB possessing hematopoietic progenitor cells (HPC) was reported by Knudtzon in 1974, where in vitro cultured UCB cells showed increased concentration of colony-forming cells [11]. In 1982, Nakahata and Ogawa demonstrated the capability of UCB colony-forming cells to generate mono- and multipotential hemopoietic progenitors, which indicated the presence of more primitive HPC in UCB [12]. In the same year, a group of leading scientists

D. Jawdat, Ph.D.
Cord Blood Bank, King Abdullah International Medical Research Center (KAIMRC), King Saud bin Abdulaziz University for Health Sciences, Ministry of National Guard Health Affairs, P.O. Box 22490, Riyadh 11426, Saudi Arabia
e-mail: jawdatd@ngha.med.sa

E.M. Abdelalim (ed.), *Recent Advances in Stem Cells*, Stem Cell Biology and Regenerative Medicine, DOI 10.1007/978-3-319-33270-3_8

suggested a more useful role for UCB and the possibility of using it as a source of HPSC for transplantation [13]. This led to the formation of the Biocyte Corporation UCB Company to study the possibilities of UCB transplantation (UCBT). The company was founded by Boyse, Bard, Lewis Thomas, Broxmeyer, Harvey Cantor, Rodman Rockefeller, and George Strong. Broxmeyer then focused on studying UCB biology and cryopreservation, which recognized UCB as a possible source for HPSC transplantation and led to the first UCBT. Broxymeyer used the colony-forming unit (CFU) assay to validate the engraftment capability of UCB, he examined more than 100 samples before and after cryopreservation. He found that HPSC from UCB have a higher proliferative capacity when compared to bone marrow HPSC. He also showed that the number of HPSC from a single collection was comparable to the number of HPSC used in successful bone marrow transplants [14].

The first UCBT was performed in 1988, through collaboration between Gluckman and colleagues from the Hospital Saint Louis in Paris, and Broxmeyer from Indiana University School of Medicine. The patient with Fanconi anemia at that time was 5 years old. The UCB was collected from his sister at birth by Douglas at the New York University Medical Center, after the prenatal diagnosis from amniotic fluid confirmed no Fanconi anemia and HLA identical to her brother the patient. The UCB was preserved by Broxmeyer and transported to Paris for infusion after receiving the permission from the French National Ethics. The patient was conditioned with low dose of cyclophosphamide and infused with the thawed UCB without any separation or washing to avoid any extra loss of cells. The first signs of engraftment occurred on day 22 with subsequent hematological reconstitution and donor chimerism with no GVHD. The patient is currently healthy, 27 years after UCBT [15]. This successful transplant confirms that UCB is an alternative source for bone marrow; it can fully reconstitute the hematopoietic system; it can be collected at birth; and cryopreserved without losing their potency. After this successful transplant, there has been a remarkable interest in the usage of UCB as an alternative source for transplantation. Consequently, the idea of establishing an inventory to preserve UCB for future use became appealing. Thereafter, many CB banks (CBBs) have been established and over the last decade it became a popular option worldwide.

8.2 Cord Blood Banking

A CBB is a facility that preserves UCB for future use. Initially, CBBs were established by hospitals, charities, or nonprofit institutions to preserve donated CB units for anyone in need of a hematopoietic stem cell (HSC) transplant. The first cord blood bank was established in New York in 1992 under the direction of Dr. Pablo Rubinstein, after being awarded a grant from the National Institutes of Health (NIH) to establish a national CB program. Afterwards, other public banks were established to collect, process, store, and supply UCB in the United Kingdom,

France, Germany, Italy, and elsewhere. Subsequently, private organizations established CBBs for profit offering CB storage for donors or family related use, mainly as an insurance against future illnesses. Since then CBBs are classified into public and private. More recently, mixed or hybrid CBBs were established which offer a combination of public and private storage. The total cost of UCB banking is approximately $2000. Private CBBs charge approximately $1400–$2300 for collection and processing and then around $125 per year for storage. Yet charges may vary between banks according to their policy [16].

The potential advantages and disadvantages of each bank category to the general public remain controversial. Public banking is widely supported by many organizations such as the American Academy of Pediatrics, The American Society for Blood and Marrow Transplantation, and the American Congress of Obstetricians and Gynecologists. Although there are more than 22 million bone marrow donors in international registries, some patients, especially with certain race or ethnicity, only have 20–30 % chance of finding a matched unrelated bone marrow donor [17]. On the other hand, the chance of clinical usage of autologous UCB stored in private banks was estimated to be around 0.4 %. Several studies have looked into the probability of needing autologous transplant; one study estimated the probability to be between 1:20,000 and 1:200,000 [18]. Another study estimated the probability of neonates using their private stored UCB between 1:75,000 and 1:100,000. The variation in the estimates is reflected mainly by the different criteria used in each study such as age and disease [19]. Also, in the case of blood malignancies, it is unlikely that a child's own UCB will be appropriate for transplant and a unit from the public banks would be used instead.

The main advantages of using UCB for HSC transplantation is the ready availability, quick search and procurement process, safety, pain- and risk- free to the donors, long-term preservation, low risk of viral contamination and lower immunogenicity when compared to bone marrow. The less stringent HLA matching requirement increases the probability of finding a match for racial and ethnic minority patients and those with rarer HLA types [20, 21]. HPSC from UCB show higher proliferative ability than those from bone marrow and lower incidences of GVHD after transplantation. As of writing, more than 600,000 UCB units are stored in public banks, and more than 30,000 UCB units have been used for transplantation.

The process of CB banking includes donor recruitment, UCB collection, processing, testing, cryopreservation, storage, listing, search, selection, reservation, release, and distribution for administration (Fig. 8.1). Each country has its own regulation of UCB collection and storage. For example, in the United States, it is regulated by the Food and Drug Administration. In the United Kingdom, it is regulated by Human Tissue Authority. Some countries or states also require accreditation by either The American Association of Blood Banks (AABB) or The Foundation for the Accreditation of Cellular Therapy (FACT) to be legally permitted to collect and store UCB. To date, several organizations have been established such as Eurocord, The International NetCord Foundation (NetCord), and FACT, mainly to facilitate the use of UCB in transplantation, promote

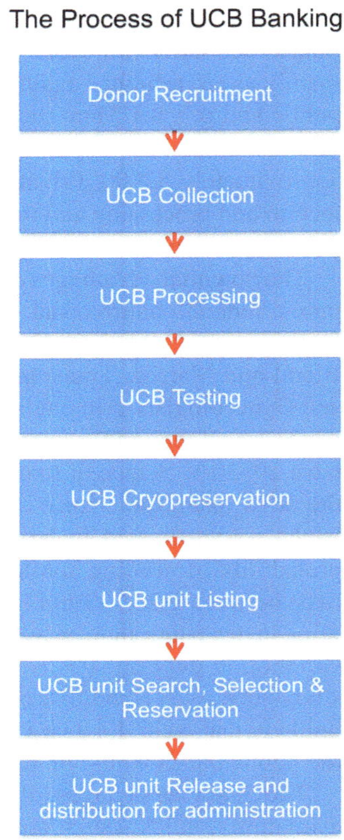

Fig. 8.1 The process of UCB Banking starts with donor recruitment, UCB collection, processing, testing, cryopreservation, storage, listing, search, selection, reservation, release, and distribution for administration

developments in clinical use of CB cells, provide standards to ensure high and uniform quality of CB units, and provide professional and public education.

Eurocord was founded by Professor Eliane Gluckman in 1995. It had been originally built as an international registry of CBT and stem cell therapies for malignant and nonmalignant hematological diseases, then diversified its activities to the field of Autoimmune Disease where it operates in association with the European Group for Blood and Marrow Transplantation (EBMT) and the "Société Française de Greffe de Moelle" (SFGM) and to collect and validate clinical data of patients transplanted. FACT is a nonprofit organization that provides standards for high quality medical and laboratory practice in cellular therapies. It was co-founded in 1996 by the International Society for Cellular Therapy (ISCT) and the American Society of Blood and Marrow Transplantation (ASBMT). FACT inspect and accredit qualified facilities after tracing the entire life of a cell product from donor selection to collection, processing, storage, release, and ultimately administration to a patient. NetCord is a nonprofit organization established in 1997. It promotes studies and research on UCB to improve cellular therapy. NetCord links CBB inventory to international registries to permit the identification of the most suitable UCB unit for each patient requiring a transplant. CBBs associated with NetCord comprise the largest source of high-quality CB grafts for patients in need of HSC transplantation. In 1999 NetCord began collaboration with FACT to promote the highest quality in CB products. Together in 2000 they published the first NetCord-FACT International Standards.

8.2.1 Donor Recruitment

CB donation starts with a donor recruitment process which can be conducted by CB bank staff, midwives, gynecologists, or nurses working in the labor and delivery clinics. During recruitment pregnant mothers become educated about UCB donation. The donation is a voluntary process and mothers have the right to refuse donation without prejudice. Prospective donor mothers must sign an informed consent form and agree to a health check questionnaire in a private interview, while fully conscious and not in active labor. The consent form clearly explains the process of donation, banking, applicable risks, discomforts, benefits, and alternatives. Signing the consent form confirms the willingness to donate UCB of the infant upon delivery, and allows a general health assessment to exclude any infectious diseases, genetic disorders, and history of malignancies within the family. The bank will then check the suitability of the prospective donor mother for UCB donation and select the donor mothers in good health for donation to reduce any risks to the mother, infant, staff, and UCB recipient. Prospective donor mother selection must comply with national legislation and regulatory requirements.

The donor mother health check questionnaire will be answered by the prospective donor mother to her best knowledge and assisted by the recruiter to explain any unclear questions. This questionnaire should include: medical history of noncommunicable diseases (hematological disorders, immunological diseases, malignancies, skin diseases, psychiatric disorders, metabolic and endocrine diseases, respiratory diseases, central nervous system diseases, renal and urinary diseases); medical history of transmissible diseases (hepatitis B virus (HBV), hepatitis C virus (HCV), human immunodeficiency virus (HIV), human T-cell lymphotropic viruses type I and II (HTLV I–II), West Nile virus, Malaria, Chagas disease, Babesiosis, Leishmaniasis, Syphilis, Gonorrhea, Tuberculosis, Prion disease, Creutzfeldt–Jakob disease); country of residence and travel history, medical and surgical intervention; immunization and vaccination; medications; blood transfusion; organ or tissue or stem cell transplantation; family history of inherited diseases; and high risk behaviors (sexual behaviors, drug abuse, detention in prison and penal institutions, tattoos, piercing and acupuncture) [22]. Signing the consent form will allow the bank's staff to access the medical record of the donor mother/infant to verify the answers within the questionnaire and to check the current pregnancy status.

8.2.2 Cord Blood Collection

At the day of donation, prospective donor mothers should be reevaluated for good health by reviewing her medical status and the current pregnancy. Mothers with any sign of current infection, evidence of illicit needle use, transfusion or hemadilution (infusion of > 2 L of fluid), evidence of genital herpes or human papilloma virus, gestational age < 34 weeks, stillborn infant or fetal malformation should be excluded from the donation process. CB collection can be done by a well-trained CBB staff, delivery physician, or midwife. At the time of delivery, the UCB assigned collector should reassess the suitability of donation based on the mother's health, infant health, and process of delivery. If abnormalities to the infant or umbilical cord or placenta appear during the delivery (abnormal umbilical cord, placental trauma, tear or malodorous, any suspicion of chorioamnionitis, abnormal health of the infant, and ABGAR score < 5) that can affect the quality or safety of the collection then the UCB should not be collected. The collection process must not start until the safe delivery of the baby and assurance of the safety of the donor mother. This should be coordinated in advance with the midwife/physician to ensure smooth and fast recovery of the UCB after delivery. It is important to collect the blood immediately after clamping the umbilical cord to avoid blood coagulation and to maximize the collecting volume. CB can be collected either ex utero or in utero from both vaginal and caesarean deliveries after safe delivery of the baby. Ex utero collection is collecting the CB after the placenta is expelled, while in in utero collection CB is collected before the placenta is expelled.

Briefly, the collection process is a venipuncture to the cord and blood drainage to a sterile bag within 5 min. However, due to the high risk of contamination from the vaginal fluid or colon derived fluid the umbilical cord needs to be thoroughly cleaned and disinfected. The umbilical cord should be clamped 3–5 cm above the umbilicus, then swabbed with chlorhexidine. A 4–8 $inch^2$ area should be disinfected for 10 s using povidone iodine, then alcohol gauze. After approximately 5 s, a needle should be introduced into the umbilical cord vein. The needle is connected to a collection bag. It is recommended to withdraw the first 2–3 mL to remove any contaminated blood from the needle puncture; this is applicable for any collection bag supplied with sampling satellite bag. This blood is usually used for any labor and delivery requested tests on the UCB.

During collection the collecting bag should be lowered to increase the blood flow by gravity and gently mixed with the anticoagulants present in the collection bag to prevent clotting of the collected blood. If during collection vessel wall puncture, clotting or vein collapse occurs, a new puncture site should be disinfected and scrubbed for a second needle puncture. Each bank has its own volume threshold. However a minimum of 40 mL should be collected for potential future clinical use. After a successful collection, UCB will be transported to a lab for processing within 48 h. From the time of collection until the time of processing the UCB should be monitored for time, temperature, and humidity according to the bank's policy and procedure.

8.2.3 Donor Mother Testing

A donor mother sample must be collected within 7 days of delivery and transported to the processing lab for communicable disease testing (Hepatitis B surface antigen, anti-hepatitis B core antibodies, anti-hepatitis C antibodies, anti-HIV 1/2 antibodies, HTLV I–II, cytomegalovirus (CMV), Syphilis and nucleic acid testing) and for future testing if required. A serum sample DNA sample from the birth mother should be stored in the bank for future testing. To maintain the confidentiality of the donor mother and infant, a standard identifier should be used to ensure international consistency to support the transfer, traceability, and transplantation. It is highly recommended to use the international identification, the global standard for the terminology, identification, coding, and labeling of medical products of human origin, organized by the International Council for Commonality in Blood Banking Automation (ICCBBA) [23]. The CBB should maintain indefinite linkage between the UCB unit, donor mother, and the donor infant records.

8.2.4 Cord Blood Processing and Cryopreservation

The HPSC population resides within the mononuclear cell fraction of the collected CB. For that different strategies have been utilized by CBBs to assure maximum recovery of this cell fraction. Two methods can be used to process UCB prior to cryopreservation. The first method is based on red blood cell reduction, using centrifugation and density gradient medium such as hetastarch to isolate buffy coat enriched mononuclear cells. The reduced final UCB volume of around 20 mL is then cryopreserved using 5 mL of 50 % dimethyl sulfoxide (DMSO). The second method is based on plasma removal and the whole remaining cellular part including red blood cells, white blood cells, and HPSC is cryopreserved. The majority of CBBs use the red blood cell reduction method, mainly to reduce the amount of red blood cells within the stored product, as it has been shown that red blood cells can negatively affect cell viability and potency after thawing [24]. Also this method is economically more efficient for banks in terms of storage space and uses less DMSO which is toxic to blood cells if exposed for more than 30 min before freezing or after thawing [25]. Therefore DMSO is immediately removed or diluted after UCB thawing before transplantation. On the other hand, the plasma removal method requires more storage space and consumes more DMSO during cryopreservation. It is considered cheaper in terms of processing but more expensive to store and more complicated to thaw [26]. Before an UCB unit is cryopreserved, it is recommended to be tested for sterility, TNC and CD34+ count, viability, and CFU potency. A minimum of 800×10^6 TNC within the final product prior to cryopreservation is recommended for potential clinical use.

In order to store UCB units for long-term periods, DMSO is added immediately after processing under cold condition in a final 10 % concentration. After that, the unit is frozen under controlled rate temperature (1–3° per min). This process will maintain cell viability and avoids intracellular ice crystal formation. Although some banks are still utilizing the "dump freezing" technique, which is freezing a unit under uncontrolled conditions at −80 °C for 2–3 h before transfer into the final storage location. This may affect cell viability and potency. The final frozen product can either be stored in liquid or vapor phase nitrogen for up to 20 years without significant effect on cell viability and function as previously reported by Broxmeyer [27].

8.2.5 Cord Blood Unit Listing

After a UCB unit is stored it should remain under quarantine status and not listed for search until a full review of the donation's record is complete to ensure the safety and quality of the unit. A donation's record includes donor mother suitability, infant health, collection process and unit's acceptance for processing, testing, cryopreservation, and storage. Listing CB units for search request could be within a single center, or a group of selected organizations, nationally, or internationally. To register UCB units on a database that is accessible by international cancer centers, the bank should meet certain accreditations or standards such as FACT or AABB.

8.2.6 Cord Blood Unit Search, Selection, and Reservation

Once CB transplantation is indicated, a CB unit search can be initiated to find a compatible unit of an appropriate cell dose from the listed CB units within a bank or registry. A search request should include at a minimum: Transplant Center name and address, requesting physician name, expected transplant date, expected date for CB unit delivery to the Transplant Center, requester name and request date, patient name and medical record number or ID, date of birth/age, sex and ethnicity, ABO/Rh blood group, molecular HLA typing for HLA-A, -B, -C, -DRB1, and -DQB1 genes, patient's weight, disease diagnosis and phase. Several banks use for HLA-A, -B, -C, -DRB1, and -DQB1 using all ten alleles while others only base their search on HLA-A, -B, and -DRB1. The search will reveal a list of UCB units from which the best 6–8 units will be presented to the Transplant Center for final selection. The order of the units within the search list depends on the HLA degree match and cell dose starting with 10/10 (6/6) HLA matching level, then 9/10 (5/6) and finally 8/10 (4/6) prioritizing HLA-DRB1 match. In each HLA matching level the units are ordered based on the TNC content, from highest to lowest. After the Transplant Center receives the list of the CB units, the transplant physician will select the most appropriate unit based on Transplant Center criteria and preference.

The transplant physician usually requests the bank to reserve the selected unit for further confirmatory testing including HLA typing, CFU potency, cell enumeration, and viability. The second best unit is also selected to be reserved in case of double UCB transplant or as a backup for a single UCBT. The cord blood bank or registry can provide assistance to the transplant physician in the selection process if required.

8.2.7 Cord Blood Unit Release and Distribution for Administration

Once a reservation request is received at a CBB, the bank will reserve the selected unit(s) and review the CBU report which should include donor/infant eligibility, CB unit and maternal transmissible disease markers test results for HIV 1/2, HTLV I/II, Hepatitis B, Hepatitis C, syphilis, and CMV, sterility test, blood group, infant donor sex, ethnicity, 6-month donor follow-up findings and, confirmatory testing on the CB unit attached segment for HLA typing, CFU, TNC and CD34+ count to ensure the data provided is correct and meets all requirements for CB unit shipment.

8.3 Advantages of Using Umbilical Cord Blood Stem Cells

CB has many advantages as an attractive HPSC source for transplantation purposes compared to bone marrow and peripheral blood HPSC. CB collection is a safe and simple procedure without causing pain or medical risks to the mother or the newborn baby, as it does not interfere with the delivery; CB is collected, tested, and long-term preserved in advance and thus readily available for anyone in need in the future with a shorter searching time when compared to unrelated donors for bone marrow transplants.

CB is highly enriched with more primitive HSCs than bone marrow and peripheral blood [28]. The percentage of surface expressing CD34 cells in CB is approximately 0.02–1.43 %, 0.5–5 % in bone marrow, and < 0.01 % in peripheral blood. The percentage of $CD34^{+}CD38^{-}$ cells (cells mainly in the G_0 phase) and $CD34^{+}$ $HLA\text{-}DR^{-}$ cells in CB is 4 % and only 1 % in bone marrow [29].

CB cells have higher proliferative capacity than bone marrow and peripheral blood; they are capable of longer hematopoiesis and can produce large numbers of long-term repopulating stem cells. A study by Mok et al., showed that the numbers of BFU-E, CFU-GM, and CFU-GEMM in CB units were at least five times more than in bone marrow [30].

CB cells have decreased immune reactivity due to the immaturity of the immune system, half of the B lymphocyte subpopulation are immature with a phenotype $CD19^{+}$ $CD5^{+}$, most of the T lymphocytes are $CD3^{-}$ $CD8^{-}$, which is a T cell precursor. This immaturity of the effector cells decreases the alloreactivity of the lymphocytes and therefore reduces the risk of GVHD [31]; CB transplants is thus less stringent in HLA matching requirement which increases the probability of finding a match for racial and ethnic minority patients and those with rarer HLA types [20, 21].

Up to date more than 600,000 UCB units are stored in public banks, and more than 30,000 UCB units have been used for transplantation.

8.4 Umbilical Cord Blood Clinical Applications

8.4.1 Pediatric Cord Blood Transplantation

After the success of the first UCBT, investigators and clinicians became more confident in the use of UCB. A study in 1995 by Wagner describes results on children with malignant and nonmalignant disorders receiving sibling UCBT with 0–1 mismatches. Engraftment at day 50 was 85 %, acute GVHD was 3 %, and survival rate at 1.6 years was 72 %. Primary graft failure occurred in 15 % of patients. Wagner subsequently in 1996 demonstrated the outcomes of unrelated UCBT with either HLA matched or 1–3 HLA mismatches. Engraftment at day 50 was 100 %, acute GVHD was 11 %, and survival rate at 6 months was 65 % [32]. In 1997 Gluckman reported the Eurocord registry experience in related and unrelated UCBT. For recipients of related UCBT, engraftment at day 60 was 79 %, acute GVHD was 18 %, and survival rate at 1 year was 55 %. For recipients of unrelated UCBT, engraftment at day 60 was 89 %, acute GVHD was 32 %, and survival rate at 1 year was 31 % [33]. Baker and colleagues compared in 2001 receiving 0–3 HLA mismatched UCBT with recipients of unrelated matched BMT. The survival rate of mismatched UCBT was similar to the BMT group. However, the engraftment time was poorly affected by the number of mismatches. Eapen and colleagues compared children receiving HLA matched and mismatched unrelated UCBT with HLA matched and mismatched unrelated BMT. Results indicated delayed engraftment and increased TRM with UCBT with low cell dose and leukemia-free survival was the same among the groups [34].

The first prospective study was a multicenter known as the COBLT published in 2008 by Kurtzberg et al. presenting the outcome of unrelated UCBT in 191 pediatric patients with hematological malignancies. Median time to neutrophil and platelet engraftment was 27 and 173 days, respectively. Graft failure occurred in 11 % of patients and the 2 year OS was 42 % [35]. Subsequently, several investigators emphasized the importance of cell dose and HLA on engraftment and TRM. Wagner et al. showed that receiving 0–2 HLA mismatches with a cell dose of 1.7×10^5 resulted in improved outcomes [36]. Few other studies showed that receiving a TNC dose more than 3.7×10^7 had a better chance of engraftment and survival. As a result the importance of HLA matching and cell dose was clearly highlighted. Thus, a minimum cell dose for UCBT was established and having more than 3/6 HLA mismatches was not recommended.

8.4.2 Adult Cord Blood Transplantation

Initially, UCBT was seen in children only due to the small volume of cells that was thought not enough for a successful engraftment in adult patients. However, due to the promising results in pediatrics UCBT was also established in adults. Most of the early retrospective studies showed poor outcome compared to pediatric though most of these patients received low doses of UCB, even lower than what was recommended for pediatric UCBT.

Laughlin and colleagues in 2001 have conducted a study on the engraftment and survival in adults with malignant and nonmalignant hematological disorders, receiving unrelated UCBT. The median time of neutrophils and platelet engraftment was 27 and 99 days, respectively. Graft failure occurred in 10 % and OS was 26 %. The cell dose of infused TNC was only 1.6×10^7/kg with 0–3 HLA mismatches [37]. Another study by Rocha compared the outcome of unrelated UCBT to matched bone marrow recipients in patients with acute leukemia. Acute GVHD was lower in the UCBT group but the time of neutrophils engraftment in UCBT was significantly delayed, primary graft failure occurred in 20 % patients vs. 7 % patients that received BMT. Chronic GVHD, relapse, TRM, and overall survival were not different between the two groups. If we look at the cell dose infused, TNC in UCBT (2.3×10^7/kg) was much lower than for BMT (2.9×10^8/kg) which could be the reason for this outcome [38]. Eapen et al. presented a similar study comparing UCBT with BMT and peripheral blood progenitor cell recipients. Again the rate of acute GVHD was lower in UCBT patients, but with higher TRM [39].

8.5 Limitations of Using Umbilical Cord Blood Stem cells

The use of CB in transplantation has some limitations mainly due to the low volume of blood that can be collected from the umbilical cord and placenta after delivery, which affects the numbers of TNC and CD34 within a CBU. Major challenges of using CB includes delayed engraftment; increased risk of graft failure; transplant related mortality; lack of donor lymphocytes for immune therapy; and the variability in the standards between different CBBs around the world reflecting cell recovery after thawing and overall quality of the CB units. Many efforts focused on improving CB transplantation outcomes. Several strategies have been developed to increase the number of HPC in a single CBU and to accelerate engraftment. The two main approaches that have been used are expanding the HPSC ex vivo before transplantation and modulating the HSPC functionality to increase the homing to the bone marrow niche after transplantation.

8.5.1 Cord Blood Ex Vivo Expansion

Different methods have been studied to mediate HPSC expansion. An early study using a combination of cytokines such as SCF, IL-3, IL-6 thrombopoietin, and GCS-F showed an increase in the number of TNC and CD34 but did not affect the time of engraftment [40]. Another method was tried using tetra-ethylenepentamine (TEPA), a copper chelator, which was suggested to block HPSC maturation and therefore reduce the rate of differentiation. Culturing CB cells with cytokines plus TEPA shown a high fold of expansion in TNC with no difference in engraftment but with a higher than expected rate of GVHD [41]. A more successful approach was achieved using two donor CBUs also known as 'double cord'. In this method the patient receives either two unmanipulated CBUs in which outcomes are comparable to bone marrow transplants or one expanded CBU and one unmanipulated unit. Receiving two unmanipulated CBUs is being used as an alternative to a single CBU mainly for adult CB transplantation when cell dosage is low.

Another approach is using mesenchymal stromal cells (MSCs), as they secrete many cytokines and ligands that are important for HSPC growth and expansion. This approach is the best ex vivo niche model as perivascular niches exist in the bone marrow and MSC have been suggested to rise from prevascular cells in the bone marrow. Several preclinical studies show a great expansion of UCB mononuclear cells when cultured with MSC, which resulted in 6–20-fold increase in TNC, 8–37-fold increase in CD34+ cells, and 3–200-fold increase in CFU potency. A clinical study using UCB after MSC-mediated expansion was conducted recently. All patients received an expanded UCB unit either derived from family members or from third party donors in addition to an unmanipulated UCB unit. The expanded unit showed 12-fold increase in TNC, 30-fold increase in CD34+ cells, and a 17-fold increase in CFU potency. The median time of engraftment was 15 days for patient who received expanded unit from family and 23 days for patients who received expanded unit from third party. Chimerism data showed unmanipulated UCB unit was responsible for long-term engraftment but expanded unit can engraft but mostly at the earlier time frame [42].

A recent approach for ex vivo expansion is the use of Nicotinamide, a form of vitamin B3 that can inhibit the function of SIRT1, a prototypical sirtuin family member, through its oxidation effect on nicotinamide adenine dinucleotide (NAD). SIRT1 has several biological effects on cell activities and its inhibition has been shown to highly affect HSC differentiation and facilitate expansion of HPC. This approach is still very recent, only one clinical trail has been conducted with 11 patients which showed that Nicotinamide can induce a 486-fold expansion in TNC and 72-fold expansion in CD34. The median time of engraftment was 13 days [43].

Two or double UCBT (dUCBT) are highly recommended as a strategy to increase cell dose and engraftment when the number of TNC in a single UCB is not enough. A study by Barker presents the outcome of adult patients with hematologic malignancy receiving two cords with 0–2 mismatches and a median TNC dose of 3.5×10^7/kg. The median time of neutrophils engraftment was 23 days, no graft failure, acute GVHD was 65 %, and 1 year DFS was 57 % [44]. In 2009, MacMillan conducted a comparative study between single UCBT and dUCBT. Chronic GVHD was similar in both groups while acute GVHD was higher in patients with dUCBT but the rate of TRM was lower in patients with dUCBT (24 vs. 39 %) [45]. A prospective study by Kindwall-Keller also comparing single UCBT vs. dUCBT was conducted in 2012. The cell dose of TNC was 2.5×10^7/kg in single UCBT and combined 3.0×10^7/kg in dUCBT. All grafts had a 0–2 HLA mismatches. The median time of neutrophils engraftment was 25 days in the single cord group and 23 days in the double cord group. The median time of platelet engraftment was 39 days in the single cord group and 57 days in the double cord group. No difference acute GVHD. Overall survival at 60 months was 26 % in the single cord group and 39 % in the double cord group [46]. The reason for contrasting results between single and double cord in adult patients is not clear but could be due the transplant center, patient condition, patient age, and conditioning. In pediatric patients comparing single cord to double cord showed no difference in overall survival and increased rate of GVHD after dUCBT.

8.5.2 Cord Blood Homing to Their Niches

Some strategies have focused on UCB HSPC homing to their niche to improve the time of engraftment. One of the first attempts was injecting the UCB directly into the bone marrow. Clinical trials have shown reduced rates of GVHD and good rates of engraftment but the median time was more than 20 days [47–49]. It is well established that chemokine stromal cell derived factor 1 (SDF1), secreted by bone marrow stromal cells, is an important mediator of HSPC homing to the bone marrow [50, 51]. Cell surface protein dipeptidyl peptidase 4 (DPP4) is a negative regulator of SDF1, which can reduce the ability of SDF1 to recruit HPC to the bone marrow. Inhibiting DPP4 has been shown to increase homing of hematopoietic cells in animal models [52]. A recent clinical trial using Sitagliptin, a DPP4 inhibitor, showed around 80 % reduction of DPP4 activity but did not markedly improve the time of neutrophil engraftment [53]. Two more recent approaches have been used to mediate UCB HSPC homing. In one approach they used complement fragment 3a (C3a) which was earlier reported to enhance CD34 cells migration toward SDF1 in vitro [54]. In the clinical trial they primed UCB cells with C3a before transplantation. However, the results of engraftment were not much different from the control patients which might be due to the concentration of C3a or other factors that need to be optimized [55]. In the other approach, they used a long-acting form of prostaglandin E2 (PGE2). Several animal studies have demonstrated enhanced UCB engraftment and homing by PGE2 [56]. However, a clinical trial using PGE2- primed UCB did not show a difference in time of engraftment to control patients. Subsequently, optimizing time, temperature, and media showed a slight advantage of engraftment but needs to be confirmed with further studies [57]. To date, using UCB expansion strategies have shown better results in terms of time to engraftment however homing strategies might still have important roles in future application.

8.6 Cord Blood and Hypoxic-Ischemic Encephalopathy

Hypoxic-ischemic encephalopathy (HIE) is an injury to the brain caused by oxygen deprivation in newborn infants, and a leading cause of death or severe impairment such as epilepsy, developmental delay, motor impairment, neurodevelopmental delay, and cognitive impairment among infants. Hypothermia is currently the standard therapy to treat newborns with HIE worldwide. Unfortunately, more than 30 % of infants treated with this cooling approach die or develop neurological and functional impairment [58, 59]. Stem cells have great potential in regenerative therapy in a variety of diseases including neurological disorders. Several in vitro studies have shown that UCB cells can differentiate into cells with characteristics of neurons, oligodendrocytes, astrocytes, and microglial cells [60, 61]. In addition, UCB has been clinically proven to prevent neurological deterioration in patients with Krabbe disease [62] and Hurler syndrome [63]. Also having the advantage of UCB being readily available after birth compared to other stem cell sources, encourages investigators to conduct studies on autologous CB infusion in neonates with HIE. This is particularly important for HIE therapy, where timing plays an important factor as shown with hypothermia.

A recent clinical trial has been conducted on infants with HIE receiving autologous CB. In this study infants receiving autologous CB infusions with hypothermia have been compared with infants receiving hypothermia alone. The results showed similar hospital outcomes, which includes mortality, oral feeds, and discharge. The 1 year outcome survival using Bayley III scores was over 85 in 74 % of CB and hypothermia recipients and 41 % of hypothermia recipients alone [64]. This confirms the safety and feasibility of autologous CB infusions for HIE neonates. However, a Phase II study is needed to provide further data on the feasibility and efficacy of this approach.

8.7 Cord Blood and Cerebral Palsy

Cerebral palsy (CP) is a general term for a group of neurological conditions caused by brain injury that affects movement and coordination. In most cases, CP occurs during or shortly after birth. The symptoms usually become apparent during the first years of a child's life, which include muscle stiffness, uncontrolled body movements, and coordination problems. There are several methods available to treat many of its symptoms however; there is no cure for CP. A clinical trial using allogeneic UCBT has been conducted on children with CP. In this study UCB was administered concomitant with recombinant human erythropoietin (rhEPO) to boost the efficacy of UCB, as it has neurotrophic effects. Ninety-six children with CP were randomly assigned to the pUCB group, which received allogeneic UCB potentiated with rhEPO; the EPO group, which received rhEPO and placebo UCB; and the Control group, which received placebo UCB and placebo rhEPO. Scales after 6 months showed that the pUCB group had significantly higher mental and motor scores compared to the other groups which suggest potential benefits of this approach [65]. However, allogeneic UCBT requires immunosuppression of the child, which can cause inflammatory and neurotoxic side effects and may reduce therapeutic efficacy. A few studies were conducted using autologous CBT on children with CP. In 2011, Papadopoulos reported a case where two toddlers presented with spastic diplegia received autologous CBT with G-CSF and hyperbaric oxygen therapy. The two toddlers improved significantly in motor ability after transplant. Another UCBT was reported in a child after severe global hypoxic-ischemic brain damage caused by cardiac arrest. The boy presented quadriplegic CP on the day of CB infusion and showed beneficial therapeutic effects few weeks after the transplant [66]. In a cohort study by Lee and colleagues on 20 children with CP, only 5/20 children showed neurological improvement [67]. The study included different types of CP and children ranging from 23 to 91 months of age which might be the reason for this discrepancy in efficacy as it seemed that younger patients responded better to treatment as well as different types of CP. Therefore, more clinical trials are necessary to define which type of patients will potentially benefit from such procedure.

8.8 Cord Blood and HIV Infection

So far the only cure for HIV/AIDS patients was seen after receiving hematopoietic cell transplantation (HCT). This accomplishment was demonstrated by Hütter et al. [68], in an HIV patient who received HCT using peripheral blood stem cells from an HLA-matched donor who had a CCR5-Δ32/Δ32 mutation. CCR5 is a co-receptor for HIV entry into CCR5 CD4 T cells and carrying a homozygous depletion of a 32 bp in the CCR5 gene confers a natural resistance to HIV. After the HCT, the patient has remained without any evidence of HIV infection for more than 8 years after discontinuation of antiretroviral drug therapy. Identifying HLA-matched CCR5-Δ32/Δ32 adult donors who are also homozygous for CCR5-Δ32 allele is not readily feasible as the prevalence of this mutation is less than 1 %. HCT from UCB on the other hand can be much more easily accomplished due to the less stringent HLA matching requirement. After this successful HCT, an inventory of cryopreserved CCR5-Δ32/Δ32 UCB units was developed at StemCyte international Cord Blood Center. However, only a few attempts were so far conducted using UCB as a cure for HIV with rather poor clinical outcomes due to cancer or post-transplant infections [69, 70]. Nevertheless, HCT from CCR5-Δ32/Δ32 UCB still remains a promising option to cure HIV.

8.9 Conclusion and Future Perspectives

In recent years UCB has become an alternative source of HPSC to peripheral blood and bone marrow for allogeneic HSC transplantation. The main advantages of using UCB for HSC transplantation is the ready availability, quick search and procurement process, safety, long-term preservation, high proliferative ability, low immunogenicity and lower incidences of GVHD after transplantation when compared to bone marrow and peripheral blood. Since the first CB transplantation many CBBs have been established worldwide. The full process of CB banking includes donor recruitment, UCB collection, processing, testing, cryopreservation, storage, listing, search, selection, reservation, release, and distribution for administration. Unfortunately, variations exist between CBBs in handling CB, which highly reflects on the quality of the CB units stored and availability for transplantation. However, having certain accreditations like FACT, for example, can provide some assurance about the quality of the CB unit to the transplant centers. To date, UCB has shown successful results in clinical applications in treating many malignant and nonmalignant diseases. Higher doses of cells are recommended to decrease the rates of graft failure. In Adults, results seem promising especially with double cord infusion. I personally anticipate that the use of CB will continue to grow not only in the field of HPSC transplantation but also in the field of immunotherapy and regenerative medicine. CB has the advantage of containing several subpopulations of non-hematopoietic cells, such as MSC and endothelial progenitor cells that have great potential to be used in therapy to treat many diseases including diabetes and neurological disorders. Although the use of CB has not increased in the last 2 years mainly due to the use of haploidentical donor transplants, I still believe that CB is still new and a full understanding of its potential is not yet developed. Much remains to be learned and understood to be able to take full advantage of these ready-for-use cells.

References

1. Rocha V, et al. Comparison of outcomes of unrelated bone marrow and umbilical cord blood transplants in children with acute leukemia. Blood. 2001;97(10):2962–71.
2. Laughlin MJ, et al. Outcomes after transplantation of cord blood or bone marrow from unrelated donors in adults with leukemia. N Engl J Med. 2004;351(22):2265–75.
3. Woodard P, et al. Unrelated donor bone marrow transplantation for myelodysplastic syndrome in children. Biol Blood Marrow Transplant. 2011;17(5):723–8.
4. Ruggeri A, et al. Umbilical cord blood transplantation for children with thalassemia and sickle cell disease. Biol Blood Marrow Transplant. 2011;17(9):1375–82.
5. Gluckman E, et al. Results of unrelated cord blood transplant in Fanconi anemia patients: risk factor analysis for engraftment and survival. Biol Blood Marrow Transplant. 2007;13 (9):1073–82.
6. Tsuji Y, et al. Hematopoietic stem cell transplantation for 30 patients with primary immunodeficiency diseases: 20 years experience of a single team. Bone Marrow Transplant. 2006;37 (5):469–77.

7. Gratwohl A, Baldomero H. European survey on clinical use of cord blood for hematopoietic and non-hematopoietic indications. Transfus Apher Sci. 2010;42(3):265–75.
8. Sutherland DR, Keating A. The CD34 antigen: structure, biology, and potential clinical applications. J Hematother. 1992;1(2):115–29.
9. Sutherland DR, et al. Sensitive detection and enumeration of CD34+ cells in peripheral and cord blood by flow cytometry. Exp Hematol. 1994;22(10):1003–10.
10. Zarrabi M, et al. Potential uses for cord blood mesenchymal stem cells. Cell J. 2014;15 (4):274–81.
11. Knudtzon S. In vitro growth of granulocytic colonies from circulating cells in human cord blood. Blood. 1974;43(3):357–61.
12. Nakahata T, Ogawa M. Hemopoietic colony-forming cells in umbilical cord blood with extensive capability to generate mono- and multipotential hemopoietic progenitors. J Clin Invest. 1982;70(6):1324–8.
13. Leary AG, Ogawa M. Blast cell colony assay for umbilical cord blood and adult bone marrow progenitors. Blood. 1987;69(3):953–6.
14. Broxmeyer HE, et al. Human umbilical cord blood as a potential source of transplantable hematopoietic stem/progenitor cells. Proc Natl Acad Sci U S A. 1989;86(10):3828–32.
15. Gluckman E, et al. Hematopoietic reconstitution in a patient with Fanconi's anemia by means of umbilical-cord blood from an HLA-identical sibling. N Engl J Med. 1989;321(17):1174–8.
16. Ballen K. Challenges in umbilical cord blood stem cell banking for stem cell reviews and reports. Stem Cell Rev. 2010;6(1):8–14.
17. Sullivan MJ. Banking on cord blood stem cells. Nat Rev Cancer. 2008;8(7):555–63.
18. Kline RM. Whose blood is it, anyway? Sci Am. 2001;284(4):42–9.
19. Rosenthal J, et al. Hematopoietic cell transplantation with autologous cord blood in patients with severe aplastic anemia: an opportunity to revisit the controversy regarding cord blood banking for private use. Pediatr Blood Cancer. 2011;56(7):1009–12.
20. Barker JN, et al. Availability of cord blood extends allogeneic hematopoietic stem cell transplant access to racial and ethnic minorities. Biol Blood Marrow Transplant. 2010;16 (11):1541–8.
21. Arcese W, et al. Clinical use of allogeneic hematopoietic stem cells from sources other than bone marrow. Haematologica. 1998;83(2):159–82.
22. Standars, T.F.f.t.A.o.C.T.F. http://www.factwebsite.org/
23. Origin, I.-T.G.I.S.f.M.P.o.H. https://www.iccbba.org/
24. Solves P, et al. A new automatic device for routine cord blood banking: critical analysis of different volume reduction methodologies. Cytotherapy. 2009;11(8):1101–7.
25. Akel S, et al. Current thawing and infusion practice of cryopreserved cord blood: the impact on graft quality, recipient safety, and transplantation outcomes. Transfusion. 2014;54 (11):2997–3009.
26. Young W. Plasma-depleted versus red cell-reduced umbilical cord blood. Cell Transplant. 2014;23(4–5):407–15.
27. Broxmeyer HE, et al. Hematopoietic stem/progenitor cells, generation of induced pluripotent stem cells, and isolation of endothelial progenitors from 21- to 23.5-year cryopreserved cord blood. Blood. 2011;117(18):4773–7.
28. Smogorzewska EM, Barsky LW, Crooks GM, Wienberg KI. Purification of hematopoietic stem cells from human bone marrow and umbilical cord blood. Cent Eur J Immunol. 1997;22:232–9.
29. Stojko R, Witek A. Umbilical cord blood—a perfect source of stem cells? Ginekol Pol. 2005;76(6):491–7.
30. Mok JO, Byun JH, Kim SJ, Jeon JW, Won JH, Baick SH, Suh WS, Hong DS, Park HS. Comparison of the clonogenicity and percentage of CD34 positive cells in each source of hematopoietic stem cells. Korean J Blood Marrow Transplant. 1996;1:97–106.
31. Rocha V, et al. Graft-versus-host disease in children who have received a cord-blood or bone marrow transplant from an HLA-identical sibling. Eurocord and International Bone Marrow Transplant Registry Working Committee on Alternative Donor and Stem Cell Sources. N Engl J Med. 2000;342(25):1846–54.

32. Wagner JE, et al. Allogeneic sibling umbilical-cord-blood transplantation in children with malignant and non-malignant disease. Lancet. 1995;346(8969):214–9.
33. Gluckman E, et al. Outcome of cord-blood transplantation from related and unrelated donors. Eurocord Transplant Group and the European Blood and Marrow Transplantation Group. N Engl J Med. 1997;337(6):373–81.
34. Barker JN, et al. Survival after transplantation of unrelated donor umbilical cord blood is comparable to that of human leukocyte antigen-matched unrelated donor bone marrow: results of a matched-pair analysis. Blood. 2001;97(10):2957–61.
35. Kurtzberg J, et al. Results of the cord blood transplantation study (COBLT): clinical outcomes of unrelated donor umbilical cord blood transplantation in pediatric patients with hematologic malignancies. Blood. 2008;112(10):4318–27.
36. Wagner JE, et al. Transplantation of unrelated donor umbilical cord blood in 102 patients with malignant and nonmalignant diseases: influence of CD34 cell dose and HLA disparity on treatment-related mortality and survival. Blood. 2002;100(5):1611–8.
37. Laughlin MJ, et al. Hematopoietic engraftment and survival in adult recipients of umbilical-cord blood from unrelated donors. N Engl J Med. 2001;344(24):1815–22.
38. Rocha V, et al. Transplants of umbilical-cord blood or bone marrow from unrelated donors in adults with acute leukemia. N Engl J Med. 2004;351(22):2276–85.
39. Eapen M, Wagner JE. Transplant outcomes in acute leukemia. I. Semin Hematol. 2010;47 (1):46–50.
40. Shpall EJ, et al. Transplantation of ex vivo expanded cord blood. Biol Blood Marrow Transplant. 2002;8(7):368–76.
41. de Lima M, et al. Transplantation of ex vivo expanded cord blood cells using the copper chelator tetraethylenepentamine: a phase I/II clinical trial. Bone Marrow Transplant. 2008;41 (9):771–8.
42. de Lima M, et al. Cord-blood engraftment with ex vivo mesenchymal-cell coculture. N Engl J Med. 2012;367(24):2305–15.
43. Horwitz ME, et al. Umbilical cord blood expansion with nicotinamide provides long-term multilineage engraftment. J Clin Invest. 2014;124(7):3121–8.
44. Barker JN, et al. Transplantation of 2 partially HLA-matched umbilical cord blood units to enhance engraftment in adults with hematologic malignancy. Blood. 2005;105(3):1343–7.
45. MacMillan ML, et al. Acute graft-versus-host disease after unrelated donor umbilical cord blood transplantation: analysis of risk factors. Blood. 2009;113(11):2410–5.
46. Kindwall-Keller TL, et al. Prospective study of one- vs two-unit umbilical cord blood transplantation following reduced intensity conditioning in adults with hematological malignancies. Bone Marrow Transplant. 2012;47(7):924–33.
47. Rocha V, et al. Unrelated cord blood transplantation: outcomes after single-unit intrabone injection compared with double-unit intravenous injection in patients with hematological malignancies. Transplantation. 2013;95(10):1284–91.
48. Brunstein CG, et al. Intra-BM injection to enhance engraftment after myeloablative umbilical cord blood transplantation with two partially HLA-matched units. Bone Marrow Transplant. 2009;43(12):935–40.
49. Frassoni F, et al. The intra-bone marrow injection of cord blood cells extends the possibility of transplantation to the majority of patients with malignant hematopoietic diseases. Best Pract Res Clin Haematol. 2010;23(2):237–44.
50. Aiuti A, et al. The chemokine SDF-1 is a chemoattractant for human CD34+ hematopoietic progenitor cells and provides a new mechanism to explain the mobilization of CD34+ progenitors to peripheral blood. J Exp Med. 1997;185(1):111–20.
51. Kim CH, Broxmeyer HE. In vitro behavior of hematopoietic progenitor cells under the influence of chemoattractants: stromal cell-derived factor-1, steel factor, and the bone marrow environment. Blood. 1998;91(1):100–10.
52. Christopherson 2nd KW, et al. CD26 inhibition on CD34+ or lineage- human umbilical cord blood donor hematopoietic stem cells/hematopoietic progenitor cells improves long-term engraftment into NOD/SCID/Beta2null immunodeficient mice. Stem Cells Dev. 2007;16 (3):355–60.

53. Farag SS, et al. In vivo DPP-4 inhibition to enhance engraftment of single-unit cord blood transplants in adults with hematological malignancies. Stem Cells Dev. 2013;22(7):1007–15.
54. Reca R, et al. Functional receptor for C3a anaphylatoxin is expressed by normal hematopoietic stem/progenitor cells, and C3a enhances their homing-related responses to SDF-1. Blood. 2003;101(10):3784–93.
55. Brunstein CG, et al. Complement fragment 3a priming of umbilical cord blood progenitors: safety profile. Biol Blood Marrow Transplant. 2013;19(10):1474–9.
56. North TE, et al. Prostaglandin E2 regulates vertebrate haematopoietic stem cell homeostasis. Nature. 2007;447(7147):1007–11.
57. Cutler C, et al. Prostaglandin-modulated umbilical cord blood hematopoietic stem cell transplantation. Blood. 2013;122(17):3074–81.
58. Gluckman PD, et al. Selective head cooling with mild systemic hypothermia after neonatal encephalopathy: multicentre randomised trial. Lancet. 2005;365(9460):663–70.
59. Shankaran S, et al. Whole-body hypothermia for neonates with hypoxic-ischemic encephalopathy. N Engl J Med. 2005;353(15):1574–84.
60. Sanchez-Ramos JR, et al. Expression of neural markers in human umbilical cord blood. Exp Neurol. 2001;171(1):109–15.
61. Buzanska L, et al. Human cord blood-derived cells attain neuronal and glial features in vitro. J Cell Sci. 2002;115(Pt 10):2131–8.
62. Escolar ML, et al. Transplantation of umbilical-cord blood in babies with infantile Krabbe's disease. N Engl J Med. 2005;352(20):2069–81.
63. Staba SL, et al. Cord-blood transplants from unrelated donors in patients with Hurler's syndrome. N Engl J Med. 2004;350(19):1960–9.
64. Cotten CM, et al. Feasibility of autologous cord blood cells for infants with hypoxic-ischemic encephalopathy. J Pediatr. 2014;164(5):973–9.
65. Min K, et al. Umbilical cord blood therapy potentiated with erythropoietin for children with cerebral palsy: a double-blind, randomized, placebo-controlled trial. Stem Cells. 2013;31 (3):581–91.
66. Jensen A, Hamelmann E. First autologous cell therapy of cerebral palsy caused by hypoxic-ischemic brain damage in a child after cardiac arrest-individual treatment with cord blood. Case Rep Transplant. 2013;951827(10):15.
67. Lee YH, et al. Safety and feasibility of countering neurological impairment by intravenous administration of autologous cord blood in cerebral palsy. J Transl Med. 2012;10 (58):1479–5876.
68. Hutter G, et al. Long-term control of HIV by CCR5 Delta32/Delta32 stem-cell transplantation. N Engl J Med. 2009;360(7):692–8.
69. Duarte RF, et al. CCR5 Delta32 homozygous cord blood allogeneic transplantation in a patient with HIV: a case report. Lancet HIV. 2015;2(6):e236–42.
70. Hutter G. More on shift of HIV tropism in stem-cell transplantation with CCR5 delta32/ delta32 mutation. N Engl J Med. 2014;371(25):2437–8. doi:10.1056/NEJMc1412279#SA1.

Chapter 9
Interactions Between Multipotential Stromal Cells (MSCs) and Immune Cells During Bone Healing

Jehan J. El-Jawhari, Elena Jones, Dennis McGonagle, and Peter V. Giannoudis

9.1 Introduction

Human bone has a unique structure formed of outer dense layer of cortical bone responsible for the weight bearing function. The outer bone is covered by the periosteum that has a contributing role in the osteogenesis and the removal of the periosteum delays significantly the bone repair [1]. The inner part of the bone is a mesh-like cancellous bone containing bone marrow (BM) where various cell types including multipotential stromal cells (MSCs) exist [2]. The first description of MSCs was as colony-forming unit fibroblasts with capability to generate a new bone in ectopic sites [3]. Later on, they were renamed as mesenchymal stem cells [4]. According to the International Society of Cell Therapy (ISCT), MSCs are defined as plastic adherent cells, which do not express hematopoietic lineage markers CD45, CD34, CD14 or CD11b, CD79 alpha, CD19 and HLA-DR, but they express surface molecules CD90, CD73, CD105. Thirdly, MSCs are able to differentiate into osteoblasts, adipoblasts and chondroblasts [5].

There are many tissues where MSCs can exist in skeleton including the periosteum, bone, BM, muscles, tendons, ligaments and adipose tissues [6]. In animal models, MSCs can migrate from BM into blood then circulate and home to the injury site where they can be active in repairing tissues [7]. The most common and best-characterised source of MSCs is BM. The surface molecule CD271 is currently considered as a distinctive and selective marker for human BM and bone MSCs [8, 9]. Interestingly, the periosteum contains MSCs with chondrogenic and

J.J. El-Jawhari • E. Jones (✉) • D. McGonagle • P.V. Giannoudis
Leeds Institute of Rheumatic and Musculoskeletal Medicine, St. James University Hospital, University of Leeds, Room 5.24, Clinical Sciences Building, LS9 7TF Leeds, UK

NIHR, Leeds Biomedical Research Unit, Chapel Allerton Hospital, University of Leeds, LS7 4SA Leeds, UK
e-mail: E.Jones@leeds.ac.uk

E.M. Abdelalim (ed.), *Recent Advances in Stem Cells*, Stem Cell Biology and Regenerative Medicine, DOI 10.1007/978-3-319-33270-3_9

osteogenic potential that is comparable to BM MSCs [10]. Furthermore, periosteal MSCs are higher in quantity relative to BM MSCs in canine models [11] but it is unknown if periosteal MSCs are similarly abundant in human.

The proliferation of MSCs is closely linked to their differentiation function. Rapidly growing MSCs have superior differentiation abilities compared to slower proliferating MSCs [12]. In addition to mesenchymal tissue differentiation, MSCs can display immunomodulatory functions, mostly suppression of the proliferation and functions of different immune cells [13]. Critically, MSCs need to be primed by inflammatory cytokines to play their immunomodulatory role [14]. With the advancement of the examination of the surface phenotype and the functional characterisation of MSCs from multiple tissue sources, the importance of MSCs as key cells in bone healing becomes better understood.

Although the bone healing is a successive process, its phases are overlapping to some-extent, inflammation, repair phase including chondrogenesis followed by ossification then finally remodelling phase. When a fracture or bone loss occurs, the injury-driven rupture of blood vessels and vasodilation causes an exudation of plasma into the surrounding tissues. Plasma-derived fibrinogen is converted into fibrin forming a haematoma, which traps various inflammatory cells and MSCs [15]. The function of inflammation is the clearance of the damaged tissue and the initiation of the repair by providing the needed cells and the appropriate cytokines and growth factors [16]. Subsequent to the inflammatory phase, the repair phase starts with the differentiation of MSCs into chondroblasts, which proliferate and differentiate, forming a cartilaginous thickened structure called soft callus. Then chondroblasts undergo hypertrophy and begin to deposit mineralised matrix and soft callus is converted into a new bone (hard) callus. This process is known as endochondral ossification leading to the formation of irregularly arranged (woven) bone. During this phase new blood vessels are formed in a process called angiogenesis. The final phase includes remodelling of woven bone into lamellar bone, i.e. normally aligned bone [17–20].

Intramembranous repair involves a direct differentiation of MSCs into osteoblasts and it usually happens when broken bone edges are perfectly aligned (direct or primary healing) [17]. In addition to MSCs, bone cells including osteoclasts and osteoblasts also play important roles in bone healing. Osteoclasts are giant multinucleated cells originated from monocyte lineage cells and express tartrate-resistant acid phosphatase. The main function of osteoclasts is bone resorption through release of the enzymes and other molecules, which degrade the bone matrix [21]. Osteoblasts are bone-forming cells originated from MSC-derived progenitors. The balance between the functions of these bone cells and immune cells helps to maintain the normal quantity and the function of the regenerating bone and is critical to determine the fate of the healing process [22]. In this chapter, the role of various immune cells, cytokines, bone cells and MSCs and their interactions during different phases of the bone healing in health and in exaggerated inflammatory milieu are reviewed (Figs. 9.1, 9.2 and 9.3, Tables 9.1 and 9.2).

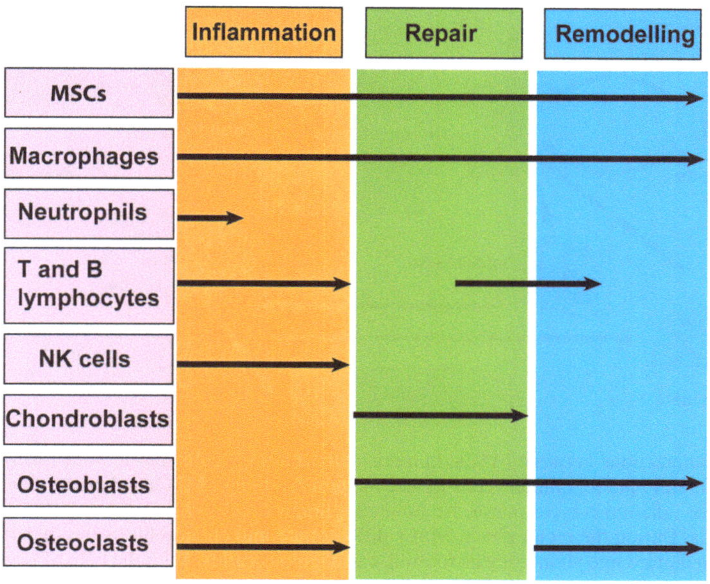

Fig. 9.1 Cells involved during three stages of secondary bone healing. MSCs are involved in the three phases of bone healing. Macrophages similarly play various roles during the whole process. Neutrophils and NK cells are known to be involved only during inflammatory phase. In contrast, B and T lymphocytes are involved in inflammatory phase then during late repair and early remodelling phase. Chondroblasts are specifically active during repair phase of the secondary healing. Osteoblasts are involved in the repair phase of the primary healing and in the remodelling phase of either secondary or primary healing. In comparison, osteoclasts are contributed in both inflammatory and remodelling phases of the repair

9.2 Inflammatory Phase

Inflammation taking place at the fracture site is caused by the damage of tissues, hypoxic and low pH environment. Inflammatory phase involves several events including the recruitment of different blood cells and release of various inflammatory chemokines and cytokines [16, 23]. Immune response is critical for physiological uncomplicated healing of fractured bone. The transfer of immune cells from young mice via BM transplantation into immune-compromised mice improves significantly the process of bone repair [24]. Furthermore, immune-compromised patients such as HIV-infected individuals show delayed or complicated healing of bone fractures [25]. Although different factors could be involved in HIV-related fragility of healing bones, immune-related mechanisms have been demonstrated. For example, serum level of both tumour necrosis factor-α (TNF-α) and the TNF receptors are increased in these patients in comparison to healthy controls [26]. Cells and molecules of innate and adaptive immune systems as well as MSCs are involved in inflammatory phase of bone healing to maintain tissue

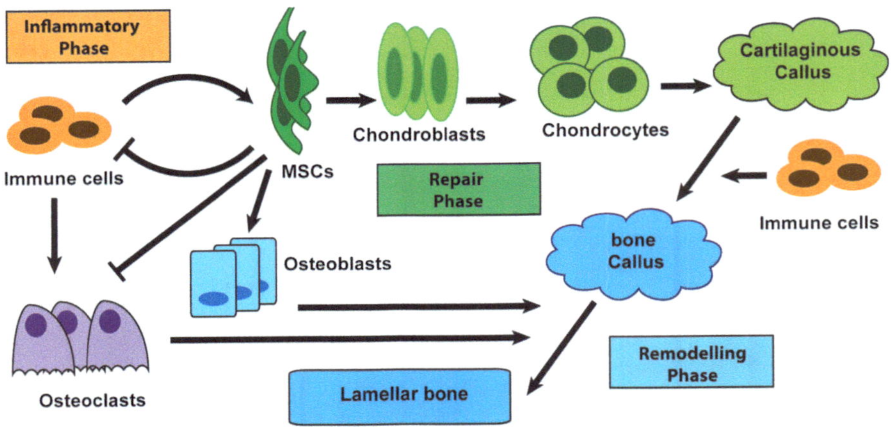

Fig. 9.2 Interactions between MSCs, immune cells and bone cells during bone healing. During the inflammatory phase, immune cells induce the proliferation of MSCs and prime them. MSCs in turn control inflammatory response. Additionally, immune cells stimulate osteoclasts to remove bone debris. During the repair phase, MSCs differentiate into chondroblasts (secondary healing), which then mature into chondrocytes forming cartilaginous callus. With the help of immune cells, cartilaginous callus converts into bone callus. Finally, the balance between osteoblasts and osteoclasts help remodelling of bone callus into lamellar bone

haemostasis through removal of the damaged cells and induction of cartilage and bone repair in addition to angiogenesis [27]. The role of different immune cells and MSCs as well as other inflammatory soluble factors are discussed below.

9.2.1 *Neutrophils*

The first cells to be recruited into hematoma at the injury site are neutrophils. In a rat model of tibia fracture, neutrophils were detected at the fracture callus on day 1 and remained for few days after the fracture [28]. In association with high level of chemokine, cytokine-induced neutrophil chemoattractant-1 (CINC-1), neutrophils migrate across the endothelium into hematoma site [29]. Neutrophils are important to eliminate the microbial infection [30]. The functions of neutrophils at the fracture site also include phagocytosis of the damaged cells and debris [27]. Although they have short life span, neutrophils play antiseptic role at the fracture site, but it remains unknown if they interact with MSCs.

9.2.2 *Macrophages and Monocytes*

Macrophages are recruited into the fracture site from the periosteum or peripheral blood [31, 32]. Macrophage-colony stimulating factor (M-CSF), which is known to target mainly macrophages [33], is expressed in the fractured bone, peaking during

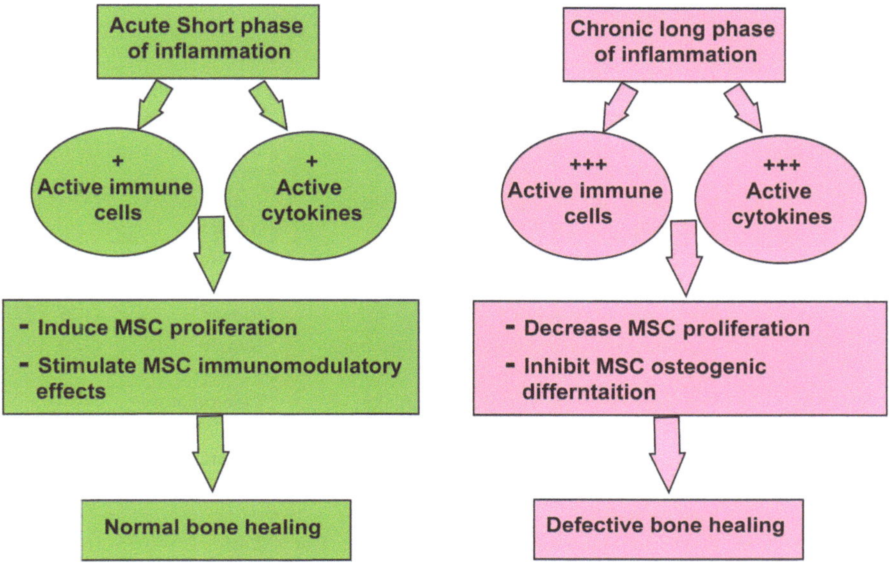

Fig. 9.3 The magnitude of inflammation affects the fate of bone healing via interactions with MSCs. A short acute inflammatory phase carried out by active cells and cytokines, helps to recruit and stimulate the proliferation of MSCs. Additionally, this inflammatory response stimulates the immunosuppressive effects of MSCs ending the inflammatory phase and progressing into normal repair phase. In contrast, uncontrolled or chronic/exaggerated inflammatory phase is associated with excessively activated cells and cytokines. These factors lead to the inhibition of proliferation and osteogenic differentiation of MSCs causing an impairment of bone healing

inflammatory phase then again when remodelling phase starts [34] indicating an involvement of the macrophages during all phases. Macrophages and platelets produce bone morphogenetic proteins (BMPs), which contribute in organising the shape of the different tissues particularly bone and cartilage [35]. BMPs are known to stimulate the proliferation of MSCs and enhance their osteogenic differentiation [36]. Another molecule, Oncostatin M, is produced by monocytes/macrophages and induces osteogenic markers, Core-binding factor alpha 1/runt-related transcription factor 2 (Cbfa1/Runx2) and alkaline phosphatase (ALP) in MSCs enhancing their differentiation into osteoblasts [37, 38]. Additionally, monocyte-derived exosomes also increase the bone-forming function of MSCs via the induction of the expression of Cbfa1/Runx2 and BMP2 in MSCs [39]. Monocytes activated by interleukin-4 (IL-4) or lipopolysaccharide (LPS) elevate the expression level of Cbfa1/Runx2 and ALP by MSCs [40]. Thus interactions between MSCs and macrophages induce the osteogenic ability of MSCs preparing for the repair phase.

Table 9.1 The role of immune cells during the bone healing

Immune cell	Role	Phase	Reference
Neutrophils	Eliminate microbial infection	Inflammatory	[30]
	Remove damaged tissue and debris	Inflammatory	[27]
Macrophages	Production of BMPs	Inflammatory/ repair	[35, 36]
	Production of Oncostatin M that stimulates MSC osteogenesis	Inflammatory/ repair	[37, 38]
	Exosomes stimulates MSC osteogenesis	Inflammatory/ repair	[39]
	Deposition of collagen I	Repair	[126, 127]
	Transition of cartilaginous callus into bone callus	Repair	[120, 121]
NK cells	Priming of immunomodulatory function of MSCs	Inflammatory	[42]
	Migration of MSCs	Inflammatory	[46]
	Production of RANKL, which induces osteo-clast formation	Inflammatory	[47]
ILCs	IL-17: osteoblast maturation, and osteogenesis of MSCs	Late inflammatory?	[63]
	IL-22: MSCs proliferation and differentiation	Late inflammatory?	[64]
T lymphocytes	Priming of immunomodulatory function of MSCs	Inflammatory	[34]
	Stimulate osteogenesis of MSCs	Inflammatory	[71]
	Production of RANKL, which induces osteo-clast formation	Inflammatory	[69, 70]
	Transition of cartilaginous callus into bone callus	Late repair	[44, 45]
Th17 cells	Stimulate MSC osteogenesis	Inflammatory	[63]
	Induce osteoblast maturation	Repair	[63]
	Transition of cartilaginous callus into bone callus	Repair	[138]
	Induce osteoclast generation	Remodelling	[154]
T reg lymphocytes	Decrease immunosuppressive effect of MSCs	Inflammatory	[73]
	Stimulate bone healing	Repair	[72]
B lymphocytes	Stimulate osteoclastogenesis	Inflammatory	[74]
	Transition of cartilaginous callus into bone callus	Late repair	[75]
	Induce death of osteoclasts	Early remodelling	[44, 45]

9.2.3 NK Cells

Natural killer (NK) cells constitute an important part of innate immune system and are divided into two functional subsets: bright CD56 (cytokine producers or regulatory NK cells) and dim CD56 (killers). NK cells can circulate and reach different

Table 9.2 The role of soluble factors during the bone healing

Soluble factor	Role	Phase	Reference
TNF-α	Migration of MSCs	Inflammatory	[87]
	Prime MSCs for immunosuppression	Inflammatory	[90]
	Regulate the functions of osteoclasts and osteoblasts	Remodelling	[44, 45]
IFN-γ	Stimulate proliferation of MSCs	Inflammatory	[92]
	Prime MSCs for immunosuppression	Inflammatory	[92]
IL-1	Prime MSCs for immunosuppression	Inflammatory	[91]
IL-17	Prime MSCs for immunosuppression	Inflammatory	[95]
	Stimulate the proliferation and osteogenesis of MSCs	Repair	[63]
	Promote osteoblast maturation	Remodelling	[63]
	Induce osteoclastogenesis	Remodelling	[153]
IL-22	The migration, proliferation and differentiation of MSCs	Inflammatory	[64]
CCR2	Increase vasculature	Inflammatory	[31]
	Recruit macrophages	And repair	
TGF-β	Suppress immune response	Inflammatory	[96, 97]
	Enhance osteogenic differentiation of MSCs	Repair	[96]
BMPs	Enhance proliferation and osteogenic differentiation of MSCs	Inflammatory/ repair	[157, 158]
	Promote osteoblast maturation	Repair	[159–161]
SDF-1	Recruitment of MSCs	Inflammatory	[83]

organs where they become activated and function to keep immune haemostasis in different tissues [41]. Up to date, little is known about the biological roles of NK cells during the bone healing. One study has described a high expression of interferon-γ (IFN-γ) in the tissues of diaphyseal regions of fractured femur in *RAG* $^{-/-}$ mice model, which lack both T and B lymphocytes [42]. As a major source of IFN-γ, this study has pointed to the importance of NK cells during bone repair. This role is assumed because NK cells produce a major priming cytokine for immunomodulatory function of MSCs, IFN-γ [42]. Yet, further research is needed to understand the magnitude of NK cell-dependent priming of MSCs. The inflammatory milieu as well as MSC-NK cell interactions could modify activated NK cell functions to increase the production of IFN-γ [43]. NK cells are also a major source of TNF-α, which has a critical role in bone repair. Mice lacking TNF-α have been shown to have defective bone generation [44, 45]. In addition to priming effects, NK cells have been shown to enhance the migration of MSCs through matrigel inserts [46].

NK cells stimulate the generation of osteoclasts through release of receptor activator of nuclear factor kappa-B ligand (RANKL) [47]. Data from in vitro studies has shown that RANKL and TNF-α also trigger monocyte differentiation into osteoclasts [48]. This suggests that NK cells can indirectly, via effect on osteoclasts, help the removal of debris and damaged tissues in physiological bone repair. In summary, NK cells can induce MSC functions including the priming and the migration via their cytokines in addition to their effect on osteoclasts all indicate their important contribution into the bone healing.

9.2.4 Innate Lymphoid Cells

Innate lymphoid cells (ILCs) are newly characterised immune cells that originate from common lymphoid progenitor but they lack lineage markers for T or B lymphocytes [49, 50]. ILCs are divided into three functionally diverse subclasses, ILCs 1, 2 and 3. NK cells are considered as a subtype of ILCs 1. ILCs have common receptors for IL-12 and IL-7 but have heterogonous functions with distinctive pattern of cytokine profiles [51, 52]. While ILCs 1 secret Th1 cell-like cytokines, TNF-α and IFN-γ [53, 54], ILCs 2 produce IL-4, IL-5, IL-9 and IL-13 similar to Th2 cells [55–57]. In contrast, ILCs 3 have similar profile to Th17 as they produce IL-17 in addition to IL-22 and M-CSF [58]. Interestingly, ILCs 3 help the regeneration of damaged inflamed intestine, thymic and lymphoid tissues via their production of IL-22 [59–61]. Furthermore, ILCs 2 play an important role in repair against viral-related damage of bronchial epithelium [62].

Compared to their role in healing of epithelial and lymphoid tissues, little is known about the role of these innate cells during the bone healing process. Interestingly, one study showed that IL-17 putatively produced by ILCs 3 could induce the expression of Cbfa1/Runx2 as well as late osteogenic marker, collagen in MSCs [63]. Although this group indicated that Th17 cells could induce osteogenesis, a similar effect of ILCs 3 can be proposed, as they are another source of IL-17 [63]. Furthermore, it has been shown that following priming with IFN-γ and TNF-α, IL-22 stimulates the migration and the proliferation as well as osteogenic differentiation of MSCs in vitro [64]. This all suggest that these innate immune cells probably work during later stage of inflammatory phase to prepare MSCs for next phase of the bone repair. However, there is a need to locate and study the functions of these ILCs within healing bone tissues.

9.2.5 T and B Lymphocytes

During inflammatory phase, the acquired immune cells, T and B lymphocytes are important in bone healing. In animal models where T and B are depleted, a defect in bone mineralisation and delayed healing has been described [65–67]. T and B lymphocytes are recruited at the bone fracture site after 3 days of injury and then reduced in numbers with the start of cartilaginous callus formation as shown in animal models [63, 68]. RANKL that is made in part by activated T lymphocytes in addition to stromal cells and NK cells, stimulates osteoclasts to remove the dead bone [69, 70].

Importantly, T lymphocytes are linked to the priming of immunomodulatory function of MSCs as T lymphocytes secret TNF-α, the cytokine that peaks during both inflammatory and repair phases [34]. Additionally, conditioned media from the cultured CD4 T lymphocytes but not CD8 T lymphocytes can induce the expression level of both early and late osteogenic markers, Cbfa1/Runx2, ALP, osteocalcin and Bone sialoprotein (BSP) by MSCs [71]. Th17 cells are positive inducers of the osteogenic potential of MSCs and IL-17 enhance osteogenic markers in MSCs both in vitro and in vivo [63]. Similarly, T regulatory lymphocytes (T reg lymphocytes) are also assumed to be involved in bone healing, as they are major source of TGF-β, which promote MSC proliferation and osteogenesis [72]. Members of TGF-β family, TGF-β2 and TGF-β3 showed maximal expression when inflammation ends and cartilage formation starts, as they play their role as immunosuppressive cytokines thus controlling the inflammation [73]. Altogether, this illustrates how T lymphocytes can enhance the osteogenic potential of MSCs in preparation to the next phase of repair.

There is some conflicting data about the role of B lymphocytes in bone repair. While it has been shown that B lymphocytes enhance osteoclast formation [74], another study showed that B lymphocytes suppressed osteoclastogenesis and promoted death of osteoclasts via TGF-β expression [75]. Furthermore, in B lymphocyte deficient mice model of tibial injury, B cells did not affect osteoblast differentiation or maturation during intramembranous ossification [76]. Remaining inconclusive, there is a need for more studies to understand if B lymphocytes have other roles during the bone repair via interactions with MSCs.

9.2.6 Multipotential Stromal Cells

9.2.6.1 Source and Recruitment

Hematoma formed soon after the bone fracture consists of granulation tissue holding various cells including MSCs [15, 77]. The origin of these MSCs could be the periosteum, BM or vascular endothelium-supporting cells, pericytes [78–80]. Periosteal-derived MSCs have been shown to form bone and cartilage with a help of BMP-2 for their differentiation [81]. In cases of open fractures where the periosteum is stripped, MSCs can be also derived from adjacent muscle tissue [82]. MSCs are recruited into the fracture site under the effect of an inflammatory chemokine, Stromal Derived Factor-1 (SDF-1) as revealed in a mouse model of femoral injury [83]. By the activation of alpha serine/threonine-protein kinase (AKT) and extracellular-signal-regulated kinases (ERK) signalling pathways, SDF-1 induces the migration of MSCs and the secretion of angiogenic factor, vascular endothelial growth factor (VEGF) [84] [85]. SDF-1 is also an important inducer for BMP-2, which activates MSCs and promotes osteogenesis [86]. Another cytokine, which mediates the invasion of MSCs into the injury site is TNF-α that acts via NF-kβ-dependent signalling pathway [87]. The multiplicity of sources of MSCs reflects the vitality of these cells in the bone repair.

9.2.6.2 The Early Role of MSCs During Inflammatory Phase

Although MSCs have been detected in fracture hematoma, their role in early phase of fracture repair is not completely clear. One in vitro study has suggested that MSCs could be involved in phagocytosis of dead cells at the fracture site. This process is associated with an increase of the expression of chemokine receptors, CXCR4 and CXCR5, by MSCs helping recruiting more MSCs into the injury site [88]. The exposure of T lymphocytes to these phagocytic MSCs could increase the expression of RANTES thus recruiting more CD4 T lymphocytes to the injury site. Furthermore, these MSCs could stimulate the differentiation of Th-17 cells that are linked to osteogenesis [88]. Another study has indicated that MSCs could induce the formation of osteoclasts with an involvement of IL-6 and M-CSF [89]. In conclusion, MSCs seem to help removal of bone debris directly or by enhancing osteoclastogenesis. Additionally, MSCs could induce further recruitment of MSCs and T lymphocytes into the fracture site.

9.2.6.3 Priming of MSCs During Early Inflammatory Stage

Inflammation-mediated priming of MSCs is critical to complete the bone healing. IFN-γ can activate the proliferation and immunosuppressive function of MSCs via the activation of the Kynurenine pathway [90]. Concomitant with IFN-γ, TNF-α or IL-1 increases the expression of adhesion molecules, ICAM-1 and VCAM-1 on MSC surface helping their contact with T lymphocytes and causing an augmented MSC-mediated inhibition of T cell proliferation [91]. It has been shown that TNF-α also helps the proliferation of MSCs and the initial priming of immunosuppressive function of MSCs via NF-kβ-dependent mechanism [92]. The inflammatory cytokine, IL-1 mediates its effect on MSCs via multiple signalling pathways including map kinase (MAK), Jun amino-terminal kinase (JNK) and NFk-β. Furthermore, the downstream activation mediated by IL-1 controls the production of immunomodulatory factors, prostaglandin 2 (PGE2) and IL-8 by MSCs [93].

Within inflammatory milieu, the activation of toll-like receptors (TLRs) on the surface of MSCs induces MSC migration, differentiation, proliferation and production of indoleamine 2,3-dioxygenase (IDO) and PGE2. The stimulation of TLR activates MAP kinase, NFk-β and PI3 kinase signalling pathways [94]. Recently, IL-17 was added to the list of priming factors that induce MSC immunomodulatory effect. IL-17 can induce the production of inducible nitric oxide synthase (iNOS) by MSCs as tested in vitro and in vivo [95].

In contrast to these priming cytokines, TGF-β can act as a counterbalancing cytokine to decrease the immunosuppressive effect of MSCs. Uniquely, TGF-β affects both immunomodulatory and repair functions of MSCs [96]. One mechanism by which TGF-β affects MSC immunomodulatory function is the decrease of iNOS expression in SMAD3-dependent manner [97]. Similarly, immunosuppressive cytokine, IL-10 abrogates the inhibitory effect of MSCs on the proliferation of CD4 and CD8 T lymphocytes [98]. However, the role of these counteracting cytokines during the inflammatory phase of bone repair is probably less evident compared to MSC priming cytokines. The expression levels of TGF-β 2 and 3 are increased during cartilaginous callus formation to help differentiation of MSCs [73]. In conclusion, MSC priming and counteracting cytokines are likely to work synergistically to prime MSCs for their immunomodulatory effects towards the transition to the repair stage of bone healing.

9.2.6.4 The Late Role of MSCs During Inflammatory Phase; Immunomodulation

The regulation of immune response within the fracture environment is critical to reduce the tissue damage and inhibit fibrosis supporting the bone regeneration [27, 34]. This important role of MSCs controlling inflammatory phase helps the transition into the next stage of bone healing process [99]. The discovery of an ability of MSCs to regulate immune systems was made in late 1990s/early 2000s by the observation that MSCs suppress the proliferation of T lymphocytes in vitro and in vivo, indicating an additional function of MSCs [100, 101]. The subsequent studies have proven that only inflammatory-primed MSCs can mediate immunomodulation of both innate and adaptive immune responses. The effect of MSCs on IL-12 or IL-15 activated NK cells includes the suppression of NK proliferation, killing and secretory functions [102, 103]. The differentiation of T lymphocytes into Th1 and Th17 subsets can be suppressed by MSCs, however MSCs promote the differentiation of T reg lymphocytes [104]. Additionally, MSCs can induce dendritic cells to trigger T reg generation via the production of IL-10 by these dendritic cells [105]. Furthermore, MSCs induce the apoptosis of T lymphocytes that trigger macrophages to secrete TGF-β inducing the expression of T reg lymphocytes [106]. Moreover, MSCs have the ability to suppress the function and the migration of B lymphocytes via the downregulation of the chemokine receptors expression, CXCR4, CXCR5 and CCR7, on the surface of B lymphocytes [107]. Overall, this indicates that MSCs interact with both innate and adaptive immune cells controlling whole inflammatory response.

The mechanisms by which MSCs exert their immunomodulatory effects are mainly related to soluble factors. The soluble immunomodulatory molecules include TGF-β, IDO, iNOS, PGE2, IL-1 receptor antagonist and tumor necrosis factor-inducible gene 6 (TSG6) [108–111]. The use of these different players by MSCs varies according to host species, tissue type or priming microenvironment of MSCs [112]. For example, mice MSCs mainly use nitric oxide (NO) to modulate immune responses, but IDO is the main player for human MSCs [112]. In summary, MSCs exert a negative feedback loop to control the inflammation at the fracture site.

9.2.7 *The Summary of Inflammatory Phase*

Under the normal condition, inflammatory phase is important initial phase of the bone healing (Fig. 9.3). Neutrophils are the first cells to arrive at the fracture site preventing sepsis. NK cells, TNF-α in addition to SDF-1 help to recruit MSCs that directly and via the activation of osteoclasts help the removal of the dead cells and debris. Other immune cells, B and T lymphocytes also stimulate the formation of osteoclasts. Inflammatory cytokines and growth factors enhance the proliferation of MSCs as well as priming of MSCs to exert their immunomodulatory effects. As a negative feedback mechanism, primed MSCs then are able to suppress the inflammatory responses and help to start the repair phase of bone healing. Nevertheless, the effects of some inflammatory cells continue to play their roles during the repair phase (Figs. 9.1 and 9.2).

9.3 Repair Phase

The repair phase includes the formation of cartilaginous callus in the secondary bone healing (endochondral ossification) from the enlarging cartilaginous tissue patches filling the bone defect site [113]. On the other hand, the primary bone healing involves the formation of hard or bone callus that happens in the absence of cartilaginous callus (intramembranous ossification) [114]. The endochondral ossification is the most common healing type and includes the degradation of cartilaginous callus, which then is replaced by the bone callus in association with the formation of new blood vasculature. The role of MSCs and immune cells as well as soluble mediators is discussed below.

9.3.1 *MSCs*

During the repair phase, MSCs proliferate and differentiate into chondroblasts that mature into chondrocytes, which deposit cartilaginous matrix [115]. Chondrocytes mature and deposit calcium granules into matrix where these granules precipitate with phosphatase forming apatite crystals under hypoxic conditions. During these events and while a mechanically rigid bone callus is forming, a high expression of osteogenic markers, procollagen-I, osteocalcin, ALP and osteonectin becomes evident [17, 116].

The second role for MSCs during this stage includes the production of VEGF under control of Cbfa1/Runx2 transcription factor [117]. BM MSCs express angiogenic factors, VEGF and angiopoietin-1 [118]. Thus, MSCs are considered the key cells initiating this phase by chondrogenic differentiation as well as induction of angiogenesis.

9.3.2 Macrophages

Macrophages are known to be involved in the intramembranous ossification during the repair phase [31, 32]. Macrophages also participate in the bone repair via the induction of angiogenesis. A significant decrease in macrophages in CCR2$^{-/-}$ mice was associated with impaired vascularisation and delayed formation of callus [31]. Macrophages are present in invading vessels during the ossification of mouse long bones [119].

Later during this phase, macrophages can efficiently secrete matrix metalloproteinases (MMPs) to break the cartilage matrix [120, 121]. MMP-9 and MMP-13 have important contribution during soft-to-hard callus conversion [122–124]. MMPs and their inhibitors help the conversion of collagen II to type I and the disturbances in the regulation of these enzymes are connected to the fracture non-union [125]. In a mouse model of tibia fracture, both resident macrophages and inflammatory circulating macrophages were shown to be vital for the deposition of collagen type I [126]. Furthermore, it has been shown that the gene expression of macrophage macrosialin protein is positively associated with the expression of collagen in fractures [127]. In summary, macrophages are active during whole repair phase working synergistically with MSCs to help deposition of collagen matrix and formation of new blood vessels.

9.3.3 T and B Lymphocytes

Although they disappear at the end of inflammatory phase and during formation of callus, T and B lymphocytes reappear during the mineralisation of cartilaginous callus and have been detected in a close contact with osteoblasts and osteoclasts [128]. Both types of adaptive immune cells are recruited into newly forming hard callus presumably via new blood vessels to produce more TNF-α, the cytokine responsible for the death of mature chondrocytes. Additionally, TNF-α stimulates the maturation of osteoblasts and osteoclasts helping the conversion from cartilage into bone [44, 45]. Overall, T and B lymphocytes have a role in the late stage of bone healing helping the transition of cartilaginous callus into bone callus. This role seems to be mediated via TNF-α to regulate the function of osteoblasts and osteoclasts.

9.3.4 Growth Factors and Cytokines

Different growth factors including platelet-derived growth factor (PDGF), TGF-β, insulin-like growth factor (IGF) and fibroblast growth factor-1 (FGF-1) promote the proliferation and the differentiation of MSCs into chondrocytes [129] [114]. Similarly, BMPs-2, 4 and 7 induce the differentiation and proliferation of MSCs [130]. Furthermore, BMPs stimulate the chondrocytes to secret extracellular matrix proteins such as collagen type II [36]. The importance of these factors has been established and it has been shown that the gene expression levels of BMPs are significantly lower in the sheep model of delayed bone union compared to controls [131]. Furthermore, the depletion of BMPs causes severe defects in the bone formation as seen in animal models, whereas the treatment with recombinant BMPs improves the fracture repair [132–134]. This indicates that multiple growth factors help chondrogenesis at the start of the repair phase.

The bone fracture needs a good vasculature. Angiopoietin-1 and -2 proteins are expressed early during healing promoting the vascularisation from periosteal capillaries [135]. VEGF is another key factor in angiogenesis and it is produced in a large quantity from MSCs and differentiated chondrocytes converting avascular soft callus into vascularised bone callus. For this process to be completed, the death of chondrocytes and the breakdown of cartilaginous callus are happened in TNF-α-dependent mechanism [136]. Importantly, TNF-α signalling in chondrocytes increases MMPs and angiopoietin coordinating the expression of the regulators of endothelial cell survival and modulators of cartilaginous destruction, the MMPs [135]. In summary, the correct balance between growth factors and cytokines produced by endothelial cells and chondrocytes is essential [137] for the transition of cartilaginous callus into vascularised bone callus helping the physiological bone repair.

Interestingly, IL-17 can suppress chondrogenic differentiation of MSCs via downregulating the expression of key chondrogenesis transcriptional factor SRY-box 9 (SOX9) and its activator cAMP-dependent protein kinase (PKA) [138]. Nam et al. have reported that an exposure of the osteoblasts to IL-17 increases the gene expression of collagen, osteocalcin and bone sialoprotein indicating enhanced maturation of osteoblasts [63]. This together shows that Th17 cells constitute an important contributing factor into the transition of chondrogenesis into osteogenesis.

9.3.5 The Summary of the Repair Phase

MSCs and other immune cells are involved in this stage (Figs. 9.1 and 9.2). MSCs differentiate into chondroblasts developing cartilaginous callus then these cells mature into chondrocytes, which help the mineralisation of cartilaginous matrix forming bone callus. The growth factors help the proliferation and the differentiation of MSCs as well as the maturation of chondrocytes. Additionally, macrophages help the deposition of cartilaginous matrix. Angiogenesis starts in this phase with a help of MSCs, macrophages and growth factors. Other immune cells, T and B lymphocytes reappear late in this phase during the mineralisation of cartilaginous callus helping the transition into bone callus aided by inflammatory cytokines TNF-α and IL-17.

9.4 Remodelling Phase

Remodelling phase includes the reinstating of the normal architecture and the orientation of the growing bone to restore its normal function. This occurs by transforming of irregular woven bone callus into lamellar bone within two steps, the resorption of mineralised bone and then the formation of new lamellar bone [139, 140]. This process is mainly dependent on the balance between osteoblast and osteoclast functions with the stimulation by BMPs [36]. Also during this phase, new blood vessel formation is continued with minimal roles for immune and other hematopoietic cells.

9.4.1 Cells

The established role for MSCs during the bone healing is the differentiation into osteoblasts at later stages of the process [141]. Osteoblast formation is tightly controlled by the influence of various growth factors and downstream signalling pathways. Under the effect of TGF-β, BMPs and IGF, MSCs differentiate into osteoblasts [142]. Furthermore, the proliferation and osteogenic differentiation of MSCs is regulated via the activation of Wnt/catenin signalling pathway [143–145]. Cyclooxygenase 2 (Cox-2) protein that induces the production of pro-inflammatory protein PGE2, can also stimulate the differentiation of MSCs into osteoblasts. Cox-2 knock out mice show delayed healing of tibia fractures [146]. Furthermore, reduced Cox2 expression with ageing is associated with a delayed bone repair as shown in a mouse model of femoral fracture [147]. MSCs have an inhibitory effect on osteoclast generation from monocytes progenitors via mechanism mediated partially by the production of Osteoprotegerin (OPG) [148]. This shows how MSCs can control the late stages of the bone remodelling and further emphasises the link between inflammation and osteogenesis.

Osteoblast progenitors mature into mid-stage of collagen-producing cells before fully maturing into osteoblasts, which also produce non-collagenous calcium and phosphate binding proteins such as osteocalcin and osteopontin forming mineralised bone [149]. Differentiated osteoblasts are involved in the matrix formation in cbfa-1/Runx-2 and Osterix-dependent mechanisms causing the formation of new lamellar bone [114, 150]. In contrast, osteoclasts are responsible for the bone resorption and they create acidic microenvironment to demineralise the bone matrix and produce enzymes, which erode the bone. The functions of osteoblasts are balanced by that of osteoclasts and the disruption in this balance leads to defective bone formation. An increase in osteoclast cell numbers and RANKL have been detected in animal model of bone non-union [151].

It has been demonstrated that Th17 cells can enhance osteoclastogenesis [152]. IL-17 enhances the differentiation of osteoblasts from MSCs as well as increases the expression of RANKL on MSCs thus promoting osteoclastogenesis when MSCs co-cultured with peripheral blood mononuclear cells (PBMCs) [153]. Although Th17 cells have not been detected in healing bone during remodelling, they are linked to osteoblast and osteoclast generation and function, highlighting their possible role in the final stage of the bone healing [154]. Additionally, macrophages are suggested to be involved in the remodelling phase by enhancement of the osteoblast activity as well as the progenitors of osteoclasts [32]. In total, inflammatory cells and IL-17 can control the balance of osteoclasts and osteoblasts, which is the main feature of the remodelling phase.

9.4.2 Soluble Factors and Cytokines

The main soluble factors that regulate the process of mineralisation of cartilaginous callus are M-CSF, RANKL and OPG. Although the early peak of RANKL is mainly derived from T lymphocytes during the inflammatory stage, its second high expression is evident during the repair/remodelling phase [34]. RANKL and M-CSF secreted by osteoblasts work to enhance the survival and the activity of osteoclasts [155, 156].

Additionally, a second elevation of pro-inflammatory cytokines, IL-6 and TNF-α, has been shown to happen later as the mineralised callus is remodelled into lamellar bone. These cytokines that are increased later on healing are expressed by MSCs and osteoblasts [34]. Overall, certain cytokines and soluble proteins are released by active osteoblasts then these factors work to induce the generation of osteoclasts thus controlling bone remodelling.

9.4.3 The Summary of Remodelling Phase of Bone Healing

Bone cells, MSCs as well as certain immune cells are the main players during remodelling phase (Figs. 9.1 and 9.2). During this phase, the hard callus formed of irregular woven bone is transformed into lamellar regular bone via maintaining the equilibrium between the activity of osteoblasts and osteoclasts. Controlling these processes, MSCs differentiate into osteoblasts and can promote osteoclastogenesis.

Th17 and macrophages regulate the balance of osteoblast and osteoclast functions. Growth factors as well as cytokines, which are produced by osteoblasts, induce the generation and the survival of osteoclasts.

9.5 Intramembranous Healing

Intramembranous healing is characterised by the direct differentiation of MSCs into osteoblasts during the repair phase. Previous evidence has shown that certain immune cells are involved in this type of healing. Bone-lining resident macrophages contribute to the intramembranous bone healing as shown in mouse tibial fracture model [126]. Furthermore, the effect of T lymphocytes seems to be extended to prepare the osteoblasts for the proliferative phase of the bone repair. It has been reported that lack of T lymphocytes in $RAG^{-/-}$ mice shows delayed maturation of osteoblasts and prolonged repair phase that further delay the remodelling phase [63]. BMPs are essential for the proliferation of MSCs and the production of alkaline phosphatase from MSCs and osteoblasts favouring bone formation [157, 158]. BMP-3, BMP-4, BMP-7 and BMP-8 are strictly expressed when the osteoblastic recruitment is most active. BMPs transduce their signal through SMAD activation and in conjunction with other signalling pathways such as Notch pathway [159–161]. These findings further demonstrate the strong link between the bone healing and immune response with a help of growth factors.

9.6 MSC-Immune Cell Interactions; Implication in Defective Bone Healing

Complications such as delayed or non-union of bone fractures could be related to systemic inflammatory diseases or fracture-related reasons including sepsis, severe soft tissue damage and multiple fractures [162]. MSCs are existed in non-union tissues, but these MSCs have an impaired function including increasing their senescence [163]. Additionally, it has been demonstrated that the number and the proliferative capacity of BM MSCs can be impaired in patients with non-union fractures compared to healthy controls [164, 165]. Furthermore, the osteogenic activity is lower compared to BM MSCs [166]. However, these non-union MSCs seem to retain their osteogenic differentiation when activated in vitro [165, 167]. Additionally, these non-union MSCs can regain a full capacity of osteogenesis if treated with BMP-2 [168]. Although, it is unknown if the changes in MSC number and function are reasons or results of non-union, injecting autologous BM MSCs into non-union site is still widely used in therapy [169]. Additionally, this indicates that the defect of non-union MSCs is related to microenvironment rather than being an intrinsic fault. Immune response is linked to bone haemostasis due to the direct effects of immune cells on osteoclasts and osteoblasts. Chronic inflammatory disorders due to systemic or local disease are always associated with bone pathology. The effects of uncontrolled inflammation including cells and cytokines are reviewed below.

9.6.1 Neutrophils

A systemic activation of neutrophils using oxygen free radicals leads to a defective healing of bone fracture as shown in rodents [170]. Additionally, an induced neutropenia in animal models of bone defects shows an enhanced osteogenic repair [171]. Although it is not clear if neutrophils interact with MSCs, an excess activation of neutrophils has a negative effect on the bone healing.

9.6.2 Macrophages

As shown in an experimental model of bone fracture in rat, an excessive activation of macrophages via systemic injection of lipopolysaccharide can reduce the secretion of BMP-2 by macrophages and results in a delayed bone healing probably via a negative effect on MSCs [157]. Monocytes and particularly those which express a high level of a co-stimulatory molecule, Osteoclast-associated receptor (OSCAR) have a greater potential to differentiate into osteoclasts via TNF-α mediated mechanism within an excessive inflammatory milieu [172]. This implies an adverse effect of activation of monocytes on the bone repair via their effects on both MSCs and osteoclasts.

9.6.3 NK Cells

Within an excessive inflammatory milieu, NK cells could play a role in the pathogenesis of delaying bone healing or even bone loss. Activated NK cells impair the survival and function of injected allogeneic or autologous MSCs and subsequently inhibit MSC-dependent therapeutic effects [102, 173–176]. NK cells also have a similar role in the pathogenesis of inflammation-related bone destruction as shown in a mouse model of arthritis and the depletion of NK cells considerably prevents the bone erosion [47]. In conclusion, activated NK cells could exert adverse effects on the bone haemostasis.

9.6.4 T and B Lymphocytes

A study comparing the abundance of cytotoxic T lymphocytes within the fracture hematoma between healing and non-healing groups of sheep has reported a predominance of T lymphocytes in the non-healing group [177]. Moreover, a mouse model of gamma delta T cell knock out has been shown an improvement in the bone healing [178]. Interestingly, the uncontrolled stimulation of B and T lymphocytes appear to be important in delayed bone healing. $RAG^{-/-}$ mice, which lack T and B cells, show an enhancement of callus mineralisation and bone remodelling and acceleration of the fracture healing [42]. These effects were associated with a lower level of pro-inflammatory cytokines, TNF-α, IFN-γ, IL-2 and IL-4 at local fracture tissues [42]. Activated T lymphocytes are known to release RANKL, which enhances osteoclast differentiation from their progenitors and consequently induce the bone lysis [156]. Similar to T lymphocytes, B lymphocytes can stimulate the generation of osteoclasts as they secret RANKL and specific autoantibodies. These autoantibodies have a high binding affinity to the surface of osteoclasts and their precursors inducing bone damage [179]. Altogether, the excess activation of these adaptive immune cells is harmful for the bone generation.

In a recent study, a positive correlation has been observed between the delayed bone repair and increase of the expression of peripheral blood terminally differentiated $CD8^+$ $CD11a^+$ T lymphocytes, which highly produce IFN-γ and TNF-α [180]. Moreover, a depletion of these $CD8^+$ T lymphocytes leads to an improvement of bone repair in an osteotomy mouse model [180]. In another study, activated Th1 cells or cytotoxic T lymphocytes were found to block osteogenic differentiation of MSCs via the effect of IFN-γ [181]. Interestingly, IL-17, which is produced by activated Th17 subset of T lymphocytes, has been linked to bone destruction in excessive inflammatory milieu [152]. These studies confirm the link between effector T lymphocytes and impaired bone healing.

In contrast to effector subsets of T lymphocytes, T reg lymphocytes have shown no suppressive effect on MSC-mediated bone formation probably because of an associated suppressive effect on IFN-γ and TNF-α. This finding was further confirmed when injected T reg lymphocytes has been shown to improve the MSC-mediated repair of bone fracture efficiently in an animal model [182]. Transplantation of syngeneic MSCs induced T reg response with a better healing compared to allogeneic MSCs, which induced Th1 response marked by the production of IFN-γ [181]. Similarly, infusion of T reg lymphocytes in calvarial defect in mice was associated with an enhancement of MSC-mediated bone healing and a reduction of the expression of TNF-α and IFN-γ [181].

In conclusion, prolonged activation of immune cells inhibits osteogenesis. Depletion of haematopoietic cells from human allograft material containing live osteocytes [183] shows no adverse immune effects upon graft implantation in vivo [184], but it is critical to study such allograft's behaviour and MSC function generally in inflammatory milieu. This will pave the way to new therapeutic solutions for non-union bone fractures.

9.6.5 Cytokines

Prolonged or uncontrolled inflammatory phase of bone repair could be destructive. There is a link between excess inflammation, e.g. in microbial infection and impaired osteogenesis [185]. Different inflammation-related cytokines and cells are linked to pathological bone healing. TNF-α mediated chronic inflammation in a diabetic mouse model has been shown to lead to the death of regenerating chondrocytes thus impairing the bone formation [186, 187]. Importantly, TNF-α has been shown to stimulate the expression of Wnt signalling pathway antagonist, Dickkopf-1 (DKK-1) that has a direct suppressive effect on the differentiation of osteoblasts. Conversely, the suppression of DKK-1 has been shown to activate the Wnt signalling pathway and induce the bone growth [188]. DKK-1 seems to suppress the OPG production and disturb OPG-RANKL balance leading to bone lysis [188]. Another role for TNF-α is to suppress nephronectin, an extracellular matrix protein that induces the development and growth of osteoblasts [189]. Additionally, TNF-α induces the production of M-CSF by BM MSCs, which in turn enhances the expression of the key osteoclastogenic cytokine receptor, RANK in the osteoclast progenitors [190]. Targeting TNF-α in these models reversed these effects and improved bone healing [187].

In chronic inflammatory milieu, TNF-α suppresses the biomarkers of MSC osteogenic differentiation via NF-kβ signalling-dependent mechanism [191]. An exposure of mouse MSCs to high doses of TNF-α and IL-1 reduced their osteogenic differentiation as shown by suppression of ALP levels compared to controls [192]. Both TNF-α and IFN-γ inhibited MSC osteogenic ability in dose-dependent manner in vitro [180]. Interestingly, an in vitro exposure to IFN-γ augmented TNF-α-mediated apoptosis of BM MSCs and suppressed their osteogenic differentiation [182, 191]. The IFN-γ-mediated inhibition of osteogenesis of MSCs was associated with increased expression levels of SMAD-6, a negative controller of bone differentiation [182]. Additionally, IFN-γ enhanced the formation of osteoclasts [193]. Another inflammatory cytokine, IL-6 mediates osteoclastogenesis and blocking of IL-6 receptor was shown to protect from bone erosion in mouse model of arthritis [194]. Similarly, osteoclast formation was significantly reduced in mouse model of arthritis where IL-1 was knocked out indicating that IL-1 has an important role in inflammation-mediated bone lysis [195].

The chronic inflammation and pathological bone formation are associated with dysregulation of BMPs and their inhibitors [35]. The gene expression of BMP antagonists (noggin and follistatin) and certain MMPs, MMP-7 and MMP-12 are higher in non-union tissues compared to that in normal healing callus [196]. In contrast, many genes are inhibited in non-union including growth factors IGF-2,

FGF-1, TGF-β2, PDGF, Wnt-induced proteins, B-catenin as well as receptors for PGE2 [197].

In summary, exaggerated or prolonged effect of inflammatory cytokines and cells have a negative effect on MSCs by inhibiting their osteogenic ability as well as a stimulatory role on osteoclasts leading to defective bone formation (Fig. 9.3).

9.7 MSC-Immune Cell Interactions; Therapeutic Implications to Fracture Repair

Animal studies and clinical trials, which used MSCs for therapeutic purposes of bone repair, indicated that the inflammation status could affect significantly the efficiency of these treatments. The magnitude of inflammation highly influences the immunomodulatory effects of MSCs [13]. High dose of IFN-γ or other priming cytokines is needed to induce the immunosuppressive function of MSCs and consequently the bone healing. In contrast, weak inflammation or low dose of IFN-γ might not be enough to prime MSCs for immunosuppressive effect, instead, it could induce the antigen presentation property in MSCs and promote the recruitment of immune cells [198, 199].

Allogeneic MSCs derived from BM, placenta and umbilical cord then implanted under the kidney capsule on collagen-based matrix did not form ectopic bone compared to syngeneic MSCs in murine recipients [200]. Similarly, cloned MSCs derived from Balb/c mice could not promote bone growth in allogeneic mice together with the suppression of osteogenic markers, Alkaline phosphatase, cbfa-1/Runx2 and osteocalcin [181]. Additionally, the chondrogenic potential of synovial MSCs transplanted into allogeneic rat with anterior meniscus defect was impaired relative to autogenic implants [201]. In these conditions, an increase of the local expression of NK cells, T and B lymphocytes as well as macrophages was detected [181, 201, 202]. In addition, a high expression level of allo-specific antibodies was demonstrated in the recipient hosts [202]. It has been proposed that Th1 response evident by increase of IFN-γ was responsible for the suppression of the bone growth [181]. It is likely that the exposure of allogeneic MSCs to the activated host immune cells leads to suppression of the functions of these MSCs and failure of the therapy.

Interestingly, autologous MSCs are susceptible for killing by cytokine-activated NK cells. This killing is related to the low level of HLA class I and to the presence of ligands for NK cell activating receptors on the surface of MSCs [102, 173–176]. Also, the activation of NK cells against MSCs is related to specific adhesion molecules [176]. In cases of GVDH, NK cells could have a negative effect on injected allogeneic MSCs, which threatens the fate of the transplant [203]. Despite these in vitro observations, it is still unknown if NK cell-mediated killing of allogeneic MSCs occurs when these MSCs used for therapy of the bone repair.

In summary, NK cell-mediated killing of allogeneic MSCs could be another mechanism causing the failure of therapeutic use of MSCs.

Allogeneic and autologous BM MSCs loaded on hydroxyapatite or β-tricalcium phosphate scaffolds then implanted in femoral defect in dogs or tibia defect in mini pigs or radius injury in rabbits, showed similar extent of the bone growth without eliciting an immune response [204–206]. Additionally, an implantation of adipose-derived MSCs loaded on matrix into ulnar defect in rabbits or added to fibrin glue to fill the mandible defect in rats showed positive bone healing results comparable to that using autologous MSCs [207, 208]. Seeding of allogeneic MSCs in β-tricalcium phosphate scaffolds implanted in dogs has been shown to elicit an inflammatory response, measured by increase of the number of T lymphocytes, similar to that induced by autologous MSCs [209]. These observations indicate that the interactions between allogeneic MSCs and recipient immune cells could be avoided if these MSCs are loaded on mineralised scaffolds thus minimising their accessibility to host immune cells.

9.8 Conclusions and Future Perspectives

Osteoimmunology is an emerging discipline exploring the relationship between inflammation and bone biology and how inflammatory signals control bone healing. Similar to the repair of muscle injuries and skin wounds where MSCs are involved in all stages of the repair [210], MSCs interact with various cells, cytokines and growth factors during the whole process of the bone fracture healing [211]. The effect of inflammation on the bone healing through interaction between MSCs and immune cells is complex. As explained, inflammatory cells and cytokines prime MSCs towards immunomodulatory function while the excess activation of the same mediators can suppress the osteogenic differentiation of MSCs. Furthermore, cytokines like IL-17 could promote or suppress osteogenesis via its dual effect on both osteoblasts and osteoclasts. Therefore a fine balance between the functions of MSCs and inflammatory mediators and cells as well as between osteoclasts and osteoblasts exists and the disturbance in these balances can lead to the complications of the bone repair such as delayed healing or fracture non-union.

Whilst the suppression of inflammation is needed for MSC differentiation to proceed, inappropriate inflammatory-mediated priming of MSCs could lead to a failure in switching off the inflammatory signals and hence to impaired progression through the bone healing stages. The ultimate goal for using MSCs in cases of bone defect or fractures should not be only be as powerful osteogenic cells but also as immune mediators controlling the inflammatory stage of bone healing. Indeed, several therapeutic approaches targeting inflammation in animal models of delayed healing have been shown successful outcomes [211]. The better understanding of MSC-immune cell interactions during the bone healing is therefore highly important in order to modulate MSC-based therapy and ultimately treat or prevent challenging cases of bone injuries.

References

1. Ozaki A, Tsunoda M, Kinoshita S, Saura R. Role of fracture hematoma and periosteum during fracture healing in rats: interaction of fracture hematoma and the periosteum in the initial step of the healing process. J Orthop Sci. 2000;5(1):64–70.
2. Schett G, Gravallese E. Bone erosion in rheumatoid arthritis: mechanisms, diagnosis and treatment. Nat Rev Rheumatol. 2012;8(11):656–64.
3. Friedenstein AJ, Chailakhjan RK, Lalykina KS. The development of fibroblast colonies in monolayer cultures of guinea-pig bone marrow and spleen cells. Cell Tissue Kinet. 1970;3(4):393–403.
4. Caplan AI. Mesenchymal stem cells. J Orthop Res. 1991;9(5):641–50.
5. Dominici M, Le Blanc K, Mueller I, Slaper-Cortenbach I, Marini F, Krause D, et al. Minimal criteria for defining multipotent mesenchymal stromal cells. The International Society for Cellular Therapy position statement. Cytotherapy. 2006;8(4):315–7.
6. Colnot C. Cell sources for bone tissue engineering: insights from basic science. Tissue Eng Part B Rev. 2011;17(6):449–57.
7. Pitchford SC, Furze RC, Jones CP, Wengner AM, Rankin SM. Differential mobilization of subsets of progenitor cells from the bone marrow. Cell Stem Cell. 2009;4(1):62–72.
8. Cuthbert R, Boxall SA, Tan HB, Giannoudis PV, McGonagle D, Jones E. Single-platform quality control assay to quantify multipotential stromal cells in bone marrow aspirates prior to bulk manufacture or direct therapeutic use. Cytotherapy. 2012;14(4):431–40.
9. Alvarez-Viejo M, Menendez-Menendez Y, Otero-Hernandez J. CD271 as a marker to identify mesenchymal stem cells from diverse sources before culture. World J Stem Cells. 2015;7(2):470–6.
10. Nakahara H, Dennis JE, Bruder SP, Haynesworth SE, Lennon DP, Caplan AI. In vitro differentiation of bone and hypertrophic cartilage from periosteal-derived cells. Exp Cell Res. 1991;195(2):492–503.
11. Kisiel AH, McDuffee LA, Masaoud E, Bailey TR, Esparza Gonzalez BP, Nino-Fong R. Isolation, characterization, and in vitro proliferation of canine mesenchymal stem cells derived from bone marrow, adipose tissue, muscle, and periosteum. Am J Vet Res. 2012;73(8):1305–17.
12. Beane OS, Fonseca VC, Cooper LL, Koren G, Darling EM. Impact of aging on the regenerative properties of bone marrow-, muscle-, and adipose-derived mesenchymal stem/stromal cells. PLoS One. 2014;9(12):e115963.
13. Wang Y, Chen X, Cao W, Shi Y. Plasticity of mesenchymal stem cells in immunomodulation: pathological and therapeutic implications. Nat Immunol. 2014;15(11):1009–16.
14. Krampera M. Mesenchymal stromal cell 'licensing': a multistep process. Leukemia. 2011;25(9):1408–14.
15. Mizuno K, Mineo K, Tachibana T, Sumi M, Matsubara T, Hirohata K. The osteogenetic potential of fracture haematoma. Subperiosteal and intramuscular transplantation of the haematoma. J Bone Joint Surg. 1990;72(5):822–9.
16. Claes L, Recknagel S, Ignatius A. Fracture healing under healthy and inflammatory conditions. Nat Rev Rheumatol. 2012;8(3):133–43.
17. Marsell R, Einhorn TA. The biology of fracture healing. Injury. 2011;42(6):551–5.
18. Nakahara H, Bruder SP, Haynesworth SE, Holecek JJ, Baber MA, Goldberg VM, et al. Bone and cartilage formation in diffusion chambers by subcultured cells derived from the periosteum. Bone. 1990;11(3):181–8.
19. Phillips AM. Overview of the fracture healing cascade. Injury. 2005;36 Suppl 3:S5–7.
20. Cottrell JA, Vales FM, Schachter D, Wadsworth S, Gundlapalli R, Kapadia R, et al. Osteogenic activity of locally applied small molecule drugs in a rat femur defect model. J Biomed Biotechnol. 2010;2010:597641.
21. Boyle WJ, Simonet WS, Lacey DL. Osteoclast differentiation and activation. Nature. 2003;423(6937):337–42.

22. Pettit AR, Ji H, von Stechow D, Muller R, Goldring SR, Choi Y, et al. TRANCE/RANKL knockout mice are protected from bone erosion in a serum transfer model of arthritis. Am J Pathol. 2001;159(5):1689–99.
23. Gerstenfeld LC, Cullinane DM, Barnes GL, Graves DT, Einhorn TA. Fracture healing as a post-natal developmental process: molecular, spatial, and temporal aspects of its regulation. J Cell Biochem. 2003;88(5):873–84.
24. Xing Z, Lu C, Hu D, Miclau 3rd T, Marcucio RS. Rejuvenation of the inflammatory system stimulates fracture repair in aged mice. J Orthop Res. 2010;28(8):1000–6.
25. Richardson J, Hill AM, Johnston CJ, McGregor A, Norrish AR, Eastwood D, et al. Fracture healing in HIV-positive populations. J Bone Joint Surg. 2008;90(8):988–94.
26. Aukrust P, Haug CJ, Ueland T, Lien E, Muller F, Espevik T, et al. Decreased bone formative and enhanced resorptive markers in human immunodeficiency virus infection: indication of normalization of the bone-remodeling process during highly active antiretroviral therapy. J Clin Endocrinol Metab. 1999;84(1):145–50.
27. Timlin M, Toomey D, Condron C, Power C, Street J, Murray P, et al. Fracture hematoma is a potent proinflammatory mediator of neutrophil function. J Trauma. 2005;58(6):1223–9.
28. Xian CJ, Zhou FH, McCarty RC, Foster BK. Intramembranous ossification mechanism for bone bridge formation at the growth plate cartilage injury site. J Orthop Res. 2004;22 (2):417–26.
29. Chung R, Cool JC, Scherer MA, Foster BK, Xian CJ. Roles of neutrophil-mediated inflammatory response in the bony repair of injured growth plate cartilage in young rats. J Leukoc Biol. 2006;80(6):1272–80.
30. Segal AW. How neutrophils kill microbes. Annu Rev Immunol. 2005;23:197–223.
31. Xing Z, Lu C, Hu D, Yu YY, Wang X, Colnot C, et al. Multiple roles for CCR2 during fracture healing. Dis Model Mech. 2010;3(7-8):451–8.
32. Wu AC, Raggatt LJ, Alexander KA, Pettit AR. Unraveling macrophage contributions to bone repair. Bonekey Rep. 2013;2:373.
33. Lacey DC, Achuthan A, Fleetwood AJ, Dinh H, Roiniotis J, Scholz GM, et al. Defining GM-CSF- and macrophage-CSF-dependent macrophage responses by in vitro models. J Immunol. 2012;188(11):5752–65.
34. Kon T, Cho TJ, Aizawa T, Yamazaki M, Nooh N, Graves D, et al. Expression of osteoprotegerin, receptor activator of NF-kappaB ligand (osteoprotegerin ligand) and related proinflammatory cytokines during fracture healing. J Bone Miner Res. 2001;16(6):1004–14.
35. Yu YY, Lieu S, Lu C, Miclau T, Marcucio RS, Colnot C. Immunolocalization of BMPs, BMP antagonists, receptors, and effectors during fracture repair. Bone. 2010;46(3):841–51.
36. Nakase T, Yoshikawa H. Potential roles of bone morphogenetic proteins (BMPs) in skeletal repair and regeneration. J Bone Miner Metab. 2006;24(6):425–33.
37. Guihard P, Danger Y, Brounais B, David E, Brion R, Delecrin J, et al. Induction of osteogenesis in mesenchymal stem cells by activated monocytes/macrophages depends on oncostatin M signaling. Stem Cells. 2012;30(4):762–72.
38. Nicolaidou V, Wong MM, Redpath AN, Ersek A, Baban DF, Williams LM, et al. Monocytes induce STAT3 activation in human mesenchymal stem cells to promote osteoblast formation. PLoS One. 2012;7(7):e39871.
39. Ekstrom K, Omar O, Graneli C, Wang X, Vazirisani F, Thomsen P. Monocyte exosomes stimulate the osteogenic gene expression of mesenchymal stem cells. PLoS One. 2013;8(9): e75227.
40. Omar OM, Graneli C, Ekstrom K, Karlsson C, Johansson A, Lausmaa J, et al. The stimulation of an osteogenic response by classical monocyte activation. Biomaterials. 2011;32 (32):8190–204.
41. Shi FD, Ljunggren HG, La Cava A, Van Kaer L. Organ-specific features of natural killer cells. Nat Rev Immunol. 2011;11(10):658–71.

42. Toben D, Schroeder I, El Khassawna T, Mehta M, Hoffmann JE, Frisch JT, et al. Fracture healing is accelerated in the absence of the adaptive immune system. J Bone Miner Res. 2011;26(1):113–24.
43. Thomas H, Jager M, Mauel K, Brandau S, Lask S, Flohe SB. Interaction with mesenchymal stem cells provokes natural killer cells for enhanced IL-12/IL-18-induced interferon-gamma secretion. Mediators Inflamm. 2014;2014:143463.
44. Gerstenfeld LC, Cho TJ, Kon T, Aizawa T, Cruceta J, Graves BD, et al. Impaired intramembranous bone formation during bone repair in the absence of tumor necrosis factor-alpha signaling. Cells Tissues Organs. 2001;169(3):285–94.
45. Gerstenfeld LC, Cho TJ, Kon T, Aizawa T, Tsay A, Fitch J, et al. Impaired fracture healing in the absence of TNF-alpha signaling: the role of TNF-alpha in endochondral cartilage resorption. J Bone Miner Res. 2003;18(9):1584–92.
46. Almeida CR, Vasconcelos DP, Goncalves RM, Barbosa MA. Enhanced mesenchymal stromal cell recruitment via natural killer cells by incorporation of inflammatory signals in biomaterials. J R Soc Interface. 2012;9(67):261–71.
47. Soderstrom K, Stein E, Colmenero P, Purath U, Muller-Ladner U, de Matos CT, et al. Natural killer cells trigger osteoclastogenesis and bone destruction in arthritis. Proc Natl Acad Sci U S A. 2010;107(29):13028–33.
48. Lam J, Takeshita S, Barker JE, Kanagawa O, Ross FP, Teitelbaum SL. TNF-alpha induces osteoclastogenesis by direct stimulation of macrophages exposed to permissive levels of RANK ligand. J Clin Invest. 2000;106(12):1481–8.
49. Spits H, Cupedo T. Innate lymphoid cells: emerging insights in development, lineage relationships, and function. Annu Rev Immunol. 2012;30:647–75.
50. Yagi R, Zhong C, Northrup DL, Yu F, Bouladoux N, Spencer S, et al. The transcription factor GATA3 is critical for the development of all IL-7Ralpha-expressing innate lymphoid cells. Immunity. 2014;40(3):378–88.
51. Spits H, Di Santo JP. The expanding family of innate lymphoid cells: regulators and effectors of immunity and tissue remodeling. Nat Immunol. 2011;12(1):21–7.
52. Artis D, Spits H. The biology of innate lymphoid cells. Nature. 2015;517(7534):293–301.
53. Fuchs A, Vermi W, Lee JS, Lonardi S, Gilfillan S, Newberry RD, et al. Intraepithelial type 1 innate lymphoid cells are a unique subset of IL-12- and IL-15-responsive IFN-gamma-producing cells. Immunity. 2013;38(4):769–81.
54. Bernink JH, Peters CP, Munneke M, te Velde AA, Meijer SL, Weijer K, et al. Human type 1 innate lymphoid cells accumulate in inflamed mucosal tissues. Nat Immunol. 2013;14 (3):221–9.
55. Price AE, Liang HE, Sullivan BM, Reinhardt RL, Eisley CJ, Erle DJ, et al. Systemically dispersed innate IL-13-expressing cells in type 2 immunity. Proc Natl Acad Sci U S A. 2010;107(25):11489–94.
56. Neill DR, Wong SH, Bellosi A, Flynn RJ, Daly M, Langford TK, et al. Nuocytes represent a new innate effector leukocyte that mediates type-2 immunity. Nature. 2010;464 (7293):1367–70.
57. Wilhelm C, Hirota K, Stieglitz B, Van Snick J, Tolaini M, Lahl K, et al. An IL-9 fate reporter demonstrates the induction of an innate IL-9 response in lung inflammation. Nat Immunol. 2011;12(11):1071–7.
58. Cupedo T, Crellin NK, Papazian N, Rombouts EJ, Weijer K, Grogan JL, et al. Human fetal lymphoid tissue-inducer cells are interleukin 17-producing precursors to RORC+ CD127+ natural killer-like cells. Nat Immunol. 2009;10(1):66–74.
59. Sawa S, Lochner M, Satoh-Takayama N, Dulauroy S, Berard M, Kleinschek M, et al. RORgammat + innate lymphoid cells regulate intestinal homeostasis by integrating negative signals from the symbiotic microbiota. Nat Immunol. 2011;12(4):320–6.
60. Dudakov JA, Hanash AM, Jenq RR, Young LF, Ghosh A, Singer NV, et al. Interleukin-22 drives endogenous thymic regeneration in mice. Science. 2012;336(6077):91–5.

61. Scandella E, Bolinger B, Lattmann E, Miller S, Favre S, Littman DR, et al. Restoration of lymphoid organ integrity through the interaction of lymphoid tissue-inducer cells with stroma of the T cell zone. Nat Immunol. 2008;9(6):667–75.
62. Monticelli LA, Sonnenberg GF, Abt MC, Alenghat T, Ziegler CG, Doering TA, et al. Innate lymphoid cells promote lung-tissue homeostasis after infection with influenza virus. Nat Immunol. 2011;12(11):1045–54.
63. Nam D, Mau E, Wang Y, Wright D, Silkstone D, Whetstone H, et al. T-lymphocytes enable osteoblast maturation via IL-17F during the early phase of fracture repair. PLoS One. 2012;7 (6):e40044.
64. Yasser El-Sherbiny AE, Evangelos MF, Richard C, Thomas B, Elena J, Dennis McG. IL-22 drives the proliferation and differentiation of human bone marrow mesenchymal stem cells (MSCs); a novel pathway that may contribute to aberrant new bone formation in human Spa and beyond. 2015 ACR/ARHP Annual Meeting. ACR Poster Session B (Innate Immunity and Rheumatic Disease Poster II), 2015
65. Askalonov AA, Gordienko SM, Avdyunicheva OE, Bondarenko AV, Voronkov SF. The role of T-system immunity in reparatory regeneration of the bone tissue in animals. J Hyg Epidemiol Microbiol Immunol. 1987;31(2):219–24.
66. Askalonov AA. Changes in some indices of cellular immunity in patients with uncomplicated and complicated healing of bone fractures. J Hyg Epidemiol Microbiol Immunol. 1981;25 (3):307–10.
67. Hauser CJ, Zhou X, Joshi P, Cuchens MA, Kregor P, Devidas M, et al. The immune microenvironment of human fracture/soft-tissue hematomas and its relationship to systemic immunity. J Trauma. 1997;42(5):895–903. discussion-4.
68. Andrew JG, Andrew SM, Freemont AJ, Marsh DR. Inflammatory cells in normal human fracture healing. Acta Orthop Scand. 1994;65(4):462–6.
69. Kong YY, Feige U, Sarosi I, Bolon B, Tafuri A, Morony S, et al. Activated T cells regulate bone loss and joint destruction in adjuvant arthritis through osteoprotegerin ligand. Nature. 1999;402(6759):304–9.
70. Connor JR, Dodds RA, James IE, Gowen M. Human osteoclast and giant cell differentiation: the apparent switch from nonspecific esterase to tartrate resistant acid phosphatase activity coincides with the in situ expression of osteopontin mRNA. J Histochem Cytochem. 1995;43 (12):1193–201.
71. Grassi F, Cattini L, Gambari L, Manferdini C, Piacentini A, Gabusi E, et al. T cell subsets differently regulate osteogenic differentiation of human mesenchymal stromal cells in vitro. J Tissue Eng Regen Med. 2013;10(4):305–14.
72. Ng F, Boucher S, Koh S, Sastry KS, Chase L, Lakshmipathy U, et al. PDGF, TGF-beta, and FGF signaling is important for differentiation and growth of mesenchymal stem cells (MSCs): transcriptional profiling can identify markers and signaling pathways important in differentiation of MSCs into adipogenic, chondrogenic, and osteogenic lineages. Blood. 2008;112(2):295–307.
73. Cho TJ, Gerstenfeld LC, Einhorn TA. Differential temporal expression of members of the transforming growth factor beta superfamily during murine fracture healing. J Bone Miner Res. 2002;17(3):513–20.
74. Manabe N, Kawaguchi H, Chikuda H, Miyaura C, Inada M, Nagai R, et al. Connection between B lymphocyte and osteoclast differentiation pathways. J Immunol. 2001;167 (5):2625–31.
75. Weitzmann MN, Cenci S, Haug J, Brown C, DiPersio J, Pacifici R. B lymphocytes inhibit human osteoclastogenesis by secretion of TGFbeta. J Cell Biochem. 2000;78(2):318–24.
76. Raggatt LJ, Alexander KA, Kaur S, Wu AC, MacDonald KPA, Pettit AR. Absence of B cells does not compromise intramembranous bone formation during healing in a tibial injury model. Am J Pathol. 2013;182(5):1501–8.
77. McKibbin B. The biology of fracture healing in long bones. J Bone Joint Surg. 1978;60-B (2):150–62.

78. Kumagai K, Vasanji A, Drazba JA, Butler RS, Muschler GF. Circulating cells with osteogenic potential are physiologically mobilized into the fracture healing site in the parabiotic mice model. J Orthop Res. 2008;26(2):165–75.
79. Malizos KN, Papatheodorou LK. The healing potential of the periosteum molecular aspects. Injury. 2005;36 Suppl 3:S13–9.
80. Colnot C, Huang S, Helms J. Analyzing the cellular contribution of bone marrow to fracture healing using bone marrow transplantation in mice. Biochem Biophys Res Commun. 2006;350(3):557–61.
81. Yu YY, Lieu S, Lu C, Colnot C. Bone morphogenetic protein 2 stimulates endochondral ossification by regulating periosteal cell fate during bone repair. Bone. 2010;47(1):65–73.
82. Liu R, Birke O, Morse A, Peacock L, Mikulec K, Little DG, et al. Myogenic progenitors contribute to open but not closed fracture repair. BMC Musculoskelet Disord. 2011;12:288.
83. Kitaori T, Ito H, Schwarz EM, Tsutsumi R, Yoshitomi H, Oishi S, et al. Stromal cell-derived factor 1/CXCR4 signaling is critical for the recruitment of mesenchymal stem cells to the fracture site during skeletal repair in a mouse model. Arthritis Rheum. 2009;60(3):813–23.
84. Liu X, Duan B, Cheng Z, Jia X, Mao L, Fu H, et al. SDF-1/CXCR4 axis modulates bone marrow mesenchymal stem cell apoptosis, migration and cytokine secretion. Protein Cell. 2011;2(10):845–54.
85. Guiducci S, Manetti M, Romano E, Mazzanti B, Ceccarelli C, Dal Pozzo S, et al. Bone marrow-derived mesenchymal stem cells from early diffuse systemic sclerosis exhibit a paracrine machinery and stimulate angiogenesis in vitro. Ann Rheum Dis. 2011;70 (11):2011–21.
86. Hosogane N, Huang Z, Rawlins BA, Liu X, Boachie-Adjei O, Boskey AL, et al. Stromal derived factor-1 regulates bone morphogenetic protein 2-induced osteogenic differentiation of primary mesenchymal stem cells. Int J Biochem Cell Biol. 2010;42(7):1132–41.
87. Bocker W, Docheva D, Prall WC, Egea V, Pappou E, Rossmann O, et al. IKK-2 is required for TNF-alpha-induced invasion and proliferation of human mesenchymal stem cells. J Mol Med. 2008;86(10):1183–92.
88. Tso GH, Law HK, Tu W, Chan GC, Lau YL. Phagocytosis of apoptotic cells modulates mesenchymal stem cells osteogenic differentiation to enhance IL-17 and RANKL expression on CD4+ T cells. Stem Cells. 2010;28(5):939–54.
89. Mbalaviele G, Jaiswal N, Meng A, Cheng L, Van Den Bos C, Thiede M. Human mesenchymal stem cells promote human osteoclast differentiation from CD34+ bone marrow hematopoietic progenitors. Endocrinology. 1999;140(8):3736–43.
90. Croitoru-Lamoury J, Lamoury FM, Caristo M, Suzuki K, Walker D, Takikawa O, et al. Interferon-gamma regulates the proliferation and differentiation of mesenchymal stem cells via activation of indoleamine 2,3 dioxygenase (IDO). PLoS One. 2011;6(2): e14698.
91. Ren G, Zhao X, Zhang L, Zhang J, L'Huillier A, Ling W, et al. Inflammatory cytokine-induced intercellular adhesion molecule-1 and vascular cell adhesion molecule-1 in mesenchymal stem cells are critical for immunosuppression. J Immunol. 2010;184(5):2321–8.
92. Dorronsoro A, Ferrin I, Salcedo JM, Jakobsson E, Fernandez-Rueda J, Lang V, et al. Human mesenchymal stromal cells modulate T-cell responses through TNF-alpha-mediated activation of NF-kappaB. Eur J Immunol. 2014;44(2):480–8.
93. Fan H, Zhao G, Liu L, Liu F, Gong W, Liu X, et al. Pre-treatment with IL-1beta enhances the efficacy of MSC transplantation in DSS-induced colitis. Cell Mol Immunol. 2012;9 (6):473–81.
94. Delarosa O, Dalemans W, Lombardo E. Toll-like receptors as modulators of mesenchymal stem cells. Front Immunol. 2012;3:182.
95. Han X, Yang Q, Lin L, Xu C, Zheng C, Chen X, et al. Interleukin-17 enhances immunosuppression by mesenchymal stem cells. Cell Death Differ. 2014;21(11):1758–68.
96. Crane JL, Cao X. Bone marrow mesenchymal stem cells and TGF-beta signaling in bone remodeling. J Clin Invest. 2014;124(2):466–72.

97. Xu C, Yu P, Han X, Du L, Gan J, Wang Y, et al. TGF-beta promotes immune responses in the presence of mesenchymal stem cells. J Immunol. 2014;192(1):103–9.
98. Renner P, Eggenhofer E, Rosenauer A, Popp FC, Steinmann JF, Slowik P, et al. Mesenchymal stem cells require a sufficient, ongoing immune response to exert their immunosuppressive function. Transplant Proc. 2009;41(6):2607–11.
99. Granero-Molto F, Weis JA, Miga MI, Landis B, Myers TJ, O'Rear L, et al. Regenerative effects of transplanted mesenchymal stem cells in fracture healing. Stem Cells. 2009;27 (8):1887–98.
100. Klyushnenkova E, Mosca JD, McIntosh KR. Human mesenchymal stem cells suppress allogeneic T cell responses in vitro: Implications for allogeneic transplantation. Blood. 1998;92(10):642a.
101. Bartholomew A, Sturgeon C, Siatskas M, Ferrer K, McIntosh K, Patil S, et al. Mesenchymal stem cells suppress lymphocyte proliferation in vitro and prolong skin graft survival in vivo. Exp Hematol. 2002;30(1):42–8.
102. Spaggiari GM, Capobianco A, Becchetti S, Mingari MC, Moretta L. Mesenchymal stem cell-natural killer cell interactions: evidence that activated NK cells are capable of killing MSCs, whereas MSCs can inhibit IL-2-induced NK-cell proliferation. Blood. 2006;107(4):1484–90.
103. Spaggiari GM, Capobianco A, Abdelrazik H, Becchetti F, Mingari MC, Moretta L. Mesenchymal stem cells inhibit natural killer-cell proliferation, cytotoxicity, and cytokine production: role of indoleamine 2,3-dioxygenase and prostaglandin E2. Blood. 2008;111 (3):1327–33.
104. Luz-Crawford P, Kurte M, Bravo-Alegria J, Contreras R, Nova-Lamperti E, Tejedor G, et al. Mesenchymal stem cells generate a CD4 + CD25 + Foxp3+ regulatory T cell population during the differentiation process of Th1 and Th17 cells. Stem Cell Res Ther. 2013;4 (3):65.
105. Deng Y, Yi S, Wang G, Cheng J, Zhang Y, Chen W, et al. Umbilical cord-derived mesenchymal stem cells instruct dendritic cells to acquire tolerogenic phenotypes through the IL-6-mediated upregulation of SOCS1. Stem Cells Dev. 2014;23(17):2080–92.
106. Akiyama K, Chen C, Wang D, Xu X, Qu C, Yamaza T, et al. Mesenchymal-stem-cell-induced immunoregulation involves FAS-ligand-/FAS-mediated T cell apoptosis. Cell Stem Cell. 2012;10(5):544–55.
107. Corcione A, Benvenuto F, Ferretti E, Giunti D, Cappiello V, Cazzanti F, et al. Human mesenchymal stem cells modulate B-cell functions. Blood. 2006;107(1):367–72.
108. Nemeth K, Leelahavanichkul A, Yuen PS, Mayer B, Parmelee A, Doi K, et al. Bone marrow stromal cells attenuate sepsis via prostaglandin E(2)-dependent reprogramming of host macrophages to increase their interleukin-10 production. Nat Med. 2009;15(1):42–9.
109. Nemeth K, Keane-Myers A, Brown JM, Metcalfe DD, Gorham JD, Bundoc VG, et al. Bone marrow stromal cells use TGF-beta to suppress allergic responses in a mouse model of ragweed-induced asthma. Proc Natl Acad Sci U S A. 2010;107(12):5652–7.
110. DelaRosa O, Lombardo E, Beraza A, Mancheno-Corvo P, Ramirez C, Menta R, et al. Requirement of IFN-gamma-mediated indoleamine 2,3-dioxygenase expression in the modulation of lymphocyte proliferation by human adipose-derived stem cells. Tissue Eng Part A. 2009;15(10):2795–806.
111. Rafei M, Campeau PM, Aguilar-Mahecha A, Buchanan M, Williams P, Birman E, et al. Mesenchymal stromal cells ameliorate experimental autoimmune encephalomyelitis by inhibiting CD4 Th17 T cells in a CC chemokine ligand 2-dependent manner. J Immunol. 2009;182(10):5994–6002.
112. Shi Y, Hu G, Su J, Li W, Chen Q, Shou P, et al. Mesenchymal stem cells: a new strategy for immunosuppression and tissue repair. Cell Res. 2010;20(5):510–8.
113. Barnes GL, Kostenuik PJ, Gerstenfeld LC, Einhorn TA. Growth factor regulation of fracture repair. J Bone Miner Res. 1999;14(11):1805–15.
114. Schindeler A, McDonald MM, Bokko P, Little DG. Bone remodeling during fracture repair: the cellular picture. Semin Cell Dev Biol. 2008;19(5):459–66.

115. Knight MN, Hankenson KD. Mesenchymal stem cells in bone regeneration. Adv Wound Care. 2013;2(6):306–16.
116. Gerstenfeld LC, Alkhiary YM, Krall EA, Nicholls FH, Stapleton SN, Fitch JL, et al. Three-dimensional reconstruction of fracture callus morphogenesis. J Histochem Cytochem. 2006;54(11):1215–28.
117. Zelzer E, Glotzer DJ, Hartmann C, Thomas D, Fukai N, Soker S, et al. Tissue specific regulation of VEGF expression during bone development requires Cbfa1/Runx2. Mech Dev. 2001;106(1–2):97–106.
118. Wu Y, Chen L, Scott PG, Tredget EE. Mesenchymal stem cells enhance wound healing through differentiation and angiogenesis. Stem Cells. 2007;25(10):2648–59.
119. Blumer MJ, Longato S, Fritsch H. Localization of tartrate-resistant acid phosphatase (TRAP), membrane type-1 matrix metalloproteinases (MT1-MMP) and macrophages during early endochondral bone formation. J Anat. 2008;213(4):431–41.
120. Huang WC, Sala-Newby GB, Susana A, Johnson JL, Newby AC. Classical macrophage activation up-regulates several matrix metalloproteinases through mitogen activated protein kinases and nuclear factor-kappaB. PLoS One. 2012;7(8):e42507.
121. Dreier R, Wallace S, Fuchs S, Bruckner P, Grassel S. Paracrine interactions of chondrocytes and macrophages in cartilage degradation: articular chondrocytes provide factors that activate macrophage-derived pro-gelatinase B (pro-MMP-9). J Cell Sci. 2001;114 (Pt 21):3813–22.
122. Colnot C, Thompson Z, Miclau T, Werb Z, Helms JA. Altered fracture repair in the absence of MMP9. Development. 2003;130(17):4123–33.
123. Kosaki N, Takaishi H, Kamekura S, Kimura T, Okada Y, Minqi L, et al. Impaired bone fracture healing in matrix metalloproteinase-13 deficient mice. Biochem Biophys Res Commun. 2007;354(4):846–51.
124. McDonald MM, Morse A, Mikulec K, Peacock L, Baldock PA, Kostenuik PJ, et al. Matrix metalloproteinase-driven endochondral fracture union proceeds independently of osteoclast activity. J Bone Miner Res. 2013;28(7):1550–60.
125. Fajardo M, Liu CJ, Ilalov K, Egol KA. Matrix metalloproteinases that associate with and cleave bone morphogenetic protein-2 in vitro are elevated in hypertrophic fracture nonunion tissue. J Orthop Trauma. 2010;24(9):557–63.
126. Alexander KA, Chang MK, Maylin ER, Kohler T, Muller R, Wu AC, et al. Osteal macrophages promote in vivo intramembranous bone healing in a mouse tibial injury model. J Bone Miner Res. 2011;26(7):1517–32.
127. Hankemeier S, Grassel S, Plenz G, Spiegel HU, Bruckner P, Probst A. Alteration of fracture stability influences chondrogenesis, osteogenesis and immigration of macrophages. J Orthop Res. 2001;19(4):531–8.
128. Konnecke I, Serra A, El Khassawna T, Schlundt C, Schell H, Hauser A, et al. T and B cells participate in bone repair by infiltrating the fracture callus in a two-wave fashion. Bone. 2014;64:155–65.
129. Mountziaris PM, Mikos AG. Modulation of the inflammatory response for enhanced bone tissue regeneration. Tissue Eng Part B Rev. 2008;14(2):179–86.
130. Chen G, Deng C, Li YP. TGF-beta and BMP signaling in osteoblast differentiation and bone formation. Int J Biol Sci. 2012;8(2):272–88.
131. Lienau J, Schmidt-Bleek K, Peters A, Weber H, Bail HJ, Duda GN, et al. Insight into the molecular pathophysiology of delayed bone healing in a sheep model. Tissue Eng Part A. 2010;16(1):191–9.
132. Hak DJ, Makino T, Niikura T, Hazelwood SJ, Curtiss S, Reddi AH. Recombinant human BMP-7 effectively prevents non-union in both young and old rats. J Orthop Res. 2006;24 (1):11–20.
133. Tsuji K, Bandyopadhyay A, Harfe BD, Cox K, Kakar S, Gerstenfeld L, et al. BMP2 activity, although dispensable for bone formation, is required for the initiation of fracture healing. Nat Genet. 2006;38(12):1424–9.

134. Bandyopadhyay A, Tsuji K, Cox K, Harfe BD, Rosen V, Tabin CJ. Genetic analysis of the roles of BMP2, BMP4, and BMP7 in limb patterning and skeletogenesis. PLoS Genet. 2006;2(12):e216.
135. Lehmann W, Edgar CM, Wang K, Cho TJ, Barnes GL, Kakar S, et al. Tumor necrosis factor alpha (TNF-alpha) coordinately regulates the expression of specific matrix metalloproteinases (MMPS) and angiogenic factors during fracture healing. Bone. 2005;36(2):300–10.
136. Aizawa T, Kon T, Einhorn TA, Gerstenfeld LC. Induction of apoptosis in chondrocytes by tumor necrosis factor-alpha. J Orthop Res. 2001;19(5):785–96.
137. Wan C, Shao J, Gilbert SR, Riddle RC, Long F, Johnson RS, et al. Role of HIF-1alpha in skeletal development. Ann N Y Acad Sci. 2010;1192:322–6.
138. Kondo M, Yamaoka K, Sonomoto K, Fukuyo S, Oshita K, Okada Y, et al. IL-17 inhibits chondrogenic differentiation of human mesenchymal stem cells. PLoS One. 2013;8(11):e79463.
139. Mulari MT, Qu Q, Harkonen PL, Vaananen HK. Osteoblast-like cells complete osteoclastic bone resorption and form new mineralized bone matrix in vitro. Calcif Tissue Int. 2004;75(3):253–61.
140. Teitelbaum SL. Bone resorption by osteoclasts. Science. 2000;289(5484):1504–8.
141. Taguchi K, Ogawa R, Migita M, Hanawa H, Ito H, Orimo H. The role of bone marrow-derived cells in bone fracture repair in a green fluorescent protein chimeric mouse model. Biochem Biophys Res Commun. 2005;331(1):31–6.
142. James AW. Review of signaling pathways governing MSC osteogenic and adipogenic differentiation. Scientifica. 2013;2013:684736.
143. De Boer J, Wang HJ, Van Blitterswijk C. Effects of Wnt signaling on proliferation and differentiation of human mesenchymal stem cells. Tissue Eng. 2004;10(3–4):393–401.
144. Baksh D, Tuan RS. Canonical and non-canonical Wnts differentially affect the development potential of primary isolate of human bone marrow mesenchymal stem cells. J Cell Physiol. 2007;212(3):817–26.
145. Cawthorn WP, Bree AJ, Yao Y, Du B, Hemati N, Martinez-Santibanez G, et al. Wnt6, Wnt10a and Wnt10b inhibit adipogenesis and stimulate osteoblastogenesis through a beta-catenin-dependent mechanism. Bone. 2012;50(2):477–89.
146. Zhang X, Schwarz EM, Young DA, Puzas JE, Rosier RN, O'Keefe RJ. Cyclooxygenase-2 regulates mesenchymal cell differentiation into the osteoblast lineage and is critically involved in bone repair. J Clin Invest. 2002;109(11):1405–15.
147. Naik AA, Xie C, Zuscik MJ, Kingsley P, Schwarz EM, Awad H, et al. Reduced COX-2 expression in aged mice is associated with impaired fracture healing. J Bone Miner Res. 2009;24(2):251–64.
148. Oshita K, Yamaoka K, Udagawa N, Fukuyo S, Sonomoto K, Maeshima K, et al. Human mesenchymal stem cells inhibit osteoclastogenesis through osteoprotegerin production. Arthritis Rheum. 2011;63(6):1658–67.
149. Walsh NC, Gravallese EM. Bone remodeling in rheumatic disease: a question of balance. Immunol Rev. 2010;233(1):301–12.
150. Chen Y, Whetstone HC, Lin AC, Nadesan P, Wei Q, Poon R, et al. Beta-catenin signaling plays a disparate role in different phases of fracture repair: implications for therapy to improve bone healing. PLoS Med. 2007;4(7):e249.
151. Laird RK, Pavlos NJ, Xu J, Brankov B, White B, Fan Y, et al. Bone allograft non-union is related to excessive osteoclastic bone resorption: a sheep model study. Histol Histopathol. 2006;21(12):1277–85.
152. Sato K, Suematsu A, Okamoto K, Yamaguchi A, Morishita Y, Kadono Y, et al. Th17 functions as an osteoclastogenic helper T cell subset that links T cell activation and bone destruction. J Exp Med. 2006;203(12):2673–82.
153. Huang H, Kim HJ, Chang EJ, Lee ZH, Hwang SJ, Kim HM, et al. IL-17 stimulates the proliferation and differentiation of human mesenchymal stem cells: implications for bone remodeling. Cell Death Differ. 2009;16(10):1332–43.

154. Lee Y. The role of interleukin-17 in bone metabolism and inflammatory skeletal diseases. BMB Rep. 2013;46(10):479–83.
155. Fan X, Biskobing DM, Fan D, Hofstetter W, Rubin J. Macrophage colony stimulating factor down-regulates MCSF-receptor expression and entry of progenitors into the osteoclast lineage. J Bone Miner Res. 1997;12(9):1387–95.
156. Kong YY, Yoshida H, Sarosi I, Tan HL, Timms E, Capparelli C, et al. OPGL is a key regulator of osteoclastogenesis, lymphocyte development and lymph-node organogenesis. Nature. 1999;397(6717):315–23.
157. Champagne CM, Takebe J, Offenbacher S, Cooper LF. Macrophage cell lines produce osteoinductive signals that include bone morphogenetic protein-2. Bone. 2002;30(1):26–31.
158. Bhat A, Wooten RM, Jayasuriya AC. Secretion of growth factors from macrophages when cultured with microparticles. J Biomed Mater Res A. 2013;101(11):3170–80.
159. Stewart A, Guan H, Yang K. BMP-3 promotes mesenchymal stem cell proliferation through the TGF-beta/activin signaling pathway. J Cell Physiol. 2010;223(3):658–66.
160. Guo X, Wang XF. Signaling cross-talk between TGF-beta/BMP and other pathways. Cell Res. 2009;19(1):71–88.
161. Lin GL, Hankenson KD. Integration of BMP, Wnt, and notch signaling pathways in osteoblast differentiation. J Cell Biochem. 2011;112(12):3491–501.
162. Bhandari M, Tornetta 3rd P, Sprague S, Najibi S, Petrisor B, Griffith L, et al. Predictors of reoperation following operative management of fractures of the tibial shaft. J Orthop Trauma. 2003;17(5):353–61.
163. Bajada S, Marshall MJ, Wright KT, Richardson JB, Johnson WE. Decreased osteogenesis, increased cell senescence and elevated Dickkopf-1 secretion in human fracture non union stromal cells. Bone. 2009;45(4):726–35.
164. Seebach C, Henrich D, Tewksbury R, Wilhelm K, Marzi I. Number and proliferative capacity of human mesenchymal stem cells are modulated positively in multiple trauma patients and negatively in atrophic nonunions. Calcif Tissue Int. 2007;80(4):294–300.
165. Mathieu M, Rigutto S, Ingels A, Spruyt D, Stricwant N, Kharroubi I, et al. Decreased pool of mesenchymal stem cells is associated with altered chemokines serum levels in atrophic nonunion fractures. Bone. 2013;53(2):391–8.
166. Bajada S, Harrison PE, Ashton BA, Cassar-Pullicino VN, Ashammakhi N, Richardson JB. Successful treatment of refractory tibial nonunion using calcium sulphate and bone marrow stromal cell implantation. J Bone Joint Surg. 2007;89(10):1382–6.
167. Tawonsawatruk T, Kelly M, Simpson H. Evaluation of native mesenchymal stem cells from bone marrow and local tissue in an atrophic nonunion model. Tissue Eng Part C Methods. 2014;20(6):524–32.
168. Qu G, von Schroeder HP. The osteogenic potential of pseudoarthrosis tissue and bone from human scaphoid non-unions. J Hand Surg Eur Vol. 2008;33(4):449–56.
169. Gomez-Barrena E, Rosset P, Lozano D, Stanovici J, Ermthaller C, Gerbhard F. Bone fracture healing: cell therapy in delayed unions and nonunions. Bone. 2015;70:93–101.
170. Gokturk E, Turgut A, Baycu C, Gunal I, Seber S, Gulbas Z. Oxygen-free radicals impair fracture healing in rats. Acta Orthop Scand. 1995;66(5):473–5.
171. Grogaard B, Gerdin B, Reikeras O. The polymorphonuclear leukocyte: has it a role in fracture healing? Arch Orthop Trauma Surg. 1990;109(5):268–71.
172. Herman S, Muller RB, Kronke G, Zwerina J, Redlich K, Hueber AJ, et al. Induction of osteoclast-associated receptor, a key osteoclast costimulation molecule, in rheumatoid arthritis. Arthritis Rheum. 2008;58(10):3041–50.
173. Crop MJ, Korevaar SS, de Kuiper R, IJzermans JN, van Besouw NM, Baan CC, et al. Human mesenchymal stem cells are susceptible to lysis by CD8(+) T cells and NK cells. Cell Transplant. 2011;20(10):1547–59.
174. Gotherstrom C, Lundqvist A, Duprez IR, Childs R, Berg L, le Blanc K. Fetal and adult multipotent mesenchymal stromal cells are killed by different pathways. Cytotherapy. 2011;13(3):269–78.

175. Sotiropoulou PA, Perez SA, Gritzapis AD, Baxevanis CN, Papamichail M. Interactions between human mesenchymal stem cells and natural killer cells. Stem Cells. 2006;24 (1):74–85.
176. Poggi A, Prevosto C, Massaro AM, Negrini S, Urbani S, Pierri I, et al. Interaction between human NK cells and bone marrow stromal cells induces NK cell triggering: role of NKp30 and NKG2D receptors. J Immunol. 2005;175(10):6352–60.
177. Schmidt-Bleek K, Schell H, Schulz N, Hoff P, Perka C, Buttgereit F, et al. Inflammatory phase of bone healing initiates the regenerative healing cascade. Cell Tissue Res. 2012;347 (3):567–73.
178. Colburn NT, Zaal KJ, Wang F, Tuan RS. A role for gamma/delta T cells in a mouse model of fracture healing. Arthritis Rheum. 2009;60(6):1694–703.
179. Harre U, Georgess D, Bang H, Bozec A, Axmann R, Ossipova E, et al. Induction of osteoclastogenesis and bone loss by human autoantibodies against citrullinated vimentin. J Clin Invest. 2012;122(5):1791–802.
180. Reinke S, Geissler S, Taylor WR, Schmidt-Bleek K, Juelke K, Schwachmeyer V, et al. Terminally differentiated CD8(+) T cells negatively affect bone regeneration in humans. Sci Transl Med. 2013;5(177):177ra36.
181. Dighe AS, Yang S, Madhu V, Balian G, Cui Q. Interferon gamma and T cells inhibit osteogenesis induced by allogeneic mesenchymal stromal cells. J Orthop Res. 2013;31 (2):227–34.
182. Liu Y, Wang L, Kikuiri T, Akiyama K, Chen C, Xu X, et al. Mesenchymal stem cell-based tissue regeneration is governed by recipient T lymphocytes via IFN-gamma and TNF-alpha. Nat Med. 2011;17(12):1594–601.
183. Baboolal TG, Boxall SA, El-Sherbiny YM, Moseley TA, Cuthbert RJ, Giannoudis PV, et al. Multipotential stromal cell abundance in cellular bone allograft: comparison with fresh age-matched iliac crest bone and bone marrow aspirate. Regen Med. 2014;9 (5):593–607.
184. Kerr 3rd EJ, Jawahar A, Wooten T, Kay S, Cavanaugh DA, Nunley PD. The use of osteo-conductive stem-cells allograft in lumbar interbody fusion procedures: an alternative to recombinant human bone morphogenetic protein. J Surg Orthop Adv. 2011;20(3):193–7.
185. Struijs PA, Poolman RW, Bhandari M. Infected nonunion of the long bones. J Orthop Trauma. 2007;21(7):507–11.
186. Kayal RA, Siqueira M, Alblowi J, McLean J, Krothapalli N, Faibish D, et al. TNF-alpha mediates diabetes-enhanced chondrocyte apoptosis during fracture healing and stimulates chondrocyte apoptosis through FOXO1. J Bone Miner Res. 2010;25(7):1604–15.
187. Alblowi J, Kayal RA, Siqueira M, McKenzie E, Krothapalli N, McLean J, et al. High levels of tumor necrosis factor-alpha contribute to accelerated loss of cartilage in diabetic fracture healing. Am J Pathol. 2009;175(4):1574–85.
188. Diarra D, Stolina M, Polzer K, Zwerina J, Ominsky MS, Dwyer D, et al. Dickkopf-1 is a master regulator of joint remodeling. Nat Med. 2007;13(2):156–63.
189. Tsukasaki M, Yamada A, Suzuki D, Aizawa R, Miyazono A, Miyamoto Y, et al. Expression of POEM, a positive regulator of osteoblast differentiation, is suppressed by TNF-alpha. Biochem Biophys Res Commun. 2011;410(4):766–70.
190. Kitaura H, Zhou P, Kim HJ, Novack DV, Ross FP, Teitelbaum SL. M-CSF mediates TNF-induced inflammatory osteolysis. J Clin Invest. 2005;115(12):3418–27.
191. Huang H, Zhao N, Xu X, Xu Y, Li S, Zhang J, et al. Dose-specific effects of tumor necrosis factor alpha on osteogenic differentiation of mesenchymal stem cells. Cell Prolif. 2011;44 (5):420–7.
192. Lacey DC, Simmons PJ, Graves SE, Hamilton JA. Proinflammatory cytokines inhibit osteogenic differentiation from stem cells: implications for bone repair during inflammation. Osteoarthritis Cartilage. 2009;17(6):735–42.

193. Gao Y, Grassi F, Ryan MR, Terauchi M, Page K, Yang X, et al. IFN-gamma stimulates osteoclast formation and bone loss in vivo via antigen-driven T cell activation. J Clin Invest. 2007;117(1):122–32.
194. Axmann R, Bohm C, Kronke G, Zwerina J, Smolen J, Schett G. Inhibition of interleukin-6 receptor directly blocks osteoclast formation in vitro and in vivo. Arthritis Rheum. 2009;60 (9):2747–56.
195. Zwerina J, Redlich K, Polzer K, Joosten L, Kronke G, Distler J, et al. TNF-induced structural joint damage is mediated by IL-1. Proc Natl Acad Sci U S A. 2007;104(28):11742–7.
196. Fajardo M, Liu CJ, Egol K. Levels of expression for BMP-7 and several BMP antagonists may play an integral role in a fracture nonunion: a pilot study. Clin Orthop Relat Res. 2009;467(12):3071–8.
197. Hofmann A, Ritz U, Hessmann MH, Schmid C, Tresch A, Rompe JD, et al. Cell viability, osteoblast differentiation, and gene expression are altered in human osteoblasts from hypertrophic fracture non-unions. Bone. 2008;42(5):894–906.
198. Chan JL, Tang KC, Patel AP, Bonilla LM, Pierobon N, Ponzio NM, et al. Antigen-presenting property of mesenchymal stem cells occurs during a narrow window at low levels of interferon-gamma. Blood. 2006;107(12):4817–24.
199. Li W, Ren G, Huang Y, Su J, Han Y, Li J, et al. Mesenchymal stem cells: a double-edged sword in regulating immune responses. Cell Death Differ. 2012;19(9):1505–13.
200. Prigozhina TB, Khitrin S, Elkin G, Eizik O, Morecki S, Slavin S. Mesenchymal stromal cells lose their immunosuppressive potential after allotransplantation. Exp Hematol. 2008;36 (10):1370–6.
201. Okuno M, Muneta T, Koga H, Ozeki N, Nakagawa Y, Tsuji K, et al. Meniscus regeneration by syngeneic, minor mismatched, and major mismatched transplantation of synovial mesenchymal stem cells in a rat model. J Orthop Res. 2014;32(7):928–36.
202. Isakova IA, Lanclos C, Bruhn J, Kuroda MJ, Baker KC, Krishnappa V, et al. Allo-reactivity of mesenchymal stem cells in rhesus macaques is dose and haplotype dependent and limits durable cell engraftment in vivo. PLoS One. 2014;9(1):e87238.
203. Reinders ME, Hoogduijn MJ. NK cells and MSCs: possible implications for MSC therapy in renal transplantation. J Stem Cell Res Ther. 2014;4(2):1000166.
204. Arinzeh TL, Peter SJ, Archambault MP, van den Bos C, Gordon S, Kraus K, et al. Allogeneic mesenchymal stem cells regenerate bone in a critical-sized canine segmental defect. J Bone Joint Surg Am. 2003;85-A(10):1927–35.
205. Guo SQ, Xu JZ, Zou QM, Jiang DM. Immunological study of allogeneic mesenchymal stem cells during bone formation. J Int Med Res. 2009;37(6):1750–9.
206. Udehiya RK, Amarpal, Aithal HP, Kinjavdekar P, Pawde AM, Singh R, et al. Comparison of autogenic and allogenic bone marrow derived mesenchymal stem cells for repair of segmental bone defects in rabbits. Res Vet Sci. 2013;94(3):743–52.
207. Streckbein P, Jackel S, Malik CY, Obert M, Kahling C, Wilbrand JF, et al. Reconstruction of critical-size mandibular defects in immunoincompetent rats with human adipose-derived stromal cells. J Craniomaxillofac Surg. 2013;41(6):496–503.
208. Gu H, Xiong Z, Yin X, Li B, Mei N, Li G, et al. Bone regeneration in a rabbit ulna defect model: use of allogeneic adipose-derived stem cells with low immunogenicity. Cell Tissue Res. 2014;358(2):453–64.
209. Xie F, Teng L, Wang Q, Sun XJ, Cai L, Zeng HF, et al. Ectopic osteogenesis of allogeneic bone mesenchymal stem cells loading on beta-tricalcium phosphate in canines. Plast Reconstr Surg. 2014;133(2):142e–53.
210. Chen L, Tredget EE, Wu PY, Wu Y. Paracrine factors of mesenchymal stem cells recruit macrophages and endothelial lineage cells and enhance wound healing. PLoS One. 2008;3 (4):e1886.
211. Mountziaris PM, Spicer PP, Kasper FK, Mikos AG. Harnessing and modulating inflammation in strategies for bone regeneration. Tissue Eng Part B Rev. 2011;17(6):393–402.

Chapter 10
Bone Marrow Stromal Stem Cells for Bone Repair: Basic and Translational Aspects

Basem M. Abdallah, Asma Al-Shammary, Hany M. Khattab, Abdullah AlDahmash, and Moustapha Kassem

10.1 Introduction

Human skeletal stem cells (also known as bone marrow stromal stem cell population BMSCs, or mesenchymal stem cells) are present within the bone marrow stroma and are characterized by self-renewal capacity, clonogenicity in vitro, multipotent differentiation into mesoderm-type cells including osteoblast, adipocyte, and chondrocyte, and their ability to form bone and hematopoiesis-supporting stroma upon in vivo transplantation [1, 2]. In addition, the

B.M. Abdallah, Ph.D. (✉)
Molecular Endocrinology Laboratory (KMEB), Department of Endocrinology, Institute of Clinical Research, Odense University Hospital and University of Southern Denmark, DK-5000 Odense C, Denmark

Department of Biological Sciences, College of Science, King Faisal University, Hofuf, Saudi Arabia
e-mail: babdallah@health.sdu.dk

A. Al-Shammary
Molecular Endocrinology Laboratory (KMEB), Department of Endocrinology, Institute of Clinical Research, Odense University Hospital and University of Southern Denmark, DK-5000 Odense C, Denmark

Deanship of Scientific Research, University of Hail, Hail, Saudi Arabia

H.M. Khattab
Department of Oral Implantology and Regenerative Dental Medicine, Tokyo Medical and Dental University, Tokyo, Japan

A. AlDahmash • M. Kassem
Molecular Endocrinology Laboratory (KMEB), Department of Endocrinology, Institute of Clinical Research, Odense University Hospital and University of Southern Denmark, DK-5000 Odense C, Denmark

Stem Cell Unit, Department of Anatomy, Faculty of Medicine, King Saud University, Riyadh, Saudi Arabia

E.M. Abdelalim (ed.), *Recent Advances in Stem Cells*, Stem Cell Biology and Regenerative Medicine, DOI 10.1007/978-3-319-33270-3_10

differentiation of hBMSCs into cardiomyocytes [3], endothelial cells [4], and non-mesoderm cell lineages including neural cells [5] have been reported but not confirmed using in vivo assays.

The percentage of BMSCs subpopulation among other bone marrow mononuclear cells (MNC) is very low ranging between 0.01 and 0.001 % [6, 7]. MNBMSCs were first identified by Friedenstein and coworkers as bone marrow osteogenic stem cells with hematopoietic tissue supporting characteristics [8] and as adherent cell population with a fibroblast-like morphology. Recent lineage tracing studies in mice have revealed that bone and cartilage forming cells in the postnatal organism originate within the skeleton and not recruited from non-skeletal stromal tissues and thus the name of skeletal stem cells has been suggested to be the appropriate name for bone forming BMSC [9].

10.2 Isolation and In Vitro Expansion of hBMSCs

Traditionally, hBMSCs have been isolated from low-density MNC population of bone marrow aspirates, based on their selective adherence to plastic surfaces compared to hematopoietic cells [1, 6, 10, 11]. Disadvantages of this method include possible contamination of hematopoietic cell and the cellular heterogeneity of cultures in relation to differentiation potential. In order to isolate a homogenous population of cells with defined phenotype, several studies have used FACS-based cell sorting to enrich for hBMSCs based on the expression of one or a group of specific surface CD markers. Surface antigens including Stro-1 [12], CD271 [13], CD146 [14], SSEA4 [15], and Nestin [16] have also been used to prospectively isolate MSCs from bone marrow with tri-lineages differentiation capability. In mice, we have recently employed CD34 to identify osteoprogenitor BMSC [17]. In addition, a number of investigators employed a combination of surface markers and CD markers to phenotype BMSCs and to enrich for BMSC population. Examples of that: Stro-1+/CD106+ [18] and lin−/CD271+/CD140a- [19] that can enrich for BMSCs.

10.3 Isolation of Adult MSCs-Like Cells from Different Tissues

Populations with MSCs-like phenotype has been isolated from non-skeletal tissues including peripheral blood [20], umbilical cord blood [21], amniotic fluid [22], Wharton's jelly (connective tissue surrounds cord blood vessels) [23], synovial membranes [24], adipose tissue (AT), Lung [25], fetal liver [26], dental pulp [27, 28], and deciduous teeth [29]. Some recent studies comparing the molecular signature of these different cell populations have reported similarities but also differences related to the tissue of origin [30–33]. One significant difference is that non-skeletal MSCs are poor at forming ectopic bone when assayed in vivo.

10.4 Phenotypic Characteristics of BMSCs

hBMSCs are fusiform, fibroblast-like cells and during their initial growth in vitro, they form colonies (termed in analogy with hematopoietic stem cells (HSCs): colony forming unit-fibroblasts [CFU-f]) [10]. The in vivo location of BMSCs has been suggested to be in a perivascular niche in close association with pericytes and endothelial cells [34]. There are no specific cell surface markers that can identify MSC prospectively. However, the cultured hBMSCs have been defined based on being negative for hematopoietic and endothelial markers, e.g., CD11b, CD14, CD31, CD34, and CD45, and positive for stromal markers, e.g., CD29, CD44, CD73, CD105, CD106, CD146, and CD166 [35]. However, in practice the multipotent MSCs are usually defined in functional terms based on in vitro and in vivo differentiation assays.

The following criteria have been proposed by the International Society for Cellular Therapy to define BMSCs: (1) BMSCs must have the ability for plastic adherence during in vitro culture, (2) BMSCs should express CD73, CD90, and CD105 with no expression of hematopoietic markers such as CD14, CD45, and CD11b, and (3) these cells must have the ability to differentiate into osteoblasts, adipocytes, and chondrocytes in vitro [36]. One limitation of these criteria is that they do not distinguish multipotent stem cells from committed progenitors. Also, these criteria need revision to include newer markers that enrich for BMSC, e.g., CD146, CD271 (see above). In support of this notion, we recently demonstrated a weak association between the abovementioned criteria as determined in vitro and the ability of the cells to form in vivo ectopic bone which is the "stemness" characteristic of the cells [32] [37]. In this study, using DNA microarray analysis, we identified a predictive molecular signature for in vivo bone formation of BMSC that can be employed to select for BMSCs population with high in vivo bone forming capacity to be employed for clinical studies of bone regeneration [32].

10.5 Use of hBMSCs in Therapy

The use of hBMSCs in therapy has been based on their ability to differentiate to specific tissue forming cells, e.g., bone or cartilage. However, the initial results of preclinical and clinical trials have demonstrated low engraftment potential of the cells in vivo and thus alternative hypotheses have been proposed to explain the observed beneficial effects. The therapeutic effects of BMSCs may be mediated through their immune-modulatory functions or paracrine effects by secreting growth factors/cytokines to stimulate the recruitment and the differentiation of the residing tissue-specific stem cells [38–43]. Several studies have demonstrated that hBMSCs are hypo-immunogenic and thus allogenic hBMSCs transplantation is possible [44]. hBMSCs lack the expression of major histocompatibility complex (MHC) class II, the co-stimulatory molecules CD40, CD80 and CD86 (even after interferon-g (IFN-g) stimulation) and in addition express very little amount of MHC-I molecules on their surface [45, 46]. BMSCs were found to escape T-cell recognition and to exert anti-inflammatory effects by suppressing activated lymphocytes and T cell response to mitogens [47]. The immunomodulatory functions have encouraged using hBMSCs to reduce inflammation and thus promoting tissue repair [48] and allowed testing the cells for treatment of immune-mediated disorders such as systemic lupus erythematosus (SLE) [49] and steroid-resistant graft-versus-host disease (GvHD) [50].

10.6 Osteoblast Differentiation of BMSCs

Osteoblasts originate from BMSCs through a differentiation process that is controlled by numerous hormones and growth factors. Osteoblasts are characterized by expressing various phenotypic markers such as alkaline phosphatase (ALP) activity and synthesizing collagenous and non-collagenous bone matrix proteins, e.g., osteocalcin and osteopontin. The in vitro osteoblast differentiation process has been described as consisting of three distinct stages: (i) proliferation; (ii) lineage commitment and matrix deposition; and (iii) matrix mineralization. BMSCs under the influence of signaling molecules, e.g., bone morphogenetic protein 2 (BMP2), induce osteoblast lineage-specific transcriptional factors, e.g., Runx-2, Activating transcription factor 4 (ATF-4), and Osterix (Osx), which induce the formation of osteoprogenitors. Osteoprogenitors produce extracelluar matrix, e.g., collagen type I and increasing levels of alkaline phosphatase activity [51]. Finally, matrix maturation and mineralization takes place as the cells mature in vitro as evidenced by production of osteocalcin, osteonectin and formation of hydroxyapatite crystals. Several signaling molecules were shown to enhance osteogenic differentiation capacity of BMSCs in vitro and in vivo and thus they have been employed for enhancing bone regeneration capacity of BMSCs, e.g., BMP-2/7, insulin-like growth factor (IGF)-1, platelets-derived growth factor (PDGF), vascular endothelial growth factor (VEGF), and fibroblast growth factor (FGF) [51, 52]. Several approaches have been employed to enrich osteoblastic progenitors from BMSCs by either using in vitro treatment with osteogenic factors (e.g., BMPs or transforming growth factor [TGF]-β) [53] or by using a genetic approach for overexpression of genes that enhance osteogenic differentiation of BMSCs including Ostrix [54], Runx2 [55], and Msx2 [56]. We have employed advanced techniques of transcriptome, micro-RNA (miRNA) microarray, and quantitative proteomic analysis to identify potential factors for enhancing the in vivo bone formation capacity of BMSCs, e.g., miR-138 [57] and miRNA-34a [58]. We have also employed small molecule kinase inhibitor to enhance osteoblast differentiation and hBMSC-mediated bone formation in vitro and in vivo [59].

10.7 Limiting Factors Affecting the Clinical Use of hBMSCs

hBMSCs are promising stem cell source in regenerative medicine, however some factors are still limiting their use in the clinical applications. In the following, we will discuss two aspects of hBMSCs biology that have been examined extensively in our laboratory: in vitro replicative senescence phenotype which hinders the expansion of hBMSCs and phenotypic heterogeneity of cultured hBMSCs.

10.7.1 Replicative Senescence

In vitro replicative senescence (senescence-associated growth arrest) of hBMSCs is one of the most important characteristic phenotype that hampers the generation of a large number of cells needed for clinical applications. During long-term in vitro culture of hBMSCs, the cells exhibit reduced proliferation rate and finally enter a state of growth arrest. We found age-related decrease in the number of in vitro population doubling (PD) of hBMSCs. While hBMSCs derived from young donors can be maintained in culture for around 40 PD, hBMSCs derived from elderly donors can be grown in cultures for only 24 PD [60, 61]. However, we did not detect a donor age-related decrease in the number of CFU-Fs or in their base-line differentiation potential [7]. Replicative senescence is caused by several factors including DNA damage, accumulation of abnormal protein, or mitochondrial changes [62, 63]. We have demonstrated that telomere shortening during cell division [62] due to the lack of telomerase activity is an essential mechanism underlying the replicative senescence of hBMSCs [64].

10.7.2 Phenotypic Heterogeneity of hBMSCs

hBMSCs appear to be a relatively homogenous population of cells in relation to their morphological cellular phenotype and the expression of common cell surface markers (see above). However, clonal analysis of BMSC populations has revealed that the multipotent BMSC represents only around 20–30 % of total human MSC population [65, 66]. Similar percentages of multipotent BMSC has been reported in mice and rabbit (20 %) [67] and rabbit and guinea pig (36.8 %) [68]. Additionally, clonal analysis of Stro-1 bright VCAM-1^+ cells which contained an enriched population of human bone marrow-derived MSC revealed that only 17 % of the clones were multipotential [18]. Remaining cell populations represent a mixture of bipotential and unipotential BMSCs [69]. Studying the hBMSCs heterogeneity at single cell-derived clones in our laboratory revealed that human BMSCs contain committed progenitors with lineage-specific osteoblast differentiation capacity and in vivo bone forming ability [66]. Similarly, we have isolated and characterized from mouse BMSCs, two homogenous BMSCs cell lines with unipotent differentiation capacities of either osteoblasts or adipocytes: mBMSC^{Bone} and mBMSC ^{Adipo}, respectively [70]. Comparative microarray analysis of the transcriptome of these two cell populations resulted in identification of specific surface markers for prospective isolation of homogenous populations of osteogenic and adipogenic pre-committed cell populations [17].

10.8 Clinical Applications of hBMSCs in Bone Tissue Regeneration

Several preclinical and clinical studies have demonstrated the bone regenerative capacity of adult MSCs-based therapy for the treatment of different types of skeletal defects including cranial, oral, maxillo-facial, and long bone defects. Stem cell-biomaterial based bone tissue engineering is clinically relevant approach used for bone regeneration. In addition, both local and systemic transplantation of adult MSCs have also been reported to be efficient for the treatment of some specific bone diseases such as osteonecrosis of femur head and osteogenesis imperfecta. In the following sections, we will discuss the preclinical and the clinical applications of adult MSCs in bone regeneration (see Tables 10.1 and 10.2).

10.8.1 Bone Tissue Engineering

Stem cell-biomaterial based bone tissue engineering has been tested for enhancing bone regeneration for cranial, oral and maxillo-facial and other orthopedic reconstructions. Tissue engineering combines adult MSCs, osteo-conductive biomaterial, and osteogenic factors. In bone tissue engineering, autologous MSCs are isolated from the patients, expanded, seeded on synthetic/biological scaffold, combined with osteogenic factor(s), and subsequently implanted into the bone defect site of patients has been proposed [71].

For bone tissue regeneration, the biomaterials used should provide the following properties: (1) correct anatomic geometry that matches the bone defect, (2) osteo-conductive or osteo-inductive material for enhancing bone regenerative capacity of MSCs. (3) Owing micro/nano surface structural with highly connected and open porosity that enhance cellular adhesion, survival and proliferation and to allow cell migration, vascularization.

Table 10.1 Preclinical studies on using adult stem cells in bone regeneration

Ref.	Stem cell therapy	Bone defect model	Results
[96]	Autologous BMSCs seeded on hydroxy apatite (HA) ceramic scaffold	Critical-size tibial defect in a sheep model	BMSCs in conjunction with a HA-based material enhanced repair of critical-size tibial defects
[111]	Rat BMSCs, overexpression of BMP-2 with poly (lactide-co glycolide)/hydroxyapatite (PLAGA/HA) scaffold	SCID hind limb	Induced heterotopic bone formation in a SCID mouse model
[112]	Systemic administration of mouse BMSCs over-expressing insulin-like growth factor-I (D1-IGF-I)	Murine model	Increased percent of mineralized callus than controls at 2 weeks and average greater mineralized matrix at 4 and 6 weeks
[113]	BMSCs stably over-expressing human BMP-2 (Adv-hBMP-2) gene-transduced	Critical size tibial defects in goat	Improved healing of critical size tibial defects in goat
[114]	Dog BMSCs seeded on β-TCP scaffold	Dog with mandibular segmental defect	Enhanced bone formation and vascularization
[115]	Autologous adipose- MSCs with fibronectin-treated polylactic acid scaffold	Rabbit critical-sized skull defect	Enhanced bone formation
[116]	Rat BMSCs overexpression of BMP- with pre-mineralized silk scaffolds	Critical size mandibular bony defects	Enhanced bone formation
[101]	BMSCs and endothelial progenitor cells (EPCs) from buffy coat seeded on β-TCP granules, or autologous bone	A femoral critical sized in adult athymic rats	Significant bone formation in BMSCs and EPCs combination
[107]	Systemic transplantation of mBMSCs transduced with rAAV6-BMP2:VEGF	Segmental bone defect of the tibiae in athymic nude mice	Sufficient bone formation for healing
[108]	Systemic transplantation of BMSCs expressing BMP2 under the transcriptional control of collagen type-1alpha promoter	Osteopenic OVX mouse model	Therapeutic potential to restore bone growth
[117]	BMSCs seeded on porous calcium phosphate cement scaffold loaded with rhBMP-2	Maxillary sinus augmentation in rabbits	Promoted new bone formation
[118]	BMSCs over-expressing HIF-1α	Rat critical-sized calvarial defect	Enhanced the bone regeneration
[119]	Canine BMSCs, canine dental pulp stem cells (cDPSCs), and puppy deciduous teeth stem cells (pDTSCs), and platelet-rich plasma (PRP)	Bone mandibular defects in canine model	Stem cells from deciduous teeth, dental pulp, and bone marrow with PRP have the ability to improve bone formation
[120]	Periodontal ligament progenitor cells (PDLCs) with	Rat calvarial critical-sized defect model	Enhanced calvarial bone repair significantly

(continued)

Table 10.1 (continued)

Ref.	Stem cell therapy	Bone defect model	Results
	hydroxyapatite/extracellular matrix (HA-ECM) scaffold		
[81]	Adipose-MSCs seeded on coral scaffold	Cranial critical-sized defects in parietal bones in canine model	Improved bone regeneration
[98]	Allogeneic BMSCs or autologous BMSCs loaded onto small-sized allogeneic cancellous bone granules	Mid-shaft critical-sized segmental the of both radiuses in rabbits	Allogeneic MSCs are similar to autologous BMSCs in bone regeneration
[121]	Dental follicle stem cells	Calvarial critical-size defects in immunocompetent rats	DFSCs are capable to repair craniofacial defect
[122]	Adipose-MSCs with polyamide, poly lactic-co-glycolic, decellularized amniotic membrane scaffolds	Calvarial defect in rabbit model	New bone formation was more significant with ADMSC polyamide scaffold

Materials used for fabricating bone engineering scaffolds can be divided into (a) natural-based materials (i.e., alginate, chitosan, and hyaluronic acid derivatives, or proteins gelatine, collagen), (b) synthetic polymers (e.g., poly(ε-caprolactone) (PCL) and poly(lactide) (PLA)), and (c) ceramics including calcium phosphate ceramics such as hydroxyapatite (HA) and tricalcium phosphate (TCP) which are most commonly used in the clinic. Also, polymer-ceramic composites, such as poly (propylene fumarate)/$CaSO_4$/-TCP biodegradable and poly-e-caprolactone (PCL)/ hydroxyapatite were developed with improved properties for adhesion and survival of MSCs [51, 72, 73].

Some recent advances in designing large bone grafts for stem cell-based bone tissue engineering will be mentioned here. The use of advanced technology of 3D printing to create scaffold suitable for use in anatomically complex sites, e.g., for repair large craniofascial defects [74]. Oxygen generating scaffolds have been created to enhance vascularization and stem cell survival. This was achieved by incorporating oxygen enriched biomaterials (calcium peroxide) into fabricated polymer scaffold PGLA [75]. Functional scaffolds capable of prolonged and sustained release of bioactive molecules have been designed to create a drug delivery scaffold for enhancing stem cell adhesion and differentiation [76]. For example, osteogenic potential of BMSCs was significantly enhanced when cultured on PLGA-sintered microsphere scaffolds with controlled release of osteogenic factors including dexamethasone, ascorbic acid, and β-glycerophosphate [77].

10.8.1.1 Use of hBMSC for Craniofacial Bone Defect Regeneration

Treatment of large craniofacial bone defects is a highly invasive procedure that required 3D geometrically shaped and vascularized autologous bone

Table 10.2 Clinical studies on using adult stem cells in bone regeneration

Reference	Stem cell therapy	Bone defect	No. of patients	Clinical results
[123]	Mandibular periosteal MSCs	Maxillary sinus floor augmentation	2	Reasonable bone formation with periosteal derived osteoblast
[124]	Autologous ASCs	Traumatic calvarial defect	1	Case report: complete calvarial continuity and new bone formation after 3 months of reconstruction
[84]	BMSCs in combination with biphasic HA/β-TCP scaffold	Maxillary sinus augmentation	6	Improved bone regeneration in the floor of maxillary sinus
[125]	BMSCs and platelet-rich plasma and bone graft	Maxillary sinus augmentation	12	Significant increase in mineralized tissue around inserted implants
[92]	A combination of autologous adipose-MSCs and β-TCP and rhBMP-2	Hemi maxillectomy defect	1	Case report: induced a well-ossified bone
[104]	Autogenous bone marrow cells	Osteonecrosis of femoral head	19	Reduces delay progression of osteonecrosis and reduced femoral head, fracture incidence
[126]	bovine bone mineral (BioOss) mixed with autogenous bone or autogenous BMSCs	Maxillary sinus floor augmentation	12	Bone formation with BioOss seeded with stem cells to be superior to BioOss mixed with autogenous bone
[106]	Autogenous BMSCs	Femoral head osteonecrosis	100	BMSCs delay femoral neck osteonecrosis, deceased pain and joint symptoms
[127]	Autogenous BMSCs and Platelet rich plasma and rhPDGF	Alveolar cleft defects	3	Enhanced bone regeneration
[105]	Autologous bone marrow mononuclear cells	Osteonecrosis of femoral head	64	Delayed the progression of osteonecrosis
[88]	Autologous hBMSCs population enriched in $CD90^+$/ $CD14^+$ cells	Alveolar bone defects	24	Improved bone regeneration in craniofacial defects
[87]	Autogenous adipose-MSCs seeded on β-TCP supplemented with rhBMP-2	Cranio maxilla facial hard tissue defects	13	Successful reconstruction using adipose stem cells
[89]	Autologous hBMSCs population enriched in $CD90^+$/ $CD14^+$ cells delivered on β-TCP scaffold	Maxillary sinus defects	30	Sufficient de novo bone regeneration to stably place oral implants
[102]	Autologous hBMSCs in platelet rich plasma seeded on demineralized bone matrix allograft	Tibia non union	24	Significant reduction of healing time

transplantation. BMSCs have been used to repair bone defects of oral and maxillofacial region in many preclinical and clinical studies.

BMP2 gene-modified BMSCs and β-TCP particles were reported to promote new bone formation in rabbit maxillary sinus floor elevation model [78] and rat critical size mandibular defect model [79]. Furthermore, autologous BMSCs in combination with porous β-TCP were effective to repair alveolar bone defects in dogs with sufficient new bone support for tooth movement [80]. Allogeneic adipose-derived MSCs (ASCs) seeded on natural coral scaffold regenerated bone in cranial critical-sized defects of dog model without inducing any immune response [81]. In large animal, bone healing of noncritical-size defect in the pig mandible was augmented by local transplantation of ASCs into the defect site compared to the control group without cell treatment [82].

At the clinical level, studies that have employed both BMSCs and ASCs were used for treatment of patients with craniofacial bone defects. Human bone grafts have been produced using hBMSCs and a "biomimetic" scaffold-bioreactor system [83]. In the following, we will provide some examples (see Table 10.2). New bone formation without complications was reported in maxillary sinus elevation of six patients implanted with a combination of HA/TCP and allogenic BMSCs in posterior maxillary area [84]. hBMSCs seeded onto a resorbable collagen matrix sponge were employed to repair the alveolar cleft defects in patients with unilateral cleft lip [85]. In addition, an injectable mixture of hBMSCs/platelet-rich plasma and thrombin/calcium chloride preparations has been used for ridge augmentation and dental implant placement in humans [86]. Transplantation of 13 patients with defects in the cranio-maxillofacial skeleton at different sites with autologous ASCs seeded on β-TCP granules showed a successful bone reconstruction in ten out of 13 cases [87].

In two randomized, controlled feasibility trials, Kaigler D. et al. have used $CD90^+$/$CD14^+$ hBMSCs for treating large bone defect. In the first trial, patients requiring localized reconstruction of jawbone defects were randomized to receive into the extraction site either guided bone regeneration (GBR) (a procedure of isolating the bone defect from the surrounding connective tissue to allow new bone growth) or mixture of $CD90^+$/$CD14^+$ hBMSCs seeded on a gelatin sponge and covered by a bio-absorbable collagen. Clinical results demonstrated the advantage of hBMSCs-based therapy in promoting alveolar bone regeneration compared to GBR therapy [88]. In the second trial, 30 patients with severe bone atrophy of the upper jaw were treated either with β-TCP scaffold alone (control) or in a combination with seeded autologous $CD90^+$/$CD14^+$ hBMSCs. Follow-up over 6 months demonstrated the benefits of using stem cells therapy for generating bone with high density sufficient to stably place oral implants [89].

Large mandible bone reconstruction to support dental implants has been manufactured using customized titanium mesh filled with either autologous hBMSCs combined with autograft cancellous bone and BMP-7 [90], or ASCs combined with rhBMP-2 and β-TCP granules [91]. A composite of hASCs, rhBMP-2, and β-TCP granules has been used to reconstruct a major maxillary defect in patient [92]. Despite the limited number of patients in these studies, these reports demonstrated the regenerative capacity of MSCs to repair bone defect with minimal invasive procedure.

10.8.1.2 Use of hBMSC for Treatment of Bone Critical Size Defects and Non-healed Fractures

In several preclinical animal models, BMSCs have shown ability to enhance tissue regeneration. Implanted autologous BMSCs loaded on HA/TCP ceramics were shown to regenerate bone in critical-sized segmental defects in the femurs of adult athymic rats [93, 94], femurs of dogs [95], tibiae of sheep [96], and iliac wing of goats [97]. In a rabbit model of a critical-size radius bone defect, comparable results of bone regeneration were obtained by using either allogeneic or autologous BMSCs loaded on allogeneic cancellous granules [98]. Also a combination of gene therapy and tissue engineering has been examined in mice. Implantation of BMSCs-overexpressing BMP2 gene loaded on collagen type I biodegradable scaffold in nonunion bone fracture mouse model showed to form bone with chemical compositions and physical properties similar to native bone [99].

Vascularization of the implants is crucial for successful bone regeneration, improving vascularization at early stage of bone healing has been an area of intensive investigation in cell-based tissue engineering. To enhance vascularization of the newly formed bone, murine BMSCs were co-implanted with human umbilical vein endothelial cells (HUVECs) in fibrin/Matrigel complex to support neovascularization and bone formation in calvarial bone defect mouse model [100]. Enhanced early vascularization and bone healing have been observed in a critical-sized long bone defect in athymic rats upon transplantation with a co-culture of endothelial progenitor cells (EPCs)/BMSCs seeded on fibronectin-coated beta-TCP granules [101].

At the clinic level, a randomized controlled clinical study of patients with distal tibia fractures were injected into the site of fracture with composite graft of Ignite ICS injectable scaffold (demineralized bone matrix), sorted autologous $CD105^{+}$ BMSCs and platelet-rich plasma. Clinical data revealed enhanced fracture healing as compared to untreated control group [102]. In addition, a complex of enriched-BMSCs (by centrifugation using COBE 2991™ Cell Processor) with porous β-TCP granules was used to perform posterior spinal fusion in patients with degenerative disc disease [103]. In this study, 95.1 % cases displayed good spinal fusion results.

10.8.2 Use of hBMSC for Treatment of Osteonecrosis of the Femoral Head

Osteonecrosis of the femoral head (ONFH) is characterized by vascular ischemia resulting in apoptosis of osteoblasts and subsequently destruction of the hip joint.

Local transplantation of bone marrow cells containing adult BMSCs has been used as a less invasive therapy for the treatment of ONFH. In nonrandomized study, 19 patients with non-traumatic ONFH were treated either with a core decompression procedure (CD) (control group) or with core decompression plus autologous mononuclear bone marrow cells (BMMCs) transplantation. After 60 months of follow-up, treatment of necrotic lesion with bone marrow cells implantation was very effective in reducing pain and fractural risk [104]. Perfusion of autologous BMMCs via medial circumflex femoral artery in 62 patients with ONFH showed to be safe and effective in improving the hip function [105]. Furthermore, in a randomized study of 100 patients with early-stage ONFH, autologous expanded hBMSCs from subtrochanteric bone marrow aspirates were implanted in the femoral heads after CD procedure, while control group underwent CD procedure alone. Sixty months after surgery showed decreased pain and joint symptoms as well as delay in the progression of ONFH in cell treated group [106].

10.8.3 Systemic BMSC Transplantation

Several preclinical studies have investigated the bone regenerative capacity of genetically modified BMSCs after systemic transplantation in bone defect animal models. Kumar et al. demonstrated the capacity of genetically modified mBMSCs to expressed BMP2 and VEGF to enhance bone formation in a mouse model of segmental tibia defect after systemic transplantation [107]. Systemic transplantation of MSC-expressing BMP2 under collagen type I promoter and α-4 integrin (to enhance their homing to bone) in osteopenic ovariectomized (ovx) mouse model exerted a therapeutic potential to restore bone growth [108]. Furthermore, systemically transplanted mBMSCs-expressing insulin-like growth factor-I (IGF-I) promotes the healing of nonunion tibia fracture of insulin-receptor-substrate knockout mice. In this Irs−/− mouse model that lacking IGF/insulin signaling and the subsequent IGF-I paracrine response, the mechanism of new bone formation was found to be mediated by BMSC-IGFI through autocrine effects of IGF-I on transplanted BMSCs [109].

In the clinic, treatment of six children with severe osteogenesis imperfecta (underwent bone marrow transplantation) by systemic transplantation of allogenic health BMSCs resulted in the engraftment of BMSCs in bone, increase growth velocity in association with increased bone mineral density and no clinically significant toxicity [110].

10.9 Conclusion and Future Perspectives

Skeletal stem cell (BMSCs)-based therapy for skeletal regeneration is a novel less invasive approach that holds a great promise for replacing autologous bone grafting. Successful preclinical and clinical studies support the regenerative capacity of BMSCs for skeletal repair via both autocrine and paracrine effects. Clinical data from randomized studies demonstrated the safety and in some cased the ability of BMSC for enhancing bone tissue regeneration. In this context, the developing of osteo-conductive/inductive biodegradable micro-/nanospheres can provide adult stem cells on their biomimetic surface, with efficient 3D microenvironment enriched with growth factors. Also, engineering biomaterial with improved chemical and physical structures to prolong growth factors release can enhance the MSCs proliferation and differentiation for efficient therapy. Because of their cellular and functional heterogeneity, the regenerative capacity of transplanted MSCs can be enhanced by selecting for homogenous BMSCs with bone forming capacity. Finally, understanding the regulatory mechanisms controlling the proliferation, differentiation, and migration of BMSCs is highly relevant for their use in therapy.

Acknowledgments This work was supported by grants from Danish council for independent research (Det Frie Forskningsråd, 0602-02645B and DFF 4004-00045), Novo Nordisk Foundation (Exploratory Pre Seed Grants), NNF13OC0004192, and the Novo Nordisk foundation (2014-10309).

References

1. Abdallah BM, Kassem M. Human mesenchymal stem cells: from basic biology to clinical applications. Gene Ther. 2008;15:109–16.
2. Bianco P, Robey PG. Skeletal stem cells. Development. 2015;142:1023–7.
3. Shim WSN, Jiang S, Wong P, Tan J, Chua YL, Seng Tan Y, Sin YK, Lim CH, Chua T, Teh M, Liu TC, Sim E. Ex vivo differentiation of human adult bone marrow stem cells into cardiomyocyte-like cells. Biochem Biophys Res Commun. 2004;324:481–8.
4. Oswald J, Boxberger S, Jørgensen B, Feldmann S, Ehninger G, Bornhäuser M, Werner C. Mesenchymal stem cells can be differentiated into endothelial cells in vitro. Stem Cells. 2004;22:377–84.
5. Sanchez-Ramos J, Song S, Cardozo-Pelaez F, Hazzi C, Stedeford T, Willing A, Freeman TB, Saporta S, Janssen W, Patel N, Cooper DR, Sanberg PR. Adult bone marrow stromal cells differentiate into neural cells in vitro 5. Exp Neurol. 2000;164:247–56.
6. Rickard DJ, Kassem M, Hefferan TE, Sarkar G, Spelsberg TC, Riggs BL. Isolation and characterization of osteoblast precursor cells from human bone marrow. J Bone Miner Res. 1996;11:312–24.
7. Stenderup K, Justesen J, Eriksen EF, Rattan SI, Kassem M. Number and proliferative capacity of osteogenic stem cells are maintained during aging and in patients with osteoporosis. J Bone Miner Res. 2001;16:1120–9.
8. Friedenstein AJ, Chailakhyan RK, Gerasimov UV. Bone marrow osteogenic stem cells: in vitro cultivation and transplantation in diffusion chambers. Cell Tissue Kinet. 1987;20:263–72.
9. Kassem M, Bianco P. Skeletal stem cells in space and time. Cell. 2015;160:17–9.
10. Friedenstein AJ, Chailakhjan RK, Lalykina KS. The development of fibroblast colonies in monolayer cultures of guinea-pig bone marrow and spleen cells. Cell Tissue Kinet. 1970;3:393–403.
11. Kassem M, Mosekilde L, Rungby J, Mosekilde L, Melsen F, Eriksen EF. Formation of osteoclasts and osteoblast-like cells in long-term human bone marrow cultures. APMIS. 1991;99:262–8.

12. Gronthos S, Graves SE, Ohta S, Simmons PJ. The STRO-1+ fraction of adult human bone marrow contains the osteogenic precursors. Blood. 1994;84:4164–73.
13. Quirici N, Soligo D, Bossolasco P, Servida F, Lumini C, Deliliers GL. Isolation of bone marrow mesenchymal stem cells by anti-nerve growth factor receptor antibodies. Exp Hematol. 2002;30:783–91.
14. Sacchetti B, Funari A, Michienzi S, Di CS, Piersanti S, Saggio I, Tagliafico E, Ferrari S, Robey PG, Riminucci M, Bianco P. Self-renewing osteoprogenitors in bone marrow sinusoids can organize a hematopoietic microenvironment. Cell. 2007;131:324–36.
15. Gang EJ, Bosnakovski D, Figueiredo CA, Visser JW, Perlingeiro RC. SSEA-4 identifies mesenchymal stem cells from bone marrow. Blood. 2007;109:1743–51.
16. Mendez-Ferrer S, Michurina TV, Ferraro F, Mazloom AR, Macarthur BD, Lira SA, Scadden DT, Ma'ayan A, Enikolopov GN, Frenette PS. Mesenchymal and haematopoietic stem cells form a unique bone marrow niche. Nature. 2010;466:829–34.
17. Abdallah BM, Al-Shammary A, Skagen P, Abu Dawud R, Adjaye J, Aldahmash A, Kassem M. CD34 defines an osteoprogenitor cell population in mouse bone marrow stromal cells. Stem Cell Res. 2015;15:449–58.
18. Gronthos S, Zannettino AC, Hay SJ, Shi S, Graves SE, Kortesidis A, Simmons PJ. Molecular and cellular characterisation of highly purified stromal stem cells derived from human bone marrow. J Cell Sci. 2003;116:1827–35.
19. Li H, Ghazanfari R, Zacharaki D, Ditzel N, Isern J, Ekblom M, Méndez-Ferrer S, Kassem M, Scheding S. Low/negative expression of PDGFR-α identifies the candidate primary mesenchymal stromal cells in adult human bone marrow. Stem Cell Reports. 2014;3:965–74.
20. Kuznetsov SA, Mankani MH, Gronthos S, Satomura K, Bianco P, Robey PG. Circulating skeletal stem cells. J Cell Biol. 2001;153:1133–40.
21. Rosada C, Justesen J, Melsvik D, Ebbesen P, Kassem M. The human umbilical cord blood: a potential source for osteoblast progenitor cells. Calcif Tissue Int. 2003;72:135–42.
22. Sun H, Feng K, Hu J, Soker S, Atala A, Ma PX. Osteogenic differentiation of human amniotic fluid-derived stem cells induced by bone morphogenetic protein-7 and enhanced by nanofibrous scaffolds. Biomaterials. 2010;31:1133.
23. Karadas O, Yucel D, Kenar H, Torun Kose G, Hasirci V. Collagen scaffolds with in situ-grown calcium phosphate for osteogenic differentiation of Wharton's jelly and menstrual blood stem cells. J Tissue Eng Regen Med. 2014;8:534–45.
24. De Bari C, Dell'Accio F, Tylzanowski P, Luyten FP. Multipotent mesenchymal stem cells from adult human synovial membrane. Arthritis Rheum. 2001;44:1928–42.
25. in 't Anker PS, Noort WA, Scherjon SA, Kleijburg-van der Keur C, Kruisselbrink AB, van Bezooijen RL, Beekhuizen W, Willemze R, Kanhai HH, Fibbe WE. Mesenchymal stem cells in human second-trimester bone marrow, liver, lung, and spleen exhibit a similar immunophenotype but a heterogeneous multilineage differentiation potential. Haematologica. 2003;88:845–52.
26. Campagnoli C, Roberts IA, Kumar S, Bennett PR, Bellantuono I, Fisk NM. Identification of mesenchymal stem/progenitor cells in human first-trimester fetal blood, liver, and bone marrow 1. Blood. 2001;98:2396–402.
27. Gronthos S, Robey PG, Boyde A, Shi S. Human dental pulp stem cells (DPSCs): characterization and developmental potential. J Bone Miner Res. 2001;16:S265.
28. Otaki S, Ueshima S, Shiraishi K, Sugiyama K, Hamada S, Yorimoto M, Matsuo O. Mesenchymal progenitor cells in adult human dental pulp and their ability to form bone when transplanted into immunocompromised mice. Cell Biol Int. 2007;31(10):1191–7.
29. Miura Y, Miura M, Gronthos S, Allen MR, Cao C, Uveges TE, Bi Y, Ehirchiou D, Kortesidis A, Shi S, Zhang L. Defective osteogenesis of the stromal stem cells predisposes CD18-null mice to osteoporosis. Proc Natl Acad Sci U S A. 2005;102:14022–7.
30. Al-Nbaheen M, Vishnubalaji R, Ali D, Bouslimi A, Al-Jassir F, Megges M, Prigione A, Adjaye J, Kassem M, Aldahmash A. Human stromal (mesenchymal) stem cells from bone marrow, adipose tissue and skin exhibit differences in molecular phenotype and differentiation potential. Stem Cell Rev. 2013;9:32–43.

31. Djouad F, Bony C, Haupl T, Uze G, Lahlou N, Louis-Plence P, Apparailly F, Canovas F, Reme T, Sany J, Jorgensen C, Noel D. Transcriptional profiles discriminate bone marrow-derived and synovium-derived mesenchymal stem cells. Arthritis Res Ther. 2005;7: R1304–15.
32. Wagner W, Wein F, Seckinger A, Frankhauser M, Wirkner U, Krause U, Blake J, Schwager C, Eckstein V, Ansorge W, Ho AD. Comparative characteristics of mesenchymal stem cells from human bone marrow, adipose tissue, and umbilical cord blood. Exp Hematol. 2005;33:1402–16.
33. Vishnubalaji R, Al-Nbaheen M, Kadalmani B, Aldahmash A, Ramesh T. Comparative investigation of the differentiation capability of bone-marrow- and adipose-derived mesenchymal stem cells by qualitative and quantitative analysis. Cell Tissue Res. 2012;347:419–27.
34. Crisan M, Yap S, Casteilla L, Chen CW, Corselli M, Park TS, Andriolo G, Sun B, Zheng B, Zhang L, Norotte C, Teng PN, Traas J, Schugar R, Deasy BM, Badylak S, Buhring HJ, Giacobino JP, Lazzari L, Huard J, Peault B. A perivascular origin for mesenchymal stem cells in multiple human organs. Cell Stem Cell. 2008;3:301–13.
35. Abdallah BM, Kassem M. The use of mesenchymal (skeletal) stem cells for treatment of degenerative diseases: current status and future perspectives. J Cell Physiol. 2009;218:9–12.
36. Dominici M, Le BK, Mueller I, Slaper-Cortenbach I, Marini F, Krause D, Deans R, Keating A, Prockop D, Horwitz E. Minimal criteria for defining multipotent mesenchymal stromal cells. The International Society for cellular therapy position statement. Cytotherapy. 2006;8:315–7.
37. Abdallah BM, Ditzel N, Kassem M. Assessment of bone formation capacity using in vivo transplantation assays: procedure and tissue analysis. Methods Mol Biol. 2008;455:89–100.
38. Burchfield JS, Dimmeler S. Role of paracrine factors in stem and progenitor cell mediated cardiac repair and tissue fibrosis. Fibrogenesis Tissue Repair. 2008;1:4.
39. Gnecchi M, He H, Liang OD, Melo LG, Morello F, Mu H, Noiseux N, Zhang L, Pratt RE, Ingwall JS, Dzau VJ. Paracrine action accounts for marked protection of ischemic heart by Akt-modified mesenchymal stem cells. Nat Med. 2005;11:367–8.
40. Kinnaird T, Stabile E, Burnett MS, Shou M, Lee CW, Barr S, Fuchs S, Epstein SE. Local delivery of marrow-derived stromal cells augments collateral perfusion through paracrine mechanisms. Circulation. 2004;109:1543–9.
41. Gnecchi M, Zhang Z, Ni A, Dzau VJ. Paracrine mechanisms in adult stem cell signaling and therapy. Circ Res. 2008;103:1204–19.
42. Stastna M, Abraham MR, Van Eyk JE. Cardiac stem/progenitor cells, secreted proteins, and proteomics. FEBS Lett. 2009;583:1800–7.
43. Bianco P, Cao X, Frenette PS, Mao JJ, Robey PG, Simmons PJ, Wang CY. The meaning, the sense and the significance: translating the science of mesenchymal stem cells into medicine. Nat Med. 2013;19:35–42.
44. Pigott JH, Ishihara A, Wellman ML, Russell DS, Bertone AL. Investigation of the immune response to autologous, allogeneic, and xenogeneic mesenchymal stem cells after intra-articular injection in horses. Vet Immunol Immunopathol. 2013;156:99–106.
45. Pittenger MF, Mackay AM, Beck SC, Jaiswal RK, Douglas R, Mosca JD, Moorman MA, Simonetti DW, Craig S, Marshak DR. Multilineage potential of adult human mesenchymal stem cells 6. Science. 1999;284:143–7.
46. Tolar J, Le Blanc K, Keating A, Blazar BR. Hitting the right spot with mesenchymal stromal cells (MSCs). Stem Cells. 2010;28:1446–55.
47. Le Blanc K, Mougiakakos D. Multipotent mesenchymal stromal cells and the innate immune system. Nat Rev Immunol. 2012;12:383–96.
48. Le BK, Tammik C, Rosendahl K, Zetterberg E, Ringden O. HLA expression and immunologic properties of differentiated and undifferentiated mesenchymal stem cells. Exp Hematol. 2003;31:890–6.

49. Figueroa FE, Carrión F, Villanueva S, Khoury M. Mesenchymal stem cell treatment for autoimmune diseases: a critical review. Biol Res. 2012;45:269–77.
50. Le Blanc K, Frassoni F, Ball L, Locatelli F, Roelofs H, Lewis I, Lanino E, Sundberg B, Bernardo ME, Remberger M, Dini G, Egeler RM, Bacigalupo A, Fibbe W, Ringdén O. Mesenchymal stem cells for treatment of steroid-resistant, severe, acute graft-versus-host disease: a phase II study. Lancet. 2008;371:1579–86.
51. Arvidson K, Abdallah BM, Applegate LA, Baldini N, Cenni E, Gomez-Barrena E, Granchi D, Kassem M, Konttinen YT, Mustafa K, Pioletti DP, Sillat T, Finne-Wistrand A. Bone regeneration and stem cells. J Cell Mol Med. 2011;15:718–46.
52. Abdallah BM, Jafari A, Zaher W, Qiu W, Kassem M. Skeletal (stromal) stem cells: an update on intracellular signaling pathways controlling osteoblast differentiation. Bone. 2015;70:28–36.
53. Luu HH, Song WX, Luo X, Manning D, Luo J, Deng ZL, Sharff KA, Montag AG, Haydon RC, He TC. Distinct roles of bone morphogenetic proteins in osteogenic differentiation of mesenchymal stem cells. J Orthop Res. 2007;25:665–77.
54. Wu L, Wu Y, Lin Y, Jing W, Nie X, Qiao J, Liu L, Tang W, Tian W. Osteogenic differentiation of adipose derived stem cells promoted by overexpression of osterix. Mol Cell Biochem. 2007;301:83–92.
55. Kojima H, Uemura T. Strong and rapid induction of osteoblast differentiation by Cbfa1/Til-1 overexpression for bone regeneration. J Biol Chem. 2005;280:2944–53.
56. Ichida F, Nishimura R, Hata K, Matsubara T, Ikeda F, Hisada K, Yatani H, Cao X, Komori T, Yamaguchi A, Yoneda T. Reciprocal roles of Msx2 in regulation of osteoblast and adipocyte differentiation. J Biol Chem. 2004;279:34015–22.
57. Eskildsen T, Taipaleenmäki H, Stenvang J, Abdallah BM, Ditzel N, Nossent AY, Bak M, Kauppinen S, Kassem M. MicroRNA-138 regulates osteogenic differentiation of human stromal (mesenchymal) stem cells in vivo. Proc Natl Acad Sci U S A. 2011;108:6139–44.
58. Chen L, HolmstrØm K, Qiu W, Ditzel N, Shi K, Hokland L, Kassem M. MicroRNA-34a inhibits osteoblast differentiation and in vivo bone formation of human stromal stem cells. Stem Cells. 2014;32:902–12.
59. Jafari A, Siersbaek MS, Chen L, Qanie D, Zaher W, Abdallah BM, Kassem M. Pharmacological inhibition of protein kinase G1 enhances bone formation by human skeletal stem cells through activation of RhoA-Akt signaling. Stem Cells. 2015;33:2219–31.
60. Stenderup K, Justesen J, Clausen C, Kassem M. Aging is associated with decreased maximal life span and accelerated senescence of bone marrow stromal cells. Bone. 2003;33:919–26.
61. Kassem M, Ankersen L, Eriksen EF, Clark BF, Rattan SI. Demonstration of cellular aging and senescence in serially passaged long-term cultures of human trabecular osteoblasts. Osteoporos Int. 1997;7:514–24.
62. Rattan SIS. Aging outside the body: usefulneess of the Hayflick system. In: Kaul SC, Wadhwa R, editors. Aging of cells in and outside the body. London: Kluwer; 2003. p. 1–8.
63. Sharpless NE, DePinho RA. How stem cells age and why this makes us grow old. Nat Rev Mol Cell Biol. 2007;8:703–13.
64. Simonsen JL, Rosada C, Serakinci N, Justesen J, Stenderup K, Rattan SI, Jensen TG, Kassem M. Telomerase expression extends the proliferative life-span and maintains the osteogenic potential of human bone marrow stromal cells. Nat Biotechnol. 2002;20:592–6.
65. Kuznetsov SA, Krebsbach PH, Satomura K, Kerr J, Riminucci M, Benayahu D, Robey PG. Single-colony derived strains of human marrow stromal fibroblasts form bone after transplantation in vivo. J Bone Miner Res. 1997;12:1335–47.
66. Larsen KH, Frederiksen CM, Burns JS, Abdallah BM, Kassem M. Identifying a molecular phenotype for bone marrow stromal cells with in vivo bone forming capacity. Journal of Bone and Mineral Research. 2009;25(4):796–808.
67. Beresford JN. Osteogenic stem cells and the stromal system of bone and marrow. Clin Orthop Relat Res. 1989;240:270–80.

68. Bennett JH, Joyner CJ, Triffitt JT, Owen ME. Adipocytic cells cultured from marrow have osteogenic potential. J Cell Sci. 1991;99(Pt 1):131–9.
69. Russell KC, Phinney DG, Lacey MR, Barrilleaux BL, Meyertholen KE, O'Connor KC. In vitro high-capacity assay to quantify the clonal heterogeneity in trilineage potential of mesenchymal stem cells reveals a complex hierarchy of lineage commitment. Stem Cells. 2010;28:788–98.
70. Post S, Abdallah BM, Bentzon JF, Kassem M. Demonstration of the presence of independent pre-osteoblastic and pre-adipocytic cell populations in bone marrow-derived mesenchymal stem cells. Bone. 2008;43:32–9.
71. Petite H, Viateau V, Bensaid W, Meunier A, de Pollak C, Bourguignon M, Oudina K, Sedel L, Guillemin G. Tissue-engineered bone regeneration. Nat Biotechnol. 2000;18:959–63.
72. Cai Z-Y, Yang D-A, Zhang N, Ji C-G, Zhu L, Zhang T. Poly(propylene fumarate)/(calcium sulphate/β-tricalcium phosphate) composites: preparation, characterization and in vitro degradation. Acta Biomater. 2009;5:628–35.
73. Guarino V, Causa F, Ambrosio L. Bioactive scaffolds for bone and ligament tissue. Expert Rev Med Devices. 2007;4:405–18.
74. Temple JP, Hutton DL, Hung BP, Huri PY, Cook CA, Kondragunta R, Jia X, Grayson WL. Engineering anatomically shaped vascularized bone grafts with hASCs and 3D-printed PCL scaffolds. J Biomed Mater Res A. 2014;102:4317–25.
75. Oh SH, Ward CL, Atala A, Yoo JJ, Harrison BS. Oxygen generating scaffolds for enhancing engineered tissue survival. Biomaterials. 2009;30:757–62.
76. Huang CL, Lee WL, Loo JSC. Drug-eluting scaffolds for bone and cartilage regeneration. Drug Discov Today. 2014;19:714–24.
77. Shi X, Wang Y, Varshney RR, Ren L, Gong Y, Wang D-A. Microsphere-based drug releasing scaffolds for inducing osteogenesis of human mesenchymal stem cells in vitro. Eur J Pharm Sci. 2010;39:59–67.
78. Zhang Z. Bone regeneration by stem cell and tissue engineering in oral and maxillofacial region. Front Med. 2011;5:401–13.
79. Zhao J, Hu J, Wang S, Sun X, Xia L, Zhang X, Zhang Z, Jiang X. Combination of β-TCP and BMP-2 gene-modified bMSCs to heal critical size mandibular defects in rats. Oral Dis. 2010;16:46–54.
80. Zhang D, Chu F, Yang Y, Xia L, Zeng D, Uludağ H, Zhang X, Qian Y, Jiang X. Orthodontic tooth movement in alveolar cleft repaired with a tissue engineering bone: an experimental study in dogs. Tissue Eng Part A. 2011;17:1313–25.
81. Liu G, Zhang Y, Liu B, Sun J, Li W, Cui L. Bone regeneration in a canine cranial model using allogeneic adipose derived stem cells and coral scaffold. Biomaterials. 2013;34:2655–64.
82. Wilson SM, Goldwasser MS, Clark SG, Monaco E, Bionaz M, Hurley WL, Rodriguez-Zas S, Feng L, Dymon Z, Wheeler MB. Adipose-derived mesenchymal stem cells enhance healing of mandibular defects in the ramus of swine. J Oral Maxillofac Surg. 2012;70:e193–203.
83. Grayson WL, Fröhlich M, Yeager K, Bhumiratana S, Chan ME, Cannizzaro C, Wan LQ, Liu XS, Guo XE, Vunjak-Novakovic G. Engineering anatomically shaped human bone grafts. Proc Natl Acad Sci U S A. 2010;107:3299–304.
84. Shayesteh YS, Khojasteh A, Soleimani M, Alikhasi M, Khoshzaban A, Ahmadbeigi N. Sinus augmentation using human mesenchymal stem cells loaded into a β-tricalcium phosphate/hydroxyapatite scaffold. Oral Surg Oral Med Oral Pathol Oral Radiol Endod. 2008;106:203–9.
85. Gimbel M, Ashley RK, Sisodia M, Gabbay JS, Wasson KL, Heller J, Wilson L, Kawamoto HK, Bradley JP. Repair of alveolar cleft defects: reduced morbidity with bone marrow stem cells in a resorbable matrix. J Craniofac Surg. 2007;18:895–901.
86. Ueda M, Yamada Y, Kagami H, Hibi H. Injectable bone applied for ridge augmentation and dental implant placement: human progress study. Implant Dent. 2008;17:82–90.
87. Sándor GK, Numminen J, Wolff J, Thesleff T, Miettinen A, Tuovinen VJ, Mannerström B, Patrikoski M, Seppänen R, Miettinen S, Rautiainen M, Öhman J. Adipose stem cells used to

reconstruct 13 cases with cranio-maxillofacial hard-tissue defects. Stem Cells Transl Med. 2014;3:530–40.
88. Kaigler D, Pagni G, Park CH, Braun TM, Holman LA, Yi E, Tarle SA, Bartel RL, Giannobile WV. Stem cell therapy for craniofacial bone regeneration: a randomized, controlled feasibility trial. Cell Transplant. 2013;22:767–77.
89. Kaigler D, Avila-Ortiz G, Travan S, Taut AD, Padial-Molina M, Rudek I, Wang F, Lanis A, Giannobile WV. Bone engineering of maxillary sinus bone deficiencies using enriched CD90 + stem cell therapy: a randomized clinical trial. J Bone Miner Res. 2015;30:1206–16.
90. Warnke PH, Springer IN, Wiltfang J, Acil Y, Eufinger H, Wehmoller M, Russo PA, Bolte H, Sherry E, Behrens E, Terheyden H. Growth and transplantation of a custom vascularised bone graft in a man. Lancet. 2004;364:766–70.
91. Sándor GK, Tuovinen VJ, Wolff J, Patrikoski M, Jokinen J, Nieminen E, Mannerström B, Lappalainen O-P, Seppänen R, Miettinen S. Adipose stem cell tissue-engineered construct used to treat large anterior mandibular defect: a case report and review of the clinical application of good manufacturing practice-level adipose stem cells for bone regeneration. J Oral Maxillofac Surg. 2013;71:938–50.
92. Mesimäki K, Lindroos B, Törnwall J, Mauno J, Lindqvist C, Kontio R, Miettinen S, Suuronen R. Novel maxillary reconstruction with ectopic bone formation by GMP adipose stem cells. Int J Oral Maxillofac Surg. 2009;38:201–9.
93. Tseng SS, Lee MA, Reddi AH. Nonunions and the potential of stem cells in fracture-healing. J Bone Joint Surg Am. 2008;90:92–8.
94. Brummelkamp TR, Bernards R, Agami R. A system for stable expression of short interfering RNAs in mammalian cells 2. Science. 2002;296:550–3.
95. Bruder SP, Kraus KH, Goldberg VM, Kadiyala S. The effect of implants loaded with autologous mesenchymal stem cells on the healing of canine segmental bone defects. J Bone Joint Surg Am. 1998;80:985–96.
96. Kon E, Muraglia A, Corsi A, Bianco P, Marcacci M, Martin I, Boyde A, Ruspantini I, Chistolini P, Rocca M, Giardino R, Cancedda R, Quarto R. Autologous bone marrow stromal cells loaded onto porous hydroxyapatite ceramic accelerate bone repair in critical-size defects of sheep long bones. J Biomed Mater Res. 2000;49:328–37.
97. Kruyt MC, Dhert WJA, Yuan H, Wilson CE, van Blitterswijk CA, Verbout AJ, de Bruijn JD. Bone tissue engineering in a critical size defect compared to ectopic implantations in the goat. J Orthop Res. 2004;22:544–51.
98. Kang S-H, Chung Y-G, Oh I-H, Kim Y-S, Min K-O, Chung J-Y. Bone regeneration potential of allogeneic or autogeneic mesenchymal stem cells loaded onto cancellous bone granules in a rabbit radial defect model. Cell Tissue Res. 2014;355:81–8.
99. Tai K, Pelled G, Sheyn D, Bershteyn A, Han L, Kallai I, Zilberman Y, Ortiz C, Gazit D. Nanobiomechanics of repair bone regenerated by genetically modified mesenchymal stem cells. Tissue Eng Part A. 2008;14:1709–20.
100. Koob S, Torio-Padron N, Stark GB, Hannig C, Stankovic Z, Finkenzeller G. Bone formation and neovascularization mediated by mesenchymal stem cells and endothelial cells in critical-sized calvarial defects. Tissue Eng Part A. 2010;17:311–21.
101. Seebach C, Henrich D, Kähling C, Wilhelm K, Tami AE, Alini M, Marzi I. Endothelial progenitor cells and mesenchymal stem cells seeded onto β-TCP granules enhance early vascularization and bone healing in a critical-sized bone defect in rats. Tissue Eng Part A. 2010;16:1961–70.
102. Liebergall M, Schroeder J, Mosheiff R, Gazit Z, Yoram Z, Rasooly L, Daskal A, Khoury A, Weil Y, Beyth S. Stem cell-based therapy for prevention of delayed fracture union: a randomized and prospective preliminary study. Mol Ther. 2013;21:1631–8.
103. Gan Y, Dai K, Zhang P, Tang T, Zhu Z, Lu J. The clinical use of enriched bone marrow stem cells combined with porous beta-tricalcium phosphate in posterior spinal fusion. Biomaterials. 2008;29:3973–82.

104. Gangji V, De Maertelaer V, Hauzeur J-P. Autologous bone marrow cell implantation in the treatment of non-traumatic osteonecrosis of the femoral head: five year follow-up of a prospective controlled study. Bone. 2011;49:1005–9.
105. Mao Q, Jin H, Liao F, Xiao L, Chen D, Tong P. The efficacy of targeted intraarterial delivery of concentrated autologous bone marrow containing mononuclear cells in the treatment of osteonecrosis of the femoral head: a five year follow-up study. Bone. 2013;57:509–16.
106. Zhao D, Cui D, Wang B, Tian F, Guo L, Yang L, Liu B, Yu X. Treatment of early stage osteonecrosis of the femoral head with autologous implantation of bone marrow-derived and cultured mesenchymal stem cells. Bone. 2012;50:325–30.
107. Kumar S, Wan C, Ramaswamy G, Clemens TL, Ponnazhagan S. Mesenchymal stem cells expressing osteogenic and angiogenic factors synergistically enhance bone formation in a mouse model of segmental bone defect. Mol Ther. 2010;18:1026–34.
108. Kumar S, Nagy TR, Ponnazhagan S. Therapeutic potential of genetically modified adult stem cells for osteopenia. Gene Ther. 2010;17:105–16.
109. Granero-Moltó F, Myers TJ, Weis JA, Longobardi L, Li T, Yan Y, Case N, Rubin J, Spagnoli A. Mesenchymal stem cells expressing insulin-like growth factor-I (MSC(IGF)) promote fracture healing and restore new bone formation in Irs1 knock-out mice: analyses of MSC (IGF) autocrine and paracrine regenerative effects. Stem Cells. 2011;29:1537–48.
110. Horwitz EM, Gordon PL, Koo WKK, Marx JC, Neel MD, McNall RY, Muul L, Hofmann T. Isolated allogeneic bone marrow-derived mesenchymal cells engraft and stimulate growth in children with osteogenesis imperfecta: implications for cell therapy of bone. Proc Natl Acad Sci U S A. 2002;99:8932–7.
111. Laurencin CT, Attawia MA, Lu LQ, Borden MD, Lu HH, Gorum WJ, Lieberman JR. Poly (lactide-co-glycolide)/hydroxyapatite delivery of BMP-2-producing cells: a regional gene therapy approach to bone regeneration 1. Biomaterials. 2001;22:1271–7.
112. Shen FH, Visger JM, Balian G, Hurwitz SR, Diduch DR. Systemically administered mesenchymal stromal cells transduced with insulin-like growth factor-I localize to a fracture site and potentiate healing. J Orthop Trauma. 2002;16:651–9.
113. Xu XL, Tang T, Dai K, Zhu Z a, Guo XE, Yu C, Lou J. Immune response and effect of adenovirus-mediated human BMP-2 gene transfer on the repair of segmental tibial bone defects in goats. Acta Orthop. 2005;76:637–46.
114. He Y, Zhang Z-Y, Zhu H-G, Qiu W, Jiang X, Guo W. Experimental study on reconstruction of segmental mandible defects using tissue engineered bone combined bone marrow stromal cells with three-dimensional tricalcium phosphate. J Craniofac Surg. 2007;18:800–5.
115. Di Bella C, Farlie P, Penington AJ. Bone regeneration in a rabbit critical-sized skull defect using autologous adipose-derived cells. Tissue Eng Part A. 2008;14:483–90.
116. Jiang X, Zhao J, Wang S, Sun X, Zhang X, Chen J, Kaplan DL, Zhang Z. Mandibular repair in rats with premineralized silk scaffolds and BMP-2-modified bMSCs. Biomaterials. 2009;30:4522–32.
117. Xia L, Xu Y, Wei J, Zeng D, Ye D, Liu C, Zhang Z, Jiang X. Maxillary sinus floor elevation using a tissue-engineered bone with rhBMP-2-loaded porous calcium phosphate cement scaffold and bone marrow stromal cells in rabbits. Cells Tissues Organs. 2011;194:481–93.
118. Zou D, Zhang Z, Ye D, Tang A, Deng L, Han W, Zhao J, Wang S, Zhang W, Zhu C, Zhou J, He J, Wang Y, Xu F, Huang Y, Jiang X. Repair of critical-sized rat calvarial defects using genetically engineered bone marrow-derived mesenchymal stem cells overexpressing hypoxia-inducible factor-1α. Stem Cells. 2011;29:1380–90.
119. Yamada Y, Yamada Y, Ito K, Ito K, Nakamura S, Nakamura S, Ueda M, Ueda M, Nagasaka T, Nagasaka T. Promising cell-based therapy for bone regeneration using stem cells from deciduous teeth, dental pulp, and bone marrow. Cell Transplant. 2011;20:1003–13.
120. Tour G, Wendel M, Moll G, Tcacencu I. Bone repair using periodontal ligament progenitor cell-seeded constructs. J Dent Res. 2012;91:789–94.

121. Rezai-Rad M, Bova JF, Orooji M, Pepping J, Qureshi A, Del Piero F, Hayes D, Yao S. Evaluation of bone regeneration potential of dental follicle stem cells for treatment of craniofacial defects. Cytotherapy. 2015;17:1572–81.
122. Semyari H, Rajipour M, Sabetkish S, Sabetkish N, Abbas F, Kajbafzadeh A-M. Evaluating the bone regeneration in calvarial defect using osteoblasts differentiated from adipose-derived mesenchymal stem cells on three different scaffolds: an animal study. Cell Tissue Bank. 2016;17(1):69–83.
123. Schmelzeisen R, Schimming R, Sittinger M. Making bone: implant insertion into tissue-engineered bone for maxillary sinus floor augmentation—a preliminary report. J Craniomaxillofac Surg. 2003;31:34–9.
124. Lendeckel S, Jödicke A, Christophis P, Heidinger K, Wolff J, Fraser JK, Hedrick MH, Berthold L, Howaldt H-P. Autologous stem cells (adipose) and fibrin glue used to treat widespread traumatic calvarial defects: case report. J Craniomaxillofac Surg. 2004;32:370–3.
125. Yamada Y, Nakamura S, Ito K, Kohgo T, Hibi H, Nagasaka T, Ueda M. Injectable tissue-engineered bone using autogenous bone marrow-derived stromal cells for maxillary sinus augmentation: clinical application report from a 2–6-year follow-up. Tissue Eng Part A. 2008;14:1699–707.
126. Rickert D, Sauerbier S, Nagursky H, Menne D, Vissink A, Raghoebar GM. Maxillary sinus floor elevation with bovine bone mineral combined with either autogenous bone or autogenous stem cells: a prospective randomized clinical trial. Clin Oral Implants Res. 2011;22:251–8.
127. Behnia H, Khojasteh A, Soleimani M, Tehranchi A, Atashi A. Repair of alveolar cleft defect with mesenchymal stem cells and platelet derived growth factors: a preliminary report. J Craniomaxillofac Surg. 2012;40:2–7.

Chapter 11
Neural Crest Stem Cells: A Therapeutic Hope Machine for Neural Regeneration

Ahmed El-Hashash

11.1 Introduction

The neural crest cells (NCCs) were described for the first time by the Wilheim His, a Swiss embryologist, in 1868 as a population of cells that localize between the dorsal ectoderm and the neural tube in vertebrate during embryogenesis. NCCs are specifically localized to the dorsal margins of the closing neural folds during neurulation in vertebrates. Signaling interactions between the surface ectoderm and the neural plate induce NCC delamination through an epithelial-to-mesenchymal transition, followed by an extensive migration to different locations in the embryos, where they differentiate into different types of tissues, including the craniofacial skeleton and the peripheral nervous system (PNS) [1].

There are four NCC derivatives: the cranial NC, cardiac NC, vagal NC, and trunk NC. These four derivatives originate from different segments of the neuraxis and differentiate into different cell types. The cranial NC gives rise to smooth muscles, connective tissues, nerve ganglia, and pigment cells as well as the cartilages and bones of the head and face (Fig. 11.1). The cardiac NC plays an important role in the heart formation because it gives rise to aorticopulmonary septum and conotruncal cushions, while the vagal NC differentiates into enteric ganglia of the gut. In addition, the trunk NC differentiates into neurons and glia, secretory cells of the endocrine system and pigment cells of the skin as well as parts of the PNS [2–7]. Embryonic neural crest cells characteristically express several genetic markers, including FGF and SHH signaling elements (Fig. 11.2)

A. El-Hashash, Ph.D.
Stem Cells, Regenerative Medicine and Developmental Biology Program, Children's Hospital Los Angeles, Keck School of Medicine and Ostrow School of Dentistry, University of Southern California, Los Angeles, CA, USA
e-mail: hashash05@yahoo.co.uk

E.M. Abdelalim (ed.), *Recent Advances in Stem Cells*, Stem Cell Biology and Regenerative Medicine, DOI 10.1007/978-3-319-33270-3_11

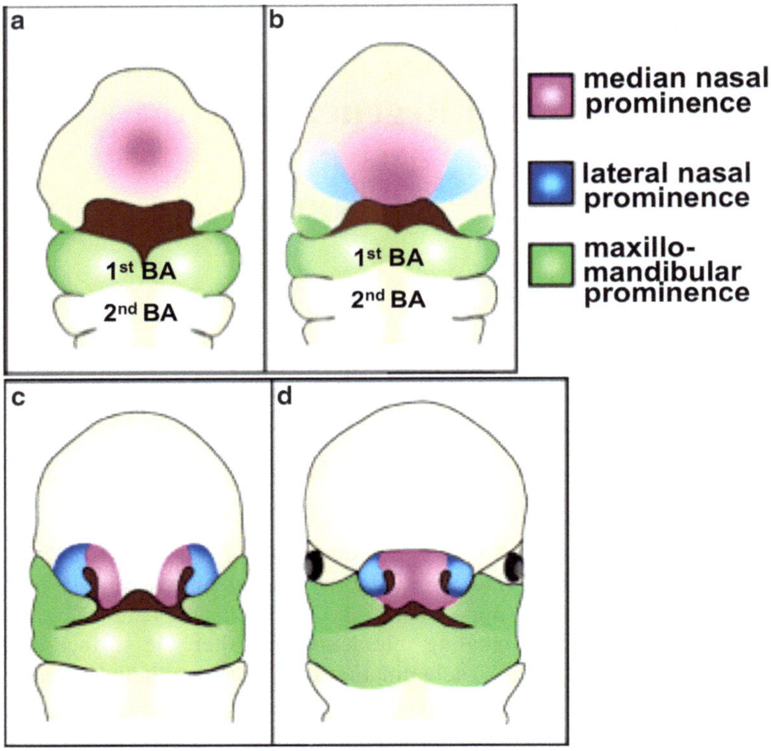

Fig. 11.1 Development of the craniofacial primordia. (**a–d**) Representations of frontal views of mouse embryos showing the prominences that give rise to the main face structures. The frontonasal prominence (*pink*) gives rise to the forehead (**a**), the middle of the nose (**b**), the philtrum of the upper lip (**c**), and the primary palate (**d**), whereas the lateral nasal prominence (*blue*) forms the sides of the nose (**b**, **d**). The NCC derived maxillo-mandibular (of the first branchial arch) prominences (*green*) give rise to the lower jaw (specifically from the mandibular prominences), to the sides of the middle and lower face, to lateral borders of the lips, and to the secondary palate (from the maxillary prominences). Adapted from Tapadia et al. [108]

11.2 The Multipotency of NCCs

Intensive studies have been carried out in the last decade on the multipotentiality and self-renewal capacities of NCCs. However, several caveats still remain, and deserve more investigations, including the description of the majority of NCCs as progenitor cells rather than true stem cells because these are only generated transiently during embryogenesis [8]. Although NCCs have the capacity to self-renew and differentiate similar to stem cells, this capacity is more limited in progenitor cells compared to stem cells [8].

Classical experiments investigating the multipotency of NCCs, by using vital dyes as cell fate and lineage-tracing markers, have demonstrated that cranial NCCs

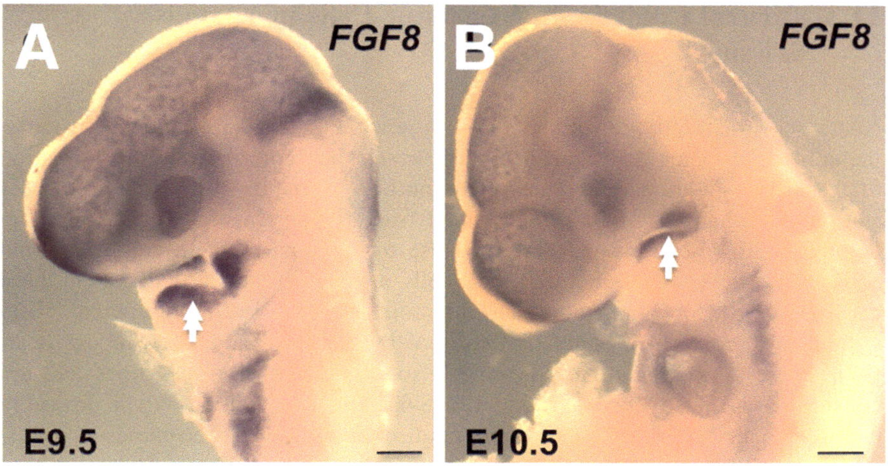

Fig. 11.2 Strong expression of FGF8 in the NCC-derived first branchial arch, and its derivatives: maxillary and mandibular processes (*double arrows* in **a–b**), as evidenced by in situ hybridization

give rise to mesectodermal precursors, which contribute to the formation of connective tissues, cartilages and bones, as well as different other types of cells. The later includes glia and both neuronal and melanocyte lineages. These studies have also shown that trunk NCCs differentiate into both neuronal and nonneuronal descendants [9, 10]. In addition, isolated individual migratory NCCs from the visceral arches of quail embryos give rise to up to four different types of cells [11]. Several other reports have also successfully demonstrated the multipotency of NCCs in both avian and mouse systems [12–14].

Little is known about the molecular mechanisms and factors that sustain the multipotency of NCCs and derivatives. However, a recent study has provided evidences about the importance of FGF8 signaling in sustaining the progenitor status and multipotency of cranial NCC-derived mesenchymal cells in vivo and in culture [15]. This study has shown that augmented FGF8 signaling in pre-migratory cranial NCCs acts to inhibit both NC cells' differentiation by maintaining their progenitor status in the craniofacial region during embryogenesis. This study has further shown that Fgf8 overexpression in cranial NCC-derived mesenchymal cells or treatment of control cells with FGF8 peptide leads to prolonged proliferation, survival, and multipotent differentiation of these cells in vitro. FGF8 signaling also inhibits osteogenesis, but stimulates adipogenesis of cranial NCC-derived mesenchymal cells in culture [15].

11.3 Neural Crest Stem/Progenitor Cells in Various Tissues

Neural crest-derived progenitors exist in several embryonic and adult tissues, including embryonic and adult hearts, in which they contribute to the formation of the aortico-pulmonary septum of the outflow tract [16–19]. Growing of presumptive cardiac NCCs that are isolated from primary neural tube explants in culture as single-cell suspensions give rise to neurons, pigment cells, Schwann cells, chondrocytes, and smooth muscle cells, suggesting the multipotency of these cardiac NCCs [16]. Other studies have identified a population of multipotent NCCs within the cardiac side population (SP) of the neonatal and adult mouse heart [17]. These side population (SP) cells also exist in other tissue types and are considered as mostly dormant and tissue-specific progenitors. When grown in culture, isolated cardiac SP cells form cardiospheres, which are spheres of proliferating cells that are similar to neurospheres and express markers of stem/progenitor cells, including nestin and musashi-1. These cardiosphere-derived cells have the ability to differentiate accordingly in each tissue they colonized, and contribute to heart repair after injury that offers an important therapeutic promise [17, 18].

In addition to the heart, NC progenitor cells also exist in both postnatal and adult murine cornea as well as in the adult murine carotid body, which is an oxygen-sensing neural organ localized to the bifurcation of the carotid artery [20–22]. A group of cells has been identified within the CB, and can form neurospheres when growing in culture. This group of cells has the ability to self-renew and differentiate into neurons such as dopaminergic neurons, and SMA+ cells in vivo and in culture [22]. The NC origin of this group of cells is confirmed by fate-mapping analysis using Wnt1-Cre-driven recombination in mice [22]. One important advantage of the ability of CB progenitors to differentiate into glomus cells, which are highly dopaminergic and are used for transplantation studies in Parkinson's disease, is the potential implication of CB progenitors for therapeutic applications in both tissue repair and engineering. Furthermore, the palatum of adult rats is another source of neural crest-derived stem/progenitor cells, and its isolated cells are called palatal NCC-related stem cells that express Sox2/Nestin neural stem cell markers as well as NCC markers such as Sox9, Twist, p75, and Slug [23].

11.4 Neural Crest Stem Cells Derived from Pluripotent Stem Cells

Embryonic stem cells (ESCs) represent an important source for neural crest stem cells (NCSCs). Multipotent NC-derived cell types have been successfully isolated from both human and murine ESCs in culture. This will facilitate and support studies on NCSCs, particularly in human, because isolation of endogenous populations of these cells is not feasible from human embryos. Other problems that face studies on NCSCs are that NC-derived multipotent progenitors isolated from adults are rare and have restricted self-renewal capacity and multipotency, compared to their embryonic counterparts. Studies on mouse embryos have demonstrated that mouse ESCs grown in culture give rise into NC-like cells expressing several NC markers, including Slug, Snail, dHand, and can differentiate into neurons of the PNS [24]. Human ESCs can give rise to NC-like cells, which have the ability to differentiate in culture into neurons, and glial cells and melanocytes [25, 26]. However, studies on the differentiation of ESCs into NCCs face some challenges. For instance, stromal cells that are used as supporting ESCs cells in culture could contaminate these cells, and the ESCs–stromal cell interactions could potentially influence ESC gene expression when growing in culture for long time. Another challenge is that ESC proliferation and differentiation in culture occur by growing cells in serum media that contain multiple unidentified growth factors. These unidentified growth factors could have a potential influence on conclusions. The problems of undefined factors in the culture medium and feeder cell-caused contamination have been sorted out by the development of research techniques for inducing the differentiation of mouse ESCs into NCCs in a serum-free monolayer culture [27]. For instance, ESCs can be induced to form NCCs expressing *Sox9/10*, *Pax3*, and *Snail* genetic markers, if they grow on laminin and in the presence of growth factors such as FGF-2 and BMP-4 in the culture medium. In addition, cells expressing markers for different cell types, including chondrocytes, osteoblasts, neurons, and adipocytes as well as both Schwann and smooth muscle cells, can be detected if ESCs are grown in the presence of differentiation media [27].

Another promising source for NCCs, particularly for regenerative medicine, is induced pluripotent stem (iPS) cells. iPS cells and subsequently their NCSCs derivatives can be derived from the patient. This can overcome major and potential problems of histocompatibility. For instance, human iPS cells and subsequently NCSCs have been used to generate melanocytes [28]. In addition, a recent study has developed a method to improve the simplicity, robustness, and efficacy to induce human NCCs from human pluripotent stem cells (hPSCs), such as human ESCs and iPS cells [29]. In this study, authors have used chemically defined medium (CDM) as the basal medium in the induction and maintenance steps. They efficiently induced human NCCs (70–80 %) from human PSCs by using a combination of both TGFβ and GSK3β inhibitors, and with a minimum growth factor (insulin) in the culture medium. The induced human NCCs characteristically express genetic markers of cranial NCCs, and stably proliferate in CDM medium that is supplemented with FGF2/EGF up to at least ten passages, as well as have the ability to differentiate into melanocytes, glia, corneal endothelial cells, and peripheral neurons [29].

11.5 Stem Cells and Neural Differentiation

In the adult organism, stem cells are enriched in organs and tissues that are characterized with a high cell turnover, including the skin and the hematopoietic bone marrow, where they are essential for renewing differentiated cell pools. Stem cells represent a great hope for the treatment of different human diseases. However, intensive research is still needed to overcome several obstacles that face the application of stem cell-based therapy in human diseases, including how to control stem cell physiology and their long-term safety. Another challenge that causes a delay of the clinical use of stem cells is the need for highly accessible tissue sources that can provide a sufficient amount of stem cells for different clinical applications, including autologous cell therapies [30–32]. Therefore, the discovery of new sources of human stem cells, in addition to understanding factors and mechanisms that control stem cell differentiation as well as evaluation of stem cell safety in vivo should be hot topics of research before the clinical use of stem cells becomes generalized.

Nerve regeneration represents one of the most demanding area for stem cell applications because of the current lack of effective therapy and treatment for many destructed nerve tissue-related conditions or diseases, including amyotrophic lateral sclerosis, both Alzheimer's and Parkinson's diseases, as well as spinal cord injury. A major medical challenge nowadays is how to regenerate the complex pattern of neuronal circuitry that forms the central nervous system (CNS) in an adult human. Another difficulty for an effective regeneration of nerve tissues is the accumulation of glial cells around a destroyed nerve tissue in order to form a fibrous glial scar.

This scar acts to suppress the penetration of growing nerve fibers and, consequently, prevents the reinnervation of the affected area [33]. Research works are being currently undertaken to sort out the problem of the glial scar in order to facilitate the penetration of growing nerve fibers. This includes glial cell transplantation in primates and rodents from the olfactory bulb that leads to a successful and functional recovery of spinal cord injury in these animal models [34, 35]. Despite its success in animal models of spinal cord injury, translation of this type of regenerative approaches to the clinic with human patients will require devising of more efficient research methods to provide a sufficient stem cell number for the treatment of human diseases/ disorders.

There are two major locations for neural stem cells (NSCs) in the adult human body: the subventricular zone of the lateral ventricles and the subgranular zone of the dentate gyrus of the hippocampus. Because both of these two areas are highly inaccessible, the expected amount of NSCs that might be obtained from them would be very low, which adds to the difficulties of using these cells in the autologous cell therapy [36, 37].

11.5.1 Mesenchymal Stem Cells as a Source of Neural Cells

Mesenchymal stem cells (MSCs) are multipotent and well-characterized human stem cells that have a mesodermal origin and are available for cell-based therapy. MSCs are ideal sources for connective tissue regeneration strategies because they are the forming precursors of most connective tissues in the body. MSCs can be isolated from multiple source tissues, including the bone marrow, umbilical cord, and adipose tissue [38].

Extensive studies have been carried out to generate neural cells from MSCs because of their abundance, and availability as well as their well-established isolation and characterization research methods [39–44]. However, transdifferentiation of MSCs to neural fates still faces important challenges and problems that need solutions before being widely accepted by the scientific community [45, 46]. For instance, the involvement of permanent genetic manipulation of MSCs by gene transfection in procedures of neural differentiation is undesirable for clinical applications [47]. In addition, the weak expression level of neural markers, which are only assessed after very short periods of several hours (after application of neural differentiation protocols), makes these markers unreliable to define neural transdifferentiation using these protocols [48]. Notably, the induction of cytoskeletal shape changes and/or apoptosis in many of the currently used protocols of neural differentiation raises a lot of doubt about whether these cells are genuine functional neural cells [48–50]. Furthermore, there is no current definitive evidence that shows the ability of transplanted MSCs to form functional synapses with neurons of the host as well as to both effectively integrate and replace neural tissues within a functional brain network.

Despite the lack of strong evidences for the transdifferentiation of mesodermal MSCs into neurons, transplanted stem cells such as MSCs can still contribute to the regeneration of nerve tissues by several other mechanisms. These include the secretion of both growth factors that stimulate cell survival and angiogenesis, and anti-inflammatory cytokines [51–54]. In addition, several studies have reported successful ameliorations of the functional outcome in animal models of neurodegenerative diseases and brain injury after transplantation of MSC to neural tissue [55–60].

Other stem cell sources exist in the adult human body and differentiate into neurons, which will help in advancing both autologous and allogeneic cell therapies. For instance, a recent study has compared the ability of CNS progenitors and enteric nervous system (ENS) progenitors to colonize the colon and differentiate into neurons [61]. They transplanted both progenitor cell populations in the postnatal colon of mice in vivo for 4 weeks before the analysis of cell migration and differentiation. They found that ENS-derived progenitors migrate further than CNS-derived cells, and also give rise to more neurons than their CNS-derived counterparts, suggesting that ENS-derived progenitors show superior migration, proliferation, and neuronal differentiation, compared with CNS progenitors within the gut environment [61].

11.5.2 Neural Differentiation of Adult (Somatic) Stem Cells and Pluripotent Stem Cells

ESCs are a major source for NSCs that can potentially be used in both cell therapy of neurodegenerative disorders/ diseases and drug screening. However, the applications of NCSCs that are derived from ESCs in these diseases/disorders are limited because of several ethical and practical considerations. Somatic stem cells represent an excellent alternative source. For instance, a study from Barbara Kaltschmidt's laboratory [62] has shown that somatic stem cells that were isolated from the human periodontium could be propagated as neurospheres in serum-free medium that underscores their cranial neural crest cell origin. This study has further shown that somatic stem cells grown in a serum-free culture medium, and in the presence of two growth factors, fibroblast growth factor-2 (FGF-2) and epidermal growth factor (EGF), give rise to a large number of nestin-positive/Sox-2-positive NCSCs, which are proliferative and migrate in response to chemokines [62].

iPS cells are another promising source for neurons. Several research laboratories have addressed questions about the potential direction of the differentiation of human induced pluripotent stem cells to form functional postmitotic neurons. For instance, a study from Lowry's laboratory [63] at University of California Los Angeles has applied the research methods used to generate motor neurons from human embryonic stem cells on human induced pluripotent stem cells. They found that human induced pluripotent stem cells have also the ability to differentiate into motor neurons, which possess prototypical electrophysiological properties, with an efficiency that is similar to human embryonic stem cells [63].

A research study by Hu and collaborators [64] has directly compared the neural differentiation capacity of human induced pluripotent stem cells versus human embryonic stem cells. This study has shown that human induced pluripotent stem cells use the same transcriptional network to generate both neuroepithelia and functionally appropriate neuronal types over the same developmental time course as human embryonic stem cells, and in response to the same set of morphogens. Human induced pluripotent stem cells, however, do these biological processes with significantly reduced efficiency and increased variability [64].

11.6 Neural Crest Stem Cells and Neural Regeneration

Finding new sources of stem cells for the repair and regeneration of nervous system is of a great hope for patients with neurodegenerative diseases/disorders, spinal cord injury, and stroke. However, the shortage of endogenous sources of NSCs in the adult body represents a major challenge for designing cell-based therapy for these diseases and injuries. NCSCs are recent emerging sources for different neural cell types. For instance, several studies have shown that hair follicle-derived NCSCs can differentiate to Schwann cells, neurons, and melanocytes, as well as contribute to the repair and regeneration of injured peripheral nerve by tissue engineering [65–70]. Skin-derived precursor cells, which are NCSCs, can also give rise to a Schwann cell-like phenotype through in vitro differentiation techniques, and are capable of myelination as well as facilitating the recovery of a focal demyelination injury [71]. Moreover, Sakaue and Sieber-Blum [72] have recently shown that ex vivo expansion of human epidermal neural crest stem cells (hEPI-NCSC) isolated from hair bulge explants, manipulating the WNT, sonic hedgehog and TGFβ signaling pathways, and exposure of the cells to pertinent growth factors lead to the formation of highly pure populations of human Schwann cells from hEPI-NCSC, without the need for genetic manipulation.

In addition, a recent research has implanted the boundary cap, which is a transient group of NCSCs located at the presumptive dorsal root transitional zone when sensory axons enter the spinal cord during development, at the site of dorsal root avulsion injury in adult rodents. This study has provided evidences that implanted NCSCs display remarkable differentiation plasticity inside the spinal cord and give rise to different types of neurons and glia [73].

11.6.1 Neural Crest-Derived Ectomesenchymal Stem Cells in Neural Regeneration

Neural crest-derived ectomesenchymal stem cells (EMSCs) are one of several stem cell sources that exist in the adult human body, and are important for cell therapies of different diseases. EMSCs are mesenchymal cells derived from the neural crest during embryogenesis, and contribute to the formation of most of craniofacial connective tissues, including craniofacial nerves, oral muscles, tongue, bones, and teeth [74, 75]. Additionally, a recent research has provided several evidences that neural crest-derived cells that reside in different adult oral tissues can differentiate into osteoblastic cells and, therefore, may be a useful cell source for bone regeneration strategies [76]. Furthermore, Abe et al. [77] have successfully developed a sphere culture system to isolate NCSCs from oral mucosa. They found that human oral mucosa stromal cells (OMSCs) form multipotent spheres, which have a self-renewal capacity and are enriched with neural crest-derived cells, as well as can generate ectopic bone tissue in vivo [77].

Recent studies have shown that tooth tissues are a rich source of EMSCs. Dental EMSCs are excellent source for neural cells because they retain a high proliferative capacity and a neural-like phenotype in culture. They are also well preserved in adult human body [78–80]. EMSCs are also enriched in dental pulp and periodontium of both deciduous and permanent teeth as well as periodontal tissues. They are essential for renewing dental pulp fibroblasts as well as for both replacing injured odontoblastic cells, if needed, and creation of a protective layer of reparative dentin [78–80]. The amount of EMSCs that can be obtained from a single tooth piece is relatively small. However, taking into account their high capacity of proliferation in culture, dental tissues represent a promising source for providing considerably sufficient amounts of EMSCs for scientific and clinical applications [81].

Both dental and periodontal EMSCs are useful sources of regeneration of nerve tissues because they preserve the phenotype and properties of NCCs. Since these dental stem cells constitutively express the genetic markers that characterize neural progenitors, even in basal culture conditions, they may preserve the intrinsic ability of redifferentiation to nerve cells [75, 82–84].

The common theme is that dental EMSCs are more closer to nerve cells than other types of stem cells, such as mesodermal MSCs that do not constitutively express neural-progenitor protein markers. This is mostly because of the common embryonic origin of dental EMSCs with the PNS, which led to the conclusion that EMSCs are more capable than other types of stem cells to genuinely differentiate into neural and glial cells, if they grow under the appropriate conditions [75, 85].

11.6.2 Dental and Periodontal Neural Crest Stem Cells in Neural Regeneration

Neuroregenerative medicine is a growing field that aims for the regeneration of lost tissues or cells due to a neurodegenerative disease. Since the available replacement alternatives for neural regeneration are very limited, stem cells are an important source for neural regeneration/neuroregenerative medicine. However, the ethical considerations, limited cellular potency, and technical difficulties represent a major challenge for using different types of stem cells, including ESCs, iPS cells, and MSCs in neuroregenerative medicine. Several recent studies have made major advances in neural regeneration using neural crest-derived stem cells. For instance, Fortino et al. [86] have successfully induced periodontal ligament stem cells (PDLSCs) derived from the neural crest into neural-like cells using a short and simple research method, thus making it easy for other neuroregenerative medicine researchers to obtain neural-like cells from PDLSC. In this research, the neuro-induction treatment included growing PDLSCs in culture for 8 days in the presence of EGF and bFGF growth factors in the culture medium [86]. Moreover, a recent study has provided evidences that in response to the neuronal inductive stimuli, dental pulp stem cells (DPSCs) cease proliferation and acquire a phenotype resembling mature neurons in dopaminergic and motor neuronal inductive media [87]. DPSCs may, therefore, represent an alternative source of stem cells for therapy-based treatments of neuronal disorders and injuries [87]. Furthermore, adult DPSCs that are isolated from third molars have the capability to differentiate into keratocytes, cells of the corneal stoma, and, therefore, are a new cellular source for corneal stromal regeneration [88].

In addition, another recent study has evaluated the effects of the combination of low-intensity pulsed ultrasound (LIPUS) and induced pluripotent stem cells-derived neural crest stem cells (iPSCs-NCSCs) on the regeneration of rat transected sciatic nerve in vivo [89]. The authors of this study have provided evidences that combination of LIPUS with iPSCs-NCSCs promote the regeneration and reconstruction of rat transected sciatic nerve and, therefore, is an efficient and cost-effective method for peripheral nerve regeneration [89].

Since they have a common origin with the nervous system, dental EMSCs are also excellent candidates for generation of neural cells/tissues for cellular therapy and applications in neuroregenerative medicine, ischemic stroke, and spinal cord trauma. These adult dental EMSCs, and their similar NCSC types in other adult human tissues, including the hair follicles and skin, are currently largely considered as a very convenient autologous stem cell source for neural repair and regeneration because of their apparent safety and easy accessibility.

When compared with other stem cell types, such as bone marrow MSCs, dental EMSCs are characterized by a high proliferation rate and, therefore, their populations can be easily expanded in a few weeks in culture [78, 84]. Other NCSC types, including those derived from the skin, have similar characteristics of high proliferative and expansion rates in culture [90, 91]. These characters are critical for using dental EMSCs for neural repair and regeneration because millions of transplanted cells are needed to repair specific damages, depending on the lesion size/volume. Dental tissues have been partly neglected in the past because they are not abundant sources for the isolation of stem cells [81].

Isolation of stem cells such as dental EMSCs from adult tissues is important for cell therapy of neural diseases/disorders. This is because it would help to obtain an autologous stem cell population, which would minimize any chance of immune rejection after transplantation [81]. Because of the extraordinary immune sensitivity of CNS, it is critical to use autologous, or patient specific cells rather than allogeneic cells from compatible human donors, when devising a cell therapy protocol for CNS repair/regeneration [81].

Devising innovative strategies for neural regeneration in human patients with neural damages in the brain or spinal cord is currently facing a big challenge because of the scarceness and non-accessibility of endogenous NSC sources in the human. NCSCs derived from dental or skin tissues are more reliable than other stem cell types for autologous cell neurotherapy, transplantation to nerve tissue, and neural regeneration because of their ease of accessibility and extraction from patients at different ages. The later includes aged patients who my not be appropriate for complicated surgery that is needed to extract fat or bone marrow tissue [85, 92–96]. The availability of dental- or skin-derived autologous NCSCs for transplantation in damaged brain or spinal cord in human patients is of a high social demand, and critical for recovery of the neural damages in these organs/tissues. This is mostly because lesions in these organs/tissues are usually quite hopeless with regard to spontaneous tissue regeneration and functional recovery [81].

The common theme is that dental EMSCs represent a privileged source for different neural cell types. They can be induced to differentiate into neural-like cells that are characterized with an abundant expression of the genetic markers for neural and glial cells, even in basal conditions and in the absence of any genetic or pharmacological manipulation in culture. Interestingly, it has been reported that dental EMSCs grown in culture exhibit neuron-like electrical activity that is characterized by the generation of action potentials as well as the expression of functional neurotransmitter receptors [85, 97]. Additionally, several studies that transplant exogenous dental EMSCs in experimental animals have demonstrated that transplanted EMSCs can survive, integrate, and adopt a neural phenotype according to their specific CNS or PNS location [84, 98, 99]. These dental EMSCs are able to secrete chemokines and neurotrophins as well as other types of paracrine factors, which are critical for the immunomodulation and survival of neighboring cells [100–102]. Furthermore, other reports have provided evidences of damage recovery in animal models of central or peripheral nervous system injury using dental and skin-derived NCSC engraftments, suggesting a promising treatment for severe and complicated neural disorders/diseases that include brain and spinal cord trauma, neurodegenerative diseases, and stroke [92, 93, 103–107].

11.7 Concluding Remarks and Future Directions

Neural crest-derived cells are considered to be stem cells that are useful for regenerative medicine strategies. Neural crest stem/progenitor cells exhibit both self-renewing capacity and multipotency, and can be isolated at embryonic stages. These cells can also be isolated from adult tissues that are easily accessible such as the adult skin. This is of a great importance because it will help to avoid the ethical issues of human embryonic stem cells, and both the ethical concerns and the immune rejection of foreign transplants. However, more in vivo studies are still needed to better understand the interactions between the transplanted NCSCs and different tissue environments. In addition, NCSCs can be derived from human embryonic stem cells, which can act as an additional and rich source for NCCs that can help to avoid the limitation of NCC quantity isolated from a single individual. However, the use of human embryonic stem cells as a source for neural crest stem/progenitor cells is still a controversial matter.

Human adult teeth and periodontium are emerging and rich sources for pluripotent NCSC populations, which are easily accessible and have several advantages that make them great candidates for clinical use, including their high proliferative capacity and multilineage differentiation potential as well as lack of both oncogenic potential and ethical concerns. Additionally, dental NCSCs are most suitable source for autologous cell therapies because of their ease isolation that does not require making a large tissue biopsy.

In addition to their current tests in different strategies for tooth/oral tissue regenerations, dental NCSCs can be widely used for repair and regeneration of neural tissues. NCSCs from dental or non-dental tissues can differentiate into neural and glial cells, as evidenced by their expression of neural/glial cell genetic markers. Current researches show successful results for using transplanted dental or non-dental NCSCs in neural regeneration that eventually leads to functional improvement in experimental animal models of brain, spinal cord, and nerve injury therapy. However, more studies are still needed to further highlight the importance of dental NCSCs as a source of neural cells that can be used for clinical cell therapy in human patients. Since the mechanisms of tissue repair/regeneration are apparently more complex and diverse than a differentiation to neurons/glia and subsequent replacement of damaged cells, more researches are also still needed to better understand how stem cells such as NCSCs can induce healing processes.

Recent studies have successfully derived neural crest stem/progenitor cells from ESCs. However, more researches on ESC-derived neural crest stem/progenitor cells are still needed to assess the capacity of these stem/progenitor cells to give rise to fully differentiated and functional cell types, particularly in vivo, using several genetic markers that can demonstrate the differentiation of these cells into specific cell types.

Finally, it is critical to carefully grow NCSCs in vitro for cell-based therapy as well as to validate the results that are obtained through in vitro cell culture in an in vivo animal model. This is of a particular importance in the view of several studies that have reported that NCSCs develop chromosomal aberrations and show downregulation of tumor-suppressor genes after several passages in culture. Therefore, it will be essential to determine the long-term stability and safety as well as both differentiation capacity and functionality of NCSCs in culture, particularly because the growth of these cells in culture is critical for their potential use in cell-based therapy and regenerative medicine.

Acknowledgments This work was supported by the American Heart Association National Scientist Grant Award [grant number 12SDG12120007], the California Institute for Regenerative Medicine [grant number TG2-01168], and the Pasadena Guild Endowment to Prof. Ahmed HK El-Hashash.

References

1. Sauka-Spengler T, Bronner-Fraser M. A gene regulatory network orchestrates neural crest formation. Nat Rev Mol Cell Biol. 2008;9:557–68.
2. Le Douarin NM, Kalcheim C. The neural crest. Cambridge: Cambridge University Press; 1999.
3. Elbalshy RM, El-Serafy S, El-Hashash AHK. The development of the neural crest in the cephalic region of Xiphophorus hellri. Egypt J Aquat Biol Fish. 2002;3:85–120.
4. El Balshy RM, El Serafy SS, El-Hashash AHK. The development of the neural crest cells in Xiphophorus helleri, a scanning electron microscopic study. Egypt J Zool. 2002;39:77.
5. El-Balshy RM, El-Serafy SS, El-Hashash AHK. The development of melanoma in the prenatal stages of Xiphophorian hybrid fishes. Egypt J Zool. 2002;39:97–123.
6. Dupin E, Sommer L. Neural crest progenitors and stem cells: from early development to adulthood. Dev Biol. 2012;366(1):83–9.
7. Trainor P, editor. Neural crest cells: evolution, development and disease. Academic Press; 2013.

8. Crane JF, Trainor PA. Neural crest stem and progenitor cells. Annu Rev Cell Dev Biol. 2006;22:267–86.
9. Bronner-Fraser M, Fraser SE. Cell lineage analysis reveals multipotency of some avian neural crest cells. Nature. 1988;335:161–4.
10. Bronner-Fraser M, Fraser S. Developmental potential of avian trunk neural crest cells in situ. Neuron. 1989;3:755–66.
11. Ito K, Sieber-Blum M. Pluripotent and developmentally restricted neural-crest-derived cells in posterior visceral arches. Dev Biol. 1993;156:191–200.
12. Calloni GW, Glavieux-Pardanaud C, Le Douarin NM, Dupin E. Sonic Hedgehog promotes the development of multipotent neural crest progenitors endowed with both mesenchymal and neural potentials. Proc Natl Acad Sci U S A. 2007;104:19879–84.
13. Calloni GW, Le Douarin NM, Dupin E. High frequency of cephalic neural crest cells shows coexistence of neurogenic, melanogenic, and osteogenic differentiation capacities. Proc Natl Acad Sci U S A. 2009;106:8947–52.
14. Motohashi T, Yamanaka K, Chiba K, et al. Neural crest cells retain their capability for multipotential differentiation even after lineage-restricted stages. Dev Dyn. 2011;240:1681–93.
15. Shao M, Liu C, Song Y, Ye W, He W, Yuan G, Gu S, Lin C, Ma L, Zhang Y, Tian W, Hu T, Chen Y. FGF8 signaling sustains progenitor status and multipotency of cranial neural crest-derived mesenchymal cells *in vivo* and *in vitro*. J Mol Cell Biol. 2015;7:441–54.
16. Youn YH, Feng J, Tessarollo L, Ito K, Sieber-Blum M. Neural crest stem cell and cardiac endothelium defects in the TrkC null mouse. Mol Cell Neurosci. 2003;24:160–70.
17. Tomita Y, Matsumura K, Wakamatsu Y, et al. Cardiac neural crest cells contribute to the dormant multipotent stem cell in the mammalian heart. J Cell Biol. 2005;170:1135–46.
18. El-Helou V, Beguin PC, Assimakopoulos J, et al. The rat heart contains a neural stem cell population; role in sympathetic sprouting and angiogenesis. J Mol Cell Cardiol. 2008;45:694–702.
19. Kirby ML, Gale TF, Stewart DE. Neural crest cells contribute to normal aorticopulmonary septation. Science. 1983;220:1059–61.
20. Yoshida S, Shimmura S, Nagoshi N, et al. Isolation of multipotent neural crest-derived stem cells from the adult mouse cornea. Stem Cells. 2006;24:2714–22.
21. Brandl C, Florian C, Driemel O, Weber BH, Morsczeck C. Identification of neural crest-derived stem cell-like cells from the corneal limbus of juvenile mice. Exp Eye Res. 2009;89:209–17.
22. Pardal R, Ortega-Saenz P, Duran R, Lopez-Barneo J. Glialike stem cells sustain physiologic neurogenesis in the adult mammalian carotid body. Cell. 2007;131:364–77.
23. Widera D, Zander C, Heidbreder M, et al. Adult palatum as a novel source of neural crest-related stem cells. Stem Cells. 2009;27:1899–910.
24. Mizuseki K, Sakamoto T, Watanabe K, et al. Generation of neural crest-derived peripheral neurons and floor plate cells from mouse and primate embryonic stem cells. Proc Natl Acad Sci U S A. 2003;100:5828–33.
25. Pomp O, Brokhman I, Ben-Dor I, Reubinoff B, Goldstein RS. Generation of peripheral sensory and sympathetic neurons and neural crest cells from human embryonic stem cells. Stem Cells. 2005;23:923–30.
26. Motohashi T, Aoki H, Chiba K, Yoshimura N, Kunisada T. Multipotent cell fate of neural crest-like cells derived from embryonic stem cells. Stem Cells. 2007;25:402–10.
27. Aihara Y, Hayashi Y, Hirata M, et al. Induction of neural crest cells from mouse embryonic stem cells in a serum-free monolayer culture. Int J Dev Biol. 2010;54:1287–94.
28. Ohta S, Imaizumi Y, Okada Y, et al. Generation of human melanocytes from induced pluripotent stem cells. PLoS One. 2011;6:e16182.
29. Fukuta M, Nakai Y, Kirino K, Nakagawa M, Sekiguchi K, Nagata S, et al. Derivation of mesenchymal stromal cells from pluripotent stem cells through a neural crest lineage using small molecule compounds with defined media. PLoS One. 2014;9(12):e112291.

30. Rama P, Matuska S, Paganoni G, Spinelli A, De Luca M, Pellegrini G. Limbal stem-cell therapy and long-term corneal regeneration. N Engl J Med. 2010;363(2):147–55.
31. Hayani A, Lampeter E, Viswanatha D, Morgan D, Salvi SN. First report of autologous cord blood transplantation in the treatment of a child with leukemia. Pediatrics. 2007;119(1): e296–300.
32. Greenow K, Clarke AR. Controlling the stem cell compartment and regeneration in vivo: the role of pluripotency pathways. Physiol Rev. 2012;92(1):75–99.
33. Sofroniew MV. Molecular dissection of reactive astrogliosis and glial scar formation. Trends Neurosci. 2009;32(12):638–47.
34. Ramón-Cueto A, Cordero M, Santos-Benito F, Avila J. Functional recovery of paraplegic rats and motor axon regeneration in their spinal cords by olfactory ensheathing glia. Neuron. 2000;25(2):425–35.
35. Ramón-Cueto A, Muñoz-Quiles C. Clinical application of adult olfactory bulb ensheathing glia for nervous system repair. Exp Neurol. 2011;229(1):181–94.
36. Ming GL, Song H. Adult neurogenesis in the mammalian brain: significant answers and significant questions. Neuron. 2011;70(4):687–702.
37. Palmer TD, Schwartz P, Taupin P, Kaspar B, Stein SA, Gage F. Progenitor cells from human brain after death. Nature. 2001;411(6833):42–3.
38. Väänänen HK. Mesenchymal stem cells. Ann Med. 2005;37(7):469–79.
39. Woodbury D, Schwarz EJ, Prockop DJ, Black I. Adult rat and human bone marrow stromal cells differentiate into neurons. J Neurosci Res. 2000;61(4):364–70.
40. Kopen GC, Prockop D, Phinney DG. Marrow stromal cells migrate throughout forebrain and cerebellum, and they differentiate into astrocytes after injection into neonatal mouse brains. Proc Natl Acad Sci U S A. 1999;96(19):10711–6.
41. Muñoz-Elias G, Marcus A, Coyne TM, Woodbury D, Black IB. Adult bone marrow stromal cells in the embryonic brain: engraftment, migration, differentiation, and long-term survival. J Neurosci. 2004;24(19):4585–95.
42. Wislet-Gendebien S, Hans G, Leprince P, Rigo J, Moonen G, Rogister B. Plasticity of cultured mesenchymal stem cells: switch from nestin-positive to excitable neuron-like phenotype. Stem Cells. 2005;23(3):392–402.
43. Cho K, Trzaska K, Greco S, et al. Neurons derived from human mesenchymal stem cells show synaptic transmission and can be induced to produce the neurotransmitter substance P by interleukin-1α. Stem Cells. 2005;23:383–91.
44. Choi CB, Cho Y, Prakash KV, et al. Analysis of neuron-like differentiation of human bone marrow mesenchymal stem cells. Biochem Biophys Res Commun. 2006;350(1):138–46.
45. Maltman DJ, Hardy SA, Przyborski SA. Role of mesenchymal stem cells in neurogenesis and nervous system repair. Neurochem Int. 2011;59(3):347–56.
46. Phinney D, Prockop DJ. Concise review: mesenchymal stem/multipotent stromal cells: the state of transdifferentiation and modes of tissue repair—current views. Stem Cells. 2007;25 (11):2896–902.
47. Dezawa M, Kanno H, Hoshino M, et al. Specific induction of neuronal cells from bone marrow stromal cells and application for autologous transplantation. J Clin Invest. 2004;113 (12):1701–10.
48. Bertani N, Malatesta P, Volpi G, Sonego P, Perris R. Neurogenic potential of human mesenchymal stem cells revisited: analysis by immunostaining, time-lapse video and microarray. J Cell Sci. 2005;118(17):3925–36.
49. Lu P, Blesch A, Tuszynski MH. Induction of bone marrow stromal cells to neurons: differentiation, transdifferentiation, or artifact? J Neurosci Res. 2004;77(2):174–91.
50. Neuhuber B, Gallo G, Howard L, Kostura L, Mackay A, Fischer I. Reevaluation of in vitro differentiation protocols for bone marrow stromal cells: disruption of actin cytoskeleton induces rapid morphological changes and mimics neuronal phenotype. J Neurosci Res. 2004;77(2):192–204.

51. Gebler A, Zabel O, Seliger B. The immunomodulatory capacity of mesenchymal stem cells. Trends Mol Med. 2012;18(2):128–34.
52. Prockop D, Oh JY. Mesenchymal stem/stromal cells (MSCs): role as guardians of inflammation. Mol Ther. 2012;20(1):14–20.
53. Crigler L, Robey RC, Asawachaicharn A, Gaupp D, Phinney DG. Human mesenchymal stem cell subpopulations express a variety of neuro-regulatory molecules and promote neuronal cell survival and neuritogenesis. Exp Neurol. 2006;198(1):54–64.
54. Phinney D, Hill K, Michelson C, et al. Biological activities encoded by the murine mesenchymal stem cell transcriptome provide a basis for their developmental potential and broad therapeutic efficacy. Stem Cells. 2006;24(1):186–98.
55. Kamada T, Koda M, Dezawa M, et al. Transplantation of human bone marrow stromal cell-derived Schwann cells reduces cystic cavity and promotes functional recovery after contusion injury of adult rat spinal cord. Neuropathology. 2011;31(1):48–58.
56. Dharmasaroja P. Bone marrow-derived mesenchymal stem cells for the treatment of ischemic stroke. J Clin Neurosci. 2009;16(1):12–20.
57. Uccelli A, Moretta L, Pistoia V. Mesenchymal stem cells in health and disease. Nat Rev Immunol. 2008;8(9):726–36.
58. Ben-Ami E, Berrih-Aknin S, Miller A. Mesenchymal stem cells as an immunomodulatory therapeutic strategy for autoimmune diseases. Autoimmun Rev. 2011;10(7):410–5.
59. Prockop DJ, Oh JY. Medical therapies with adult stem/progenitor cells (MSCs): a backward journey from dramatic results in vivo to the cellular and molecular explanations. J Cell Biochem. 2012;113(5):1460–9.
60. Chen A, Siow B, Blamire AM, Lako M, Clowry GJ. Transplantation of magnetically labeled mesenchymal stem cells in a model of perinatal brain injury. Stem Cell Res. 2010;5 (3):255–66.
61. Findlay Q, Yap KK, Bergner AJ, Young HM, Stamp LA. Enteric neural progenitors are more efficient than brain-derived progenitors at generating neurons in the colon. Am J Physiol Gastrointest Liver Physiol. 2014;307(7):G741–8.
62. Widera D, Grimm WD, Moebius JM, Mikenberg I, Piechaczek C, Gassmann G, Wolff NA, Thévenod F, Kaltschmidt C, Kaltschmidt B. Highly efficient neural differentiation of human somatic stem cells, isolated by minimally invasive periodontal surgery. Stem Cells Dev. 2007;16(3):447–60.
63. Karumbayaram S, Novitch B, Patterson M, et al. Directed differentiation of human induced pluripotent stem cells generates active motor neurons. Stem Cells. 2009;27(4):806–11.
64. Hu BY, Weick JP, Yu J, Ma LX, Zhang XQ, Thomson JA, Zhang SC. Neural differentiation of human induced pluripotent stem cells follows developmental principles but with variable potency. Proc Natl Acad Sci U S A. 2010;107(9):4335–40.
65. El Seady R, Huisman MA, Lowik CW, Frijns JH. Uncomplicated differentiation of stem cells into bipolar neurons and myelinating glia. Biochem Biophys Res Commun. 2008;376:358–62.
66. Sviderskaya EV, Easty DJ, Lawrence MA, Sanchez DP, Negulyaev YA, Patel RH, Anand P, Korchev YE, Bennett DC. Functional neurons and melanocytes induced from immortal lines of postnatal neural crest-like stem cells. FASEB J. 2009;23:3179–92.
67. Lin H, Liu F, Zhang C, Zhang Z, Guo J, Ren C, Kong Z. Pluripotent hair follicle neural crest stem-cell-derived neurons and schwann cells functionally repair sciatic nerves in rats. Mol Neurobiol. 2009;40:216–23.
68. Lin H, Liu F, Zhang C, Zhang Z, Kong Z, Zhang X, Hoffman RM. Characterization of nerve conduits seeded with neurons and Schwann cells derived from hair follicle neural crest stem cells. Tissue Eng Part A. 2011;17:1691–8.
69. Dong D, Jiang M, Xu X, Guan M, Wu J, Chen Q, Xiang L. The effects of NB-UVB on the hair follicle-derived neural crest stem cells differentiating into melanocyte lineage *in vitro*. J Dermatol Sci. 2012;66:20–8.

70. Ni Y, Zhang K, Liu X, Yang T, Wang B, Fu L, Lan A, Zhou Y. miR-21 promotes the differentiation of hair follicle-derived neural crest stem cells into Schwann cells. Neural Regen Res. 2014;9(8):828–36.
71. Grochmal J, Dhaliwal S, Stys PK, van Minnen J, Midha R. Skin-derived precursor Schwann cell myelination capacity in focal tibial demyelination. Muscle Nerve. 2014;50(2):262–72.
72. Sakaue M, Sieber-Blum M. Human epidermal neural crest stem cells as a source of Schwann cells. Development. 2015;142(18):3188–97.
73. Trolle C, Konig N, Abrahamsson N, Vasylovska S, Kozlova EN. Boundary cap neural crest stem cells homotopically implanted to the injured dorsal root transitional zone give rise to different types of neurons and glia in adult rodents. BMC Neurosci. 2014;15:60.
74. Chai Y, Jiang X, Ito Y, et al. Fate of the mammalian cranial neural crest during tooth and mandibular morphogenesis. Development. 2000;127(8):1671–9.
75. Janebodin K, Horst O, Ieronimakis N, et al. Isolation and characterization of neural crest-derived stem cells from dental pulp of neonatalmice. PLoS One. 2011;6(11):e27526.
76. Ono M, Suzawa T, Takami M, et al. Localization and osteoblastic differentiation potential of neural crest-derived cells in oral tissues of adult mice. Biochem Biophys Res Commun. 2015;464:1209–14.
77. Abe S, Yamaguchi S, Sato Y, Harada K. Sphere-derived multipotent progenitor cells obtained from human oral mucosa are enriched in neural crest cells. Stem Cells Transl Med. 2015. doi:10.5966/sctm.2015-0111.
78. Gronthos S, Mankani M, Brahim J, Robey P, Shi S. Postnatal human dental pulp stem cells (DPSCs) in vitro and in vivo. Proc Natl Acad Sci U S A. 2000;97(25):13625–30.
79. Huang GT, Gronthos S, Shi S. Mesenchymal stem cells derived from dental tissues vs. those from other sources: their biology and role in regenerative medicine. J Dent Res. 2009;88 (9):792–806.
80. Seo BM, Miura M, Gronthos S, et al. Investigation of multipotent postnatal stem cells from human periodontal ligament. Lancet. 2004;364(9429):149–55.
81. Ibarretxe G, Crende O, Aurrekoetxea M, García-Murga V, Etxaniz J, Unda F. Neural crest stem cells from dental tissues: a new hope for dental and neural regeneration. Stem Cells Int. 2012;2012:103503.
82. Gronthos S, Brahim J, Li W, et al. Stem cell properties of human dental pulp stem cells. J Dent Res. 2002;81(8):531–5.
83. Davidson RM. Neural form of voltage-dependent sodium current in human cultured dental pulp cells. Arch Oral Biol. 1994;39(7):613–20.
84. Miura M, Gronthos S, Zhao M, Lu B, Fisher L, Robey P, et al. SHED: stem cells from human exfoliated deciduous teeth. Proc Natl Acad Sci U S A. 2003;100(10):5807–12.
85. Arthur A, Rychkov G, Shi S, Koblar S, Gronthose S. Adult human dental pulp stem cells differentiate toward functionally active neurons under appropriate environmental cues. Stem Cells. 2008;26(7):1787–95.
86. Fortino VR, Chen R-S, Pelaez D, Cheung HS. Neurogenesis of neural crest derived periodontal ligament stem cells by EGF and bFGF. J Cell Physiol. 2014;229(4):479–88.
87. Chang CC, Chang KC, Tsai SJ, Chang HH, Lin CP. Neurogenic differentiation of dental pulp stem cells to neuron-like cells in dopaminergic and motor neuronal inductive media. J Formos Med Assoc. 2014;113(12):956–65.
88. Syed-Picard FN, Du Y, Lathrop KL, Mann MM, Funderburgh ML, Funderburgh JL. Dental pulp stem cells: a new cellular resource for corneal stromal regeneration. Stem Cells Transl Med. 2015;4(3):276–85.
89. Lv Y, Nan P, Chen G, Sha Y, Xia B, Yang L. In vivo repair of rat transected sciatic nerve by low-intensity pulsed ultrasound and induced pluripotent stem cells-derived neural crest stem cells. Biotechnol Lett. 2015;37(12):2497–506.
90. Toma J, McKenzie I, Bagli D, Miller FD. Isolation and characterization of multipotent skin-derived precursors from human skin. Stem Cells. 2005;23(6):727–37.

91. Wong CE, Paratore C, Dours-Zimmermann MT, et al. Neural crest-derived cells with stem cell features can be traced back to multiple lineages in the adult skin. J Cell Biol. 2006;175 (6):1005–15.
92. Amoh A, Katsuoka K, Hoffman RM. The advantages of hair follicle pluripotent stem cells over embryonic stem cells and induced pluripotent stem cells for regenerative medicine. J Dermatol Sci. 2010;60(3):131–7.
93. McKenzie IA, Biernaskie J, Toma JG, Midha R, Miller FD. Skin-derived precursors generate myelinating Schwann cells for the injured and dysmyelinated nervous system. J Neurosci. 2006;26(24):6651–60.
94. Amoh Y, Kanoh M, Niiyama S, et al. Human hair follicle pluripotent stem (hfPS) cells promote regeneration of peripheral-nerve injury: an advantageous alternative to ES and iPS cells. J Cell Biochem. 2009;107(5):1016–20.
95. Lehnhardt M, Homann H, Daigeler A, Hauser J, Palka P, Steinau H. Major and lethal complications of liposuction: a review of 72 cases in germany between 1998 and 2002. Plast Reconstr Surg. 2008;121(6):396–403.
96. Kadar K, Kiraly M, Porcsalmy B, et al. Differentiation potential of stem cells from human dental origin—promise for tissue engineering. J Physiol Pharmacol. 2009;60:167–75.
97. Király M, Porcsalmy B, Pataki A, et al. Simultaneous PKC and cAMP activation induces differentiation of human dental pulp stem cells into functionally active neurons. Neurochem Int. 2009;55(5):323–32.
98. Huang AH, Snyder BR, Cheng PH, Chan AW. Putative dental pulp-derived stem/stromal cells promote proliferation and differentiation of endogenous neural cells in the hippocampus of mice. Stem Cells. 2008;26(10):2654–63.
99. Király M, Kádár K, Horváthy DB, et al. Integration of neuronally predifferentiated human dental pulp stem cells into rat brain in vivo. Neurochem Int. 2011;59(3):371–81.
100. Pierdomenico L, Bonsi L, Calvitti M, et al. Multipotent mesenchymal stem cells with immunosuppressive activity can be easily isolated from dental pulp. Transplantation. 2005;80(6):836–42.
101. Yamaza T, Kentaro A, Chen C, et al. Immunomodulatory properties of stem cells from human exfoliated deciduous teeth. Stem Cell Res Ther. 2010;1(1):5.
102. Nosrat IV, Smith CA, Mullally P, Olson L, Nosrat CA. Dental pulp cells provide neurotrophic support for dopaminergic neurons and differentiate into neurons in vitro; implications for tissue engineering and repair in the nervous system. Eur J Neurosci. 2004;19(9):2388–98.
103. Amoh Y, Li L, Campillo R, et al. Implanted hair follicle stem cells form Schwann cells that support repair of severed peripheral nerves. Proc Natl Acad Sci U S A. 2005;102 (49):17734–8.
104. Hu YF, Gourab K, Wells C, Clewes O, Schmit BD, Sieber-Blum M. Epidermal neural crest stem cell (EPI-NCSC)—mediated recovery of sensory function in a mouse model of spinal cord injury. Stem Cell Rev. 2010;6(2):186–98.
105. Liu F, Uchugonova A, Kimura H, et al. The bulge area is the major hair follicle source of nestin-expressing pluripotent stem cells which can repair the spinal cord compared to the dermal papilla. Cell Cycle. 2011;10(5):830–9.
106. Nosrat IV, Widenfalk J, Olson L, Nosrat CA. Dental pulp cells produce neurotrophic factors, interact with trigeminal neurons in vitro, and rescue motoneurons after spinal cord injury. Dev Biol. 2001;238(1):120–32.
107. Almeida FM, Marques SA, Ramalho BD, et al. Human dental pulp cells: a new source of cell therapy in a mouse model of compressive spinal cord injury. J Neurotrauma. 2011;28 (9):1939–49.
108. Tapadia MD, Cordero DR, Helms JA. It's all in your head: new insights into craniofacial development and deformation. J Anat. 2005;207(5):461–77.

Chapter 12
Lung Stem Cells and Their Use for Patient Care: Are We There Yet?

Ahmed E. Hegab and Tomoko Betsuyaku

12.1 Introduction

Some organs require a very large "surface" for the active metabolic exchange of gases, nutrients, ions, chemicals, or water. To reduce the size of the organ, the surfaces have to be packed and folded by employing a branched morphology, thus obtaining a greater area of active surface with limited transport distance. Organs with this branched morphology include the lung, kidney, and salivary and mammary glands. However, this branched morphology produces a complex organ with several anatomical and functional compartments and regions [1, 2]. In the lung, the airways, arteries, and veins form an inverted tree-like structure. Functionally, the proximal "trunks" of the airway tree conduct the air in and out, while the distal "leaves," the alveolar units, provides the ultrathin enormous surface area required for efficient gas exchange. Another feature of the lung that adds to its unique complexity is that it is the only organ in the body that is continuously exposed to the external environment, exchanging substances with it through the very delicate alveolar epithelium. In normal healthy adult lungs, the epithelium lining the airways and alveoli has a very slow turnover. However, when this epithelium is injured, in most cases, it shows a great repair potential. This potential to repair damages to the lung indicates the presence of multiple efficient stem cells in each and every compartment of this complex organ. The identities of these stem cells have been markedly delineated over the past several years [3, 4]. This has opened the door for a whole new and wide area of research on using lung stem cells in translational and clinical experiments to improve patient care and cure lung formidable diseases.

A.E. Hegab (✉) • T. Betsuyaku
Division of Pulmonary Medicine, Department of Medicine, Keio University School of Medicine, Tokyo, Japan
e-mail: ahegab@a2.keio.jp

E.M. Abdelalim (ed.), *Recent Advances in Stem Cells*, Stem Cell Biology and Regenerative Medicine, DOI 10.1007/978-3-319-33270-3_12

12.2 Stem Cells of the Lung

Most of our knowledge regarding lung stem cells has been obtained from studying mice and to a lesser extent rats. However, there are some critical differences between the human and rodent lungs that we need to be aware of when interpreting animal data in relation to humans. Humans have more extensive submucosal glands (SMG) than mice, which extends from the trachea submucosa down to the bronchi. In mice, SMGs are restricted to the uppermost part of the trachea. Furthermore, the epithelial cellular lining of the conducting airways in humans is much more complex than in mice. In humans, it is pseudostratified columnar consisting of basal, secretory, and ciliated cells throughout the bronchi, while in rodents, the pseudostratified columnar epithelium is restricted to the trachea while the rest of the conducting airways are lined with club and ciliated cells (no basal cells) forming a simple columnar epithelium [5].

12.2.1 Lung Stem Cells; Few or Many?

In 2001, two studies described the detection of label-retaining cells (LRCs) in several distinctive areas of the airways. These were scattered cells within the SMG ducts, a few basal cells in the trachea intercartilaginous regions, and some club cells in the intrapulmonary airways in the vicinity of the neuroendocrine cells [6, 7]. Recently, there is accumulating evidence that there are two categories of stem cells in the lung, "dedicated" and "facultative" stem cells. "Dedicated" stem cells are few in number, quiescent and mostly undifferentiated, and are represented by the LRCs or other yet to be identified cells. "Facultative" stem cells exist in large numbers, and under normal conditions, they have additional functions apart from just being a stem cell. The facultative stem cells are most likely to be responsible for the maintenance of the various lung compartments during the slow turnover in homeostasis and for repairing mild and/or limited injury/damage. When the lung is severely and/or extensively damaged, the majority of the facultative stem cells are lost, and the few quiescent dedicated stem cells are called into action. They proliferate rapidly and differentiate to replace all the cells in the damaged area, restoring normal lung architecture and function within a few weeks [8, 9].

Although we know that these LCRs exist, we unfortunately do not have enough information on them to specify if they are the "dedicated" stem cells of the airways or not. New technologies are needed to isolate and characterize these cells in order to identify their role in healing the airways after various injuries. The well-characterized facultative stem cells of the lung are basal, club, and alveolar type II (ATII) cells (see Fig. 12.1).

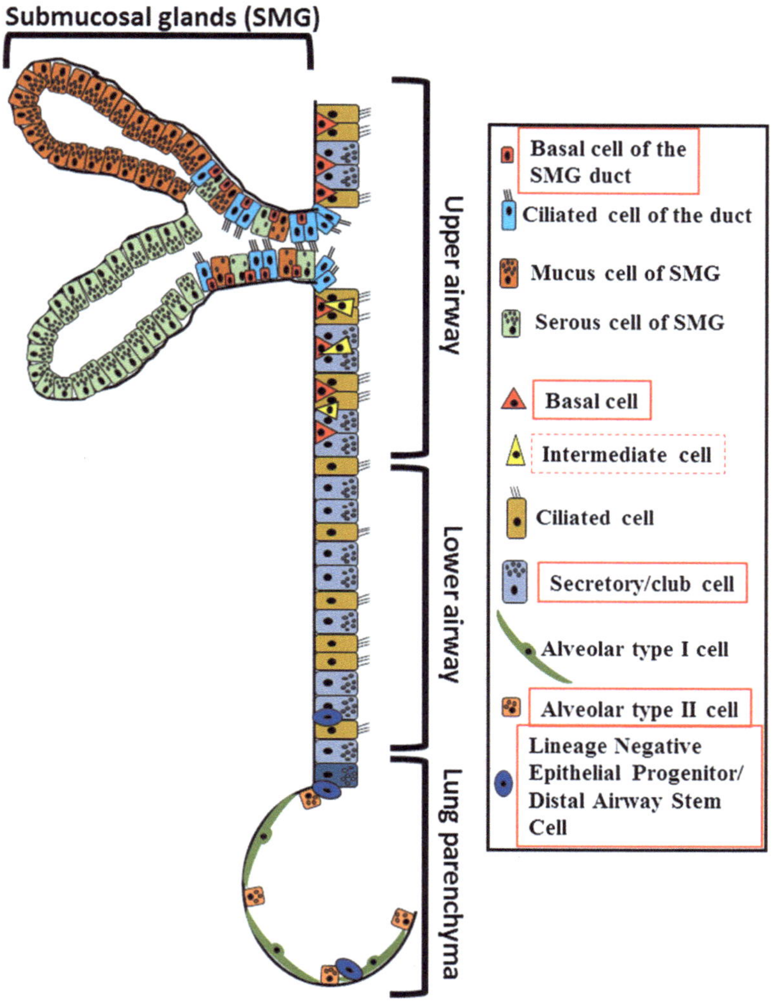

Fig. 12.1 Schematic showing the various lung epithelial and stem/progenitor cells. Cells with established stem cell role are in *red boxes*. Intermediate cells require more characterization to identify their exact role in health and diseases (*dotted red box*)

12.2.2 Basal Cells

Basal cells of the proximal airways (as well as basal cells of the skin, esophagus, and several other tissues) are identified based on their basal position and the expression of several markers including Trp-63 (p63), cytokeratins (K)5 (occasionally K14), as well as Nerve Growth Factor Receptor (NGFR), integrin alpha 6 (ITGA6), integrin beta 6 (ITGB4) and CD44 [10–12]. The current understanding is that basal cells are the main stem cells of the proximal airway. They slowly self-renew and differentiate into both club and ciliated cells during homeostasis. When the airways are exposed to an injury that spares some basal cells, these surviving basal cells undergo several cycles of rapid proliferation followed by remodeling and differentiation into secretory and ciliated cells, eventually regaining the normal structure and function of the airways [12–14]. A recent report suggested that mouse tracheal basal cells comprise two populations, a basal "stem cells" and a basal "luminal precursors". The basal stem cells maintain the epithelium during homeostasis by both self-renewal and differentiation into morphologically indistinguishable basal luminal precursors. These basal luminal precursors are widespread and relatively long-lived. They eventually differentiate into secretory cells [15]. Club cells of the proximal airways possess a limited ability to proliferate and differentiate into ciliated cells but their main source is differentiation from the basal cells [15]. It was recently reported, however, that a severe injury that depletes most of the basal cells can induce club cells to "de-differentiate" into basal cells, then proliferate and repair the damaged epithelium [16] (see Fig. 12.1).

12.2.3 Intermediate Cells

Recently, some data were published describing early progenitor cells that appear as intermediate cells during basal cell transition/differentiation into club or ciliated cells. These are marked by the expression of the transcription factor Myb in both mouse and human. Their importance comes from the finding that their numbers seem to increase in several lung pathologies including COPD and some cancers [17, 18]. Further characterization of their function and factors controlling their differentiation might provide insight into their potential role in health and disease.

12.2.4 SMGs Duct Cells

Compared to airway basal and secretory cells, our knowledge regarding how SMGs are maintained and the role of stem cells in their health and disease is limited. Hegab et al. have published several papers that identified that the cells residing at the SMG ducts are the main stem cells of the glands [10, 11, 14, 19] (see Fig. 12.1). They showed some evidence, similar to what Borthwick et al. showed before [7], that the cells at the SMG duct may contribute to the repair of the trachea surface epithelium, although this requires further confirmation. Several lung diseases like chronic bronchitis, asthma, and cystic fibrosis are characterized by SMG hyperplasia and the change in the amount, viscosity, and character of SMG secretion. Better understanding of SMG stem cells and factors that induce their hyperplasia should help advise new therapies for these pathological conditions.

12.2.5 Club and Variant Club Cells

The distal mouse airways are lined with simple columnar epithelium, which consists mainly of club and ciliated cells with a few serous and neuroendocrine cells. The current understanding is that all club cells possess an equal power to self-renew and to differentiate into ciliated cells [20] (see Fig. 12.1). However, when the airways are exposed to chemical injury with naphthalene, most of the club cells are depleted and only a few club cells survive. As these cells are located in a specific location, close to the neuroendocrine bodies and the bronchoalveolar duct junction, they were termed variant club cells [21]. These surviving cells rapidly expand and regenerate the damaged epithelium, differentiating into club and ciliated cells [20, 21]. Interestingly, LRCs comprised a subset of these variant club cells, which confirms them as the very slowly cycling stem cells of this location [6, 7]. These variant club cells do not express cytochrome p450 and express lower Scgb1a1 and higher Scgb3a2 compared to the rest of the club cells [22]. Similar to the proximal airway club cells that could, under extreme conditions, de-differentiate into basal-like cells, the distal airway club cells have also been shown to be able to differentiate into alveolar cells in response to severe injury to the alveoli with bleomycin and influenza [23], although their percentage of contribution to the repaired alveoli is thought to be limited.

12.2.6 Stem Cells of the Lung Parenchyma

Evidence has accumulated over the years that ATII cells are the main stem cells of the lung parenchymal epithelium. They self-renew and differentiate into ATI cells under homeostatic and various injuries [24–26]. All ATII cells were considered to have equal potency but recent single cell clonal analysis employing lineage tracing with multicolor, stochastic examination revealed that only some ATII cells self-renew and differentiate into ATI cells forming "renewal foci," which continue to expand over the life span of a mouse in spite of the presence of other ATII cells nearby, which do not undergo similar foci formation [27]. The question of whether all ATII cells are equal or whether some of them are more stem than others is still debatable [28]. Interestingly, ATI cells showed a previously unknown degree of plasticity by proliferating and "de-differentiating" into ATII cells during lung growth seen after partial pneumonectomy [29].

Recently, two groups published results suggesting the presence of another rare multipotent stem cell group residing in the distal lung, other than ATII cells. One group infected mouse lungs with the H1N1 influenza virus, and detected $p63^{+}K5^{+}$ cell clusters in the damaged areas. These eventually differentiated into alveolar cells and thus, they were termed distal airway stem cells (DASC) [30]. The other group injured the lung with bleomycin and showed that the alveolar cells in the fibrotic areas were not derived from preexisting ATII cells but probably from rare surfactant protein C (SPC) negative cells that were marked by the expression of ITGA6 and ITGB4, termed lineage negative epithelial progenitor cells (LNEP) [31]. Interestingly, p63, K5, ITGA6, and ITGB4 are all markers of the proximal airway basal cells, which are not known to reside in the distal lung. Both groups showed evidence that these cells possess multipotent differentiation potential towards both airway and alveolar lineages [30, 31]. Both groups then concomitantly but independently published follow-up studies that suggested that both DASC and LNEP are the same cell, or more specifically, that LNEP are more upstream multipotent cells that undergo a dynamic switch into DASC, which proliferate extensively in response to major lung damage [32, 33] (see Fig. 12.1). More extensive studies of this new distal lung multipotent stem cell population will enable us to understand how the lung repairs (or fails to repair) after severe damage like those seen in acute respiratory distress syndrome or other forms of acute lung injury.

12.3 Potential Clinical Applications Using Lung Stem Cells

Cell therapy is a type of therapy in which cells are administered to a patient with the purpose of treating a condition or helping a tissue to repair. Tissue engineering is the use of a combination of cells and an engineered natural or synthetic material to make a tissue or organ with the purpose of implanting it into a recipient to improve or replace deficient biological functions. Over the past 10 years, many groups have tried to use stem cells both for cell therapy and for the creation of engineered lung tissues, in the hope of eventually obtaining clinical benefits (see Fig. 12.2).

12.3.1 Cell Therapy

The most common pathological conditions affecting the upper airway epithelium are self-limiting viral or bacterial infections, or mild injuries caused by environmental pollution and smoke. In most cases, the airway epithelium is capable of efficient repair and only supportive treatment is required. However, chronic injury, such as those seen in heavy smokers, can result in aberrant airway epithelial repair, premalignant lesions, or progress to lung cancer.

More severe acute and massive injuries like smoke inhalation injury seen in burn patients or inhalation of industrial or warfare chemicals are known to massively injure the airway epithelium and result in major morbidity and mortality. The morbidity and mortality in these situations is usually a result of damage and ulceration of the airway epithelial lining, which results in intraluminal transudation of protein-rich liquid and/or bleeding, which later solidify and obstruct the airways and interfere with repair. The current main treatment procedures for such conditions

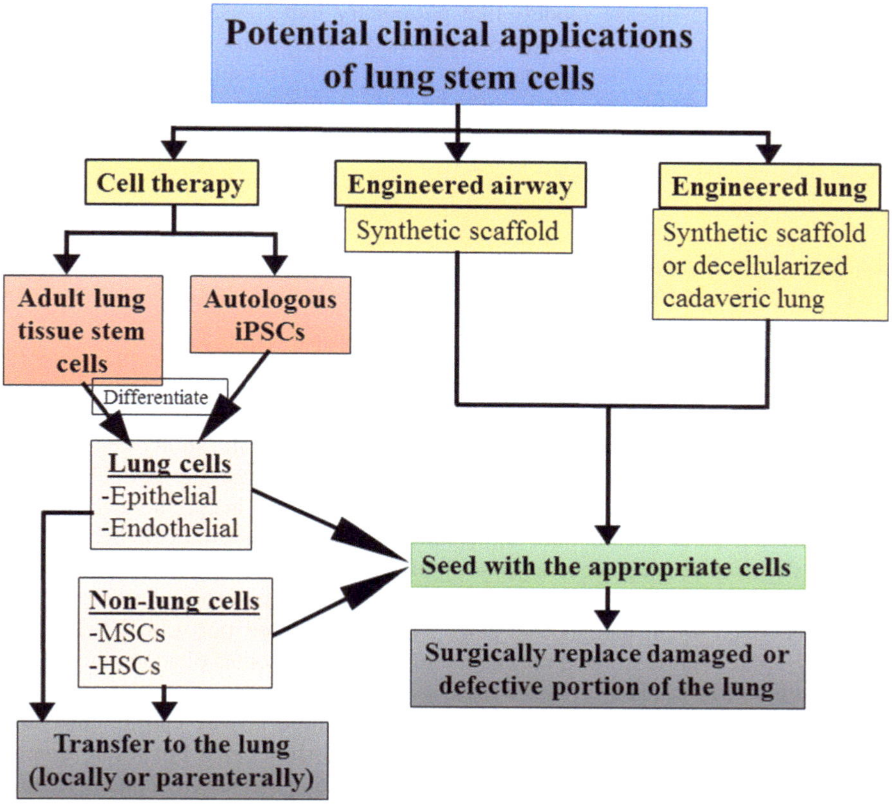

Fig. 12.2 Diagram summarizing the current effort to achieve clinical applications of the lung stem cells. *MSCs* mesenchymal stem cells, *HSCs* hematopoietic stem cells, *iPSCs* induced pluripotent stem cells

are appropriate ventilator support, vigorous bronchial cleaning to clear the cellular debris and/or blood; in addition to guarding against respiratory tract infections [34].

Obviously, this treatment protocol relies on the surviving "stem" cells to reepithelialize the denuded airways and restore the appropriate mucociliary escalator and fluid control. The idea of using "cell therapy" to treat various types of acute lung injury to aid endogenous stem cell repair is an attractive one that has many proponents.

Several early studies reported that different types of cells including hematopoietic stem cells, mesenchymal stem cells (MSC), and lung progenitor cells could engraft into the lung epithelium, endothelium, or interstitial tissues in mice after intratracheal or parental administration of cells [35]. However, later studies that used more sophisticated microscopic and analysis techniques reported that the degree of such engraftment is much less than what had been described previously [36–39]. Also, systemic administration of endothelial progenitor cells have been used to treat lung disease models like pulmonary hypertension in experimental animals although the contribution of engrafted cells versus induction of native recipient angiogenesis due to a paracrine effect of the transplanted cells remains controversial [40, 41]. Importantly, regardless of mechanisms, consistent functional improvement in pulmonary pressure had been observed and accordingly several clinical trials have been initiated [42, 43].

12.3.1.1 The Promise of Using Pluripotent and Tissue Stem Cells in Lung Cell Therapy

Pluripotent stem-cell biology is now a flourishing research area. The ability to create an embryonic stem cells (ESCs)-like cells from human body cells, the induced pluripotent stem cells (iPSCs), has made the idea of autologous cell therapy a reasonable dream. This dream will come true when we can rapidly generate the patient's own iPSCs, differentiate them into a pure and specific epithelial stem (or differentiated) airway cell population, and then use them in cell therapy. Several groups have tried to differentiate and characterize lung epithelial cells from ESCs or iPSCs with increasing success [44–47], but the purity and functional maturity of the differentiated cells remains a concern, along with the reproducibility of the protocols. Even when using these cells with unconfirmed purity and functional maturity, some reports showed improvements in animal models of acute lung injury [48] and lung fibrosis [49].

Another candidate cell type to regenerate an injured airway epithelium could potentially be the lung's own endogenous epithelial stem cells. For future human clinical applications, this may involve obtaining autologous airway epithelial stem cells from the injured patient, expanding them in vitro and then delivering them and facilitating their engraftment in the airway epithelium. However, our knowledge regarding human adult lung stem cells types, characteristics, isolation methods and methods for their expansion and activation in vitro are still very limited. Furthermore, the route of administration (intratracheal vs. systemic), the type of cells to use (epithelial, endothelial, or mesenchymal), their numbers, and any expansion and conditioning in vitro prior to administration are areas yet to be explored [50]. More research is needed to develop more efficient and rapid protocols for differentiating ESCs and iPSCs into the different lung epithelial cellular subtypes in large numbers, with purity and functional maturity. Further work is then needed to find the conditions that can enable these cells to engraft and repair acute airway epithelial injuries in animal preclinical models.

12.3.2 Tissue Engineering of the Proximal Airway

Another potential clinical application of the upper airway stem cells is the construction of a bioengineered tracheal/bronchial replacement for patients with congenital or acquired stenosis/atresia or to replace a surgically resected airway (see Fig. 12.2). Early experimental models using decellularized tracheal/bronchial allografts or synthetic scaffolds relied on the recipients stem cells from the airway portions, proximal and distal to the graft to invade the graft and recellularize it. The graft required about 2 months for epithelial regeneration [51]. Seeding the scaffold with autologous adipose-derived mesenchymal-like stem cells shortened the time of neovascularization and epithelialization from 2 months down to 2 weeks [52]. The efficiency of the scaffold was improved further by seeding it with autologous expanded chondrocytes [53], iPSC-derived chondrocytes [54], or a combination of chondrocytes and mesenchymal-like stem cells [55]. Experiments and clinical trials to obtain a synthetic scaffold seeded with the "perfect" combination of chondrocytes, fibroblasts (or MSCs), and epithelial (stem) cells to produce a bioengineered proximal airway patch or tube are currently underway [56]. Overall, a critical step in improving all of our bioengineering strategies involves obtaining a better understanding of tracheal epithelial stem cells and their interactions with the niche in order to improve the efficiency and efficacy of airway transplantation.

12.3.3 Tissue Engineering of the Lung

Currently, lung transplantation is the only treatment available for patients with end-stage lung disease refractory to other forms of treatments. Over the past 25 years, lung transplantation has improved survival and enhanced the quality of life of many of these patients. However, the shortage of suitable donor organs has resulted in the growing number of patients on the waiting list, causing many of them to die before transplantation [57]. Therefore, tissue engineering of lung segments that are suitable for transplantation is a major hope for the growing number of lung patients.

The distal lung units are both anatomically and functionally much more complex than the trachea or the bronchus. To transplant a functional bioengineered lung segment, lobe or whole lung, a combination of multiple properties needs to be achieved. These include a non-leaking anastomosis of both the vascular and air components with the rest of the circulatory and respiratory systems, an optimum viscoelastic property, a thin alveolar capillary membrane over an extensive surface area, and the correct population of cells in the right position and quantity. Currently, unlike the major advances achieved in creating a synthetic scaffold for the trachea, no satisfactory lung scaffold has been created, and thus most researchers have opted for the use of decellularized lungs as the starting scaffold. The optimum decellularized lung should maintain relative similarity to the normal lung elasticity, retain most of the normal lung matrix components, retain no cellular components, be sterile of all microorganisms and pathogens, and when seeded with stem cells, allow these cells to remain viable, differentiate into the proper phenotype and function [58]. To date, mice, rats, monkeys, pigs, and cadaveric human lungs have been examined for decellularization [59]. The recent advances in 3D printing technology, which produce reproducible and stunning controls of the printed structures, are a promising cheaper and easier-to-obtain alternative to lung decellularization [59]. Recently, the first biofabricated human air-blood tissue barrier analogue composed of endothelial and epithelial cell layers on either side of a basement membrane was engineered using a bioprinter [60].

12.4 Conclusion

In spite of the enormous advances in the fields of lung stem cells and bioengineering over the past number of years, we seem to remain years away from a widespread clinical application of stem cell therapy for patients with lung diseases. Many challenges remain, including the need for better characterization of lung stem cells and their response to various types of injuries, the need for more efficient and robust methods for differentiating ESCs and iPS cells into specific lung stem or mature epithelial populations, in addition to having a better understanding of the roles and interactions played by the stromal and niche cells to direct stem cell proliferation and differentiation. The rapidly developing field of lung tissue engineering offers great hope for patients with lung diseases but there are several problems that need to be dealt with before an engineered lung can be used for treating patients.

References

1. Hogan BL. Morphogenesis. Cell. 1999;96(2):225–33.
2. Iber D, Menshykau D. The control of branching morphogenesis. Open Biol. 2013;3(9):130088.
3. Hogan BL, Barkauskas CE, Chapman HA, Epstein JA, Jain R, Hsia CC, et al. Repair and regeneration of the respiratory system: complexity, plasticity, and mechanisms of lung stem cell function. Cell Stem Cell. 2014;15(2):123–38.
4. Lau AN, Goodwin M, Kim CF, Weiss DJ. Stem cells and regenerative medicine in lung biology and diseases. Mol Ther. 2012;20(6):1116–30.
5. Mercer RR, Russell ML, Roggli VL, Crapo JD. Cell number and distribution in human and rat airways. Am J Respir Cell Mol Biol. 1994;10(6):613–24.
6. Hong KU, Reynolds SD, Giangreco A, Hurley CM, Stripp BR. Clara cell secretory protein-expressing cells of the airway neuroepithelial body microenvironment include a label-retaining subset and are critical for epithelial renewal after progenitor cell depletion. Am J Respir Cell Mol Biol. 2001;24(6):671–81.
7. Borthwick DW, Shahbazian M, Krantz QT, Dorin JR, Randell SH. Evidence for stem-cell niches in the tracheal epithelium. Am J Respir Cell Mol Biol. 2001;24(6):662–70.
8. Li L, Clevers H. Coexistence of quiescent and active adult stem cells in mammals. Science. 2010;327(5965):542–5.
9. Rawlins EL, Hogan BL. Epithelial stem cells of the lung: privileged few or opportunities for many? Development. 2006;133(13):2455–65.

10. Hegab AE, Ha VL, Gilbert JL, Zhang KX, Malkoski SP, Chon AT, et al. Novel stem/progenitor cell population from murine tracheal submucosal gland ducts with multipotent regenerative potential. Stem Cells. 2011;29(8):1283–93.
11. Hegab AE, Ha VL, Darmawan DO, Gilbert JL, Ooi AT, Attiga YS, et al. Isolation and in vitro characterization of basal and submucosal gland duct stem/progenitor cells from human proximal airways. Stem Cells Transl Med. 2012;1(10):719–24.
12. Rock JR, Onaitis MW, Rawlins EL, Lu Y, Clark CP, Xue Y. Basal cells as stem cells of the mouse trachea and human airway epithelium. Proc Natl Acad Sci U S A. 2009;106(31):12771–5.
13. Engelhardt JF, Schlossberg H, Yankaskas JR, Dudus L. Progenitor cells of the adult human airway involved in submucosal gland development. Development. 1995;121(7):2031–46.
14. Hegab AE, Nickerson DW, Ha VL, Darmawan DO, Gomperts BN. Repair and regeneration of tracheal surface epithelium and submucosal glands in a mouse model of hypoxic-ischemic injury. Respirology. 2012;17(7):1101–13.
15. Watson JK, Rulands S, Wilkinson AC, Wuidart A, Ousset M, Van Keymeulen A, et al. Clonal dynamics reveal two distinct populations of basal cells in slow-turnover airway epithelium. Cell Rep. 2015;12(1):90–101.
16. Tata PR, Mou H, Pardo-Saganta A, Zhao R, Prabhu M, Law BM, et al. Dedifferentiation of committed epithelial cells into stem cells in vivo. Nature. 2013;503(7475):218–23.
17. Rock JR, Gao X, Xue Y, Randell SH, Kong YY, Hogan BL. Notch-dependent differentiation of adult airway basal stem cells. Cell Stem Cell. 2011;8(6):639–48.
18. Pan JH, Adair-Kirk TL, Patel AC, Huang T, Yozamp NS, Xu J, et al. Myb permits multilineage airway epithelial cell differentiation. Stem Cells. 2014;32(12):3245–56.
19. Hegab AE, Ha VL, Attiga YS, Nickerson DW, Gomperts BN. Isolation of basal cells and submucosal gland duct cells from mouse trachea. J Vis Exp. 2012;14(67):e3731.
20. Rawlins EL, Okubo T, Xue Y, Brass DM, Auten RL, Hasegawa H, et al. The role of Scgb1a1+ Clara cells in the long-term maintenance and repair of lung airway, but not alveolar, epithelium. Cell Stem Cell. 2009;4(6):525–34.
21. Giangreco A, Reynolds SD, Stripp BR. Terminal bronchioles harbor a unique airway stem cell population that localizes to the bronchoalveolar duct junction. Am J Pathol. 2002;161(1):173–82.
22. Guha A, Vasconcelos M, Cai Y, Yoneda M, Hinds A, Qian J, et al. Neuroepithelial body microenvironment is a niche for a distinct subset of Clara-like precursors in the developing airways. Proc Natl Acad Sci U S A. 2012;109(31):12592–7.
23. Zheng D, Limmon GV, Yin L, Leung NH, Yu H, Chow VT, et al. Regeneration of alveolar type I and II cells from Scgb1a1-expressing cells following severe pulmonary damage induced by bleomycin and influenza. PLoS One. 2012;7(10):e48451.
24. Adamson IY, Bowden DH. The type 2 cell as progenitor of alveolar epithelial regeneration. A cytodynamic study in mice after exposure to oxygen. Lab Invest. 1974;30(1):35–42.
25. Mason RJ, Williams MC. Type II alveolar cell. Defender of the alveolus. Am Rev Respir Dis. 1977;115(6 Pt 2):81–91.
26. Barkauskas CE, Cronce MJ, Rackley CR, Bowie EJ, Keene DR, Stripp BR, et al. Type 2 alveolar cells are stem cells in adult lung. J Clin Invest. 2013;123(7):3025–36.
27. Desai TJ, Brownfield DG, Krasnow MA. Alveolar progenitor and stem cells in lung development, renewal and cancer. Nature. 2014;507(7491):190–4.
28. Logan CY, Desai TJ. Keeping it together: pulmonary alveoli are maintained by a hierarchy of cellular programs. Bioessays. 2015;37(9):1028–37.
29. Jain R, Barkauskas CE, Takeda N, Bowie EJ, Aghajanian H, Wang Q. Plasticity of Hopx(+) type I alveolar cells to regenerate type II cells in the lung. Nat Commun. 2015;6:6727.
30. Kumar PA, Hu Y, Yamamoto Y, Hoe NB, Wei TS, Mu D, et al. Distal airway stem cells yield alveoli in vitro and during lung regeneration following H1N1 influenza infection. Cell. 2011;147(3):525–38.

31. Chapman HA, Li X, Alexander JP, Brumwell A, Lorizio W, Tan K, et al. Integrin α6β4 identifies an adult distal lung epithelial population with regenerative potential in mice. J Clin Invest. 2011;121(7):2855–62.
32. Zuo W, Zhang T, Wu DZ, Guan SP, Liew AA, Yamamoto Y, et al. p63(+)Krt5(+) distal airway stem cells are essential for lung regeneration. Nature. 2015;517(7536):616–20.
33. Vaughan AE, Brumwell AN, Xi Y, Gotts JE, Brownfield DG, Treutlein B. Lineage-negative progenitors mobilize to regenerate lung epithelium after major injury. Nature. 2015;517 (7536):621–5.
34. Rehberg S, Maybauer MO, Enkhbaatar P, Maybauer DM, Yamamoto Y, Traber DL. Pathophysiology, management and treatment of smoke inhalation injury. Expert Rev Respir Med. 2009;3(3):283–97.
35. Weiss DJ, Bertoncello I, Borok Z, Kim C, Panoskaltsis-Mortari A, Reynolds S, et al. Stem cells and cell therapies in lung biology and lung diseases. Proc Am Thorac Soc. 2011;8:223–72.
36. Chang JC, Summer R, Sun X, Fitzsimmons K, Fine A. Evidence that bone marrow cells do not contribute to the alveolar epithelium. Am J Respir Cell Mol Biol. 2005;33:335–42.
37. Kotton DN, Fabian AJ, Mulligan RC. Failure of bone marrow to reconstitute lung epithelium. Am J Respir Cell Mol Biol. 2005;33:328–34.
38. Loi R, Beckett T, Goncz KK, Suratt BT, Weiss DJ. Limited restoration of cystic fibrosis lung epithelium in vivo with adult bone marrow-derived cells. Am J Respir Crit Care Med. 2006;173:171–9.
39. Sueblinvong V, Loi R, Eisenhauer PL, Bernstein IM, Suratt BT, Spees JL, et al. Derivation of lung epithelium from human cord blood-derived mesenchymal stem cells. Am J Respir Crit Care Med. 2008;177:701–11.
40. Takahashi M, Nakamura T, Toba T, Kajiwara N, Kato H, Shimizu Y. Transplantation of endothelial progenitor cells into the lung to alleviate pulmonary hypertension in dogs. Tissue Eng. 2004;10:771–9.
41. Yoshida H, Kitaichi T, Urata M, Kurobe H, Kanbara T, Motoki T, et al. Syngeneic bone marrow mononuclear cells improve pulmonary arterial hypertension through vascular endothelial growth factor upregulation. Ann Thorac Surg. 2009;88:418–24.
42. Zhu YG, Hao Q, Monsel A, Feng XM, Lee JW. Adult stem cells for acute lung injury: remaining questions and concerns. Respirology. 2013;18(5):744–56.
43. Hayes M, Curley G, Ansari B, Laffey JG. Clinical review: stem cell therapies for acute lung injury/acute respiratory distress syndrome—hope or hype? Crit Care. 2012;16(2):205.
44. Longmire TA, Ikonomou L, Hawkins F, Christodoulou C, Cao Y, Jean JC. Efficient derivation of purified lung and thyroid progenitors from embryonic stem cells. Cell Stem Cell. 2012;10 (4):398–411.
45. Huang SX, Islam MN, O'Neill J, Hu Z, Yang YG, Chen YW, et al. Efficient generation of lung and airway epithelial cells from human pluripotent stem cells. Nat Biotechnol. 2014;32 (1):84–91.
46. Gomperts BN. Induction of multiciliated cells from induced pluripotent stem cells. Proc Natl Acad Sci U S A. 2014;111(17):6120–1.
47. Ikonomou L, Kotton DN. Derivation of endodermal progenitors from pluripotent stem cells. J Cell Physiol. 2015;230(2):246–58.
48. Wang D, Morales JE, Calame DG, Alcorn JL, Wetsel RA. Transplantation of human embryonic stem cell-derived alveolar epithelial type II cells abrogates acute lung injury in mice. Mol Ther. 2010;18(3):625–34.
49. Banerjee ER, Laflamme MA, Papayannopoulou T, Kahn M, Murry CE, Henderson Jr WR. Human embryonic stem cells differentiated to lung lineage-specific cells ameliorate pulmonary fibrosis in a xenograft transplant mouse model. PLoS One. 2012;7(3):e33165.
50. Weiss DJ. Current status of stem cells and regenerative medicine in lung biology and diseases. Stem Cells. 2014;32(1):16–25.

51. Murakawa T, Nakajima J, Motomura N, Murakami A, Takamoto S. Successful allotransplantation of cryopreserved tracheal grafts with preservation of the pars membranacea in nonhuman primates. J Thorac Cardiovasc Surg. 2002;123(1):153–60.
52. Suzuki T, Kobayashi K, Tada Y, Suzuki Y, Wada I, Nakamura T, et al. Regeneration of the trachea using a bioengineered scaffold with adipose-derived stem cells. Ann Otol Rhinol Laryngol. 2008;117(6):453–63.
53. Komura M, Komura H, Kanamori Y, Tanaka Y, Suzuki K, Sugiyama M, et al. An animal model study for tissue-engineered trachea fabricated from a biodegradable scaffold using chondrocytes to augment repair of tracheal stenosis. J Pediatr Surg. 2008;43(12):2141–6.
54. Imaizumi M, Nomoto Y, Sato Y, Sugino T, Miyake M, Wada I. Evaluation of the use of induced pluripotent stem cells (iPSCs) for the regeneration of tracheal cartilage. Cell Transplant. 2013;22(2):341–53.
55. Kobayashi K, Suzuki T, Nomoto Y, Tada Y, Miyake M, Hazama A, et al. A tissue-engineered trachea derived from a framed collagen scaffold, gingival fibroblasts and adipose-derived stem cells. Biomaterials. 2010;31(18):4855–63.
56. Haag JC, Jungebluth P, Macchiarini P. Tracheal replacement for primary tracheal cancer. Curr Opin Otolaryngol Head Neck Surg. 2013;21(2):171–7.
57. Kotsimbos T, Williams TJ, Anderson GP. Update on lung transplantation: programmes, patients and prospects. Eur Respir Rev. 2012;21(126):271–305.
58. Calle EA, Ghaedi M, Sundaram S, Sivarapatna A, Tseng MK, Niklason LE. Strategies for whole lung tissue engineering. IEEE Trans Biomed Eng. 2014;61(5):1482–96.
59. Chia HN, Wu BM. Recent advances in 3D printing of biomaterials. J Biol Eng. 2015;9:4.
60. Horváth L, Umehara Y, Jud C, Blank F, Petri-Fink A, Rothen-Rutishauser B. Engineering an in vitro air-blood barrier by 3D bioprinting. Sci Rep. 2015;5:7974.

Index

E.M. Abdelalim (ed.), *Recent Advances in Stem Cells*, Stem Cell Biology and Regenerative Medicine, DOI 10.1007/978-3-319-33270-3

MIX
Papier aus verantwortungsvollen Quellen
Paper from responsible sources
FSC® C105338

If you have any concerns about our products,
you can contact us on
ProductSafety@springernature.com

In case Publisher is established outside the EU,
the EU authorized representative is:
Springer Nature Customer Service Center GmbH
Europaplatz 3, 69115 Heidelberg, Germany

Printed by Libri Plureos GmbH
in Hamburg, Germany